Cochlear Implants

A Practical Guide

Practical Aspects of Audiology

Series Editor: Michael Martin, OBE, Royal National Institute for the Deaf, London

Audiology is a relatively new discipline, formed over the last 50 years. As with all new disciplines, the pace of research is high and standardisation or acceptance of agreed procedures and norms has been low. Examples of this may be seen in the work of the International Standards Organisation (ISO) which only in recent years has produced standards for basic audiometric test methods and given levels for masking signals in pure-tone audiometry.

While much is written on audiology, a great deal of the material concentrates on research aspects of the work. The aim of this series of books is to emphasise practical aspects of audiology and to set out clearly current practice and ways in which research might be applied.

Furthermore, an international perspective will be given to the series, in order to spread the information that is available on a world-wide scale. This will bring to the attention of practitioners and students ideas and procedures that may appear novel in their own countries but which are widely used in other parts of the world. Today, audiology is an international subject, and recognition must be given to this fact in our thinking. With the move to international standardisation, particularly in instrumentation, it is essential that we are aware of the different approaches being used.

Speech Audiometry, edited by Michael Martin, Royal National Institute for the Deaf, London.

Paediatric Audiology: 0–5 years, edited by Barry McCormick, Nottingham General Hospital, UK.

Manual of Practical Audiometry, Volume 1, edited by Stig Arlinger, Swedish Audiometry Methods Group.

Manual of Practical Audiometry, Volume 2, edited by Stig Arlinger, Swedish Audiometry Methods Group.

Cochlear Implants: A Practical Guide, edited by Huw Cooper, UCH/RNID Cochlear Implant Programme.

Tactile Aids for the Hearing Impaired, edited by Ian Summers, University of Exeter.

Cochlear Implants
A Practical Guide

Edited by

Huw Cooper, MSc

Audiological Scientist
UCH/RNID Cochlear Implant Programme

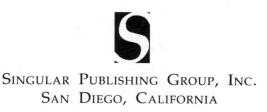

SINGULAR PUBLISHING GROUP, INC.
SAN DIEGO, CALIFORNIA

Copyright © 1991
Whurr Publishers Ltd
19b Compton Terrace, London N1 2UN

First published 1991
Reprinted 1993

Published and Distributed in the
United States and Canada by
SINGULAR PUBLISHING GROUP, INC.
4281 41st Street
San Diego, California 92105

ISBN 1-879105-32-2

Photoset by Scribe Design, Gillingham, Kent
Printed and bound in Great Britain by Athenaeum Press Ltd, Newcastle upon Tyne

Preface

My implant was a lifesaver when I was drowning in a sea of despair
Christine Harding,
Single-channel implant user

If anyone ever had the slightest doubts about the value of the cochlear implant, this quote should dispel them. The sight of Christine's face when she heard the sounds of speech for the first time after years of deafness would convince even the most sceptical observer of the huge impact this device can have on people's lives. Those of us who have had the happy experience of giving back some hearing, albeit not perfect, to people whose lives had been shattered by deafness, are convinced that we are doing something very special.

This book's purpose is made clear in its title: it is intended to be a practical guide, and I am convinced that there is a need for one. The word practical is used to underline that, throughout the book, the emphasis is on providing information that should be of practical help to all those who are actually working with cochlear implants. It is not, therefore, an attempt to bring together a set of research reports: this would be somewhat futile because research in this field is moving so fast, and so much is going on that it is better for the reader to go to any of the scientific journals in otolaryngology, audiology and hearing where the latest research is reported. A particularly useful source for background reading is provided by the proceedings of the large conferences and symposia on implants that have been held over the last 10 years, and there is a list of the major ones on page xv.

The word 'guide' is used in the title because the book is just that; it is not intended to provide the reader with everything they need to know to run an implant programme as this would be nearly impossible for one book to achieve. It should, however, be a good starting point and my hope is that all those who are involved in the application of implants, whose numbers are currently growing so rapidly, as well as those who are just interested to know more, will obtain a lot of useful information from it.

The organisation of the chapters is broadly speaking chronological, in that they cover subjects in roughly the same order as they would occur in the process starting with patient selection, going through surgery to rehabilitation and evaluation.

Mark Haggard, as Director of the Institute of Hearing Research, has been involved with research in hearing and deafness for many years and so is the ideal person to put implants into perspective and he begins the book by doing just that. The historical report by Dr Bill House and Karen Berliner from the House Ear Institute, where implants really were transformed from a scientific experiment into a viable and exciting new treatment, makes fascinating reading and reminds us how far things have come on since the early days. It is all too easy to forget that just a few years ago cochlear implants were violently opposed by some and regarded as dangerous experiments that should be banned. Dianne Mecklenburg and Ernst Lehnhardt then describe the vast amount of development and clinical work that has been done outside North America, which is so frequently overlooked.

Rich Tyler and Nancy Tye-Murray then bring us up to date with the state of the art, explain the concepts of speech processing, and give an idea of the kinds of results that we can expect to obtain with the different implant systems that are available to us now. Rich and his colleagues in Iowa are in a unique position to do this, as they have been conducting the only large-scale comparative trial of different implant systems in the world.

Although they have been established and used widely in the USA and world wide for many years now, it has taken a long time for implants to be accepted in the UK and government funding for them has only recently been forthcoming. One of the main people responsible for this achievement has been Graham Fraser. He has been the leader of a team of professionals running the implant programme at the University College Hospital, London for 7 years and, in this time, the concept of a team approach to implantation has been developed to a high level, with great success. He explains how and why this has been done in the next chapter.

The job of selecting candidates for cochlear implantation is such a huge and complex one that one chapter is not enough. After an overview of the subject in which I review the philosophies and basic criteria of selection and discuss the possibilities for predicting the results of implantation, Angela King, Paul Abbas and Carolyn Brown, Laurence McKenna and Roger Gray give detailed accounts of the four main areas of the selection process: audiology, electrophysiology, psychology and medical assessment.

Following selection, surgery is the next step and John Graham and Graeme Clark and his colleagues give clear descriptions of the latest techniques. John Graham is among the foremost otological surgeons in the UK, and has been at the forefront of the development of new surgical approaches in single-channel implants. Graeme Clark is one of the most experienced implant surgeons in the world and was instrumental in the development of the Nucleus system which is now used world wide with huge success.

The fitting and programming of the speech processor is a crucial stage in cochlear implantation and Sue Roberts explains clearly how it should be performed; her great experience in 'tuning up' hundreds of implants qualifies her probably better than anyone to do this. Training and rehabilitation is probably the most essential element in cochlear implantation, but surprisingly little is written about it or mentioned at conferences. In the next chapter, I give an introduction to the methods that are used in training of implant users and review the evidence about its benefits. Birgit Cook describes the carefully constructed and scientifically designed training programme developed by her and her colleagues in Stockholm, which is a very good example of how rehabilitation of implant users can be carried out within the context of a rehabilitational facility for the hearing impaired.

Evaluation of the results of cochlear implantation is vital for many reasons. In the majority of cases, the primary aim (but not necessarily the only one) of the implant is to enhance the ability to receive spoken communication and, in view of this, evaluation is usually mainly concerned with the assessment of speech recognition. Andy Faulkner and Theo Read give a thorough introduction to the science of speech followed by a thoughtful review of methods for assessing speech perceptual skills, and a suggestion for a core battery of tests.

There are many who see cochlear implants as having the ultimate aim of helping deaf children. There is now no doubt that even very young children can obtain enormous benefits from implants. The methods and approaches used with children are of course significantly different from those applied in adults and a very different set of skills is required. The chapters by Steve Staller and colleagues and Margery Somers give an idea of the results that are being achieved with children now, as well as an in-depth look at the methods they have developed.

The next two chapters both cover areas of benefit to cochlear implant users that have received scant attention in the past. The improvement to the implantee's own speech can often be dramatic and can make a huge difference to their self-confidence. The development of methods for objective assessment of these changes is very exciting and Theo Read is at the forefront of this area of research. Tinnitus can in many cases be just as great a problem as deafness, if not greater; the alleviation that an implant can give is sometimes the most important benefit that the implantee derives. The arrival of electrical tinnitus suppression techniques is the most exciting development in tinnitus research for many years, and offers great hope not only for deafened people, but ultimately for all tinnitus sufferers. Jonathan Hazell has been a leader in tinnitus research for a very long time, and his chapter describes some of the very latest findings.

Alison Heath, one of the first people in the UK to have an implant and a well-known figure in the deafened community, gives a fascinating and moving account of her experiences of losing her hearing and then after many years receiving a cochlear implant. Having read the rest of the chapters concerned with scientific and technical matters, her words should bring home the human element and remind the reader of the ultimate aim of all our efforts.

Huw Cooper
1991

Acknowledgements

I would like to thank all my co-authors who have put in so much hard work: it has been a pleasure working with them.

There are many others who have helped me enormously and I am very grateful to them all. First, thanks go to Mike Martin for suggesting me as editor of this book. Pat Garrett and Jeanette Sanders have given many hours of typing and their help is greatly appreciated. Theo Read has been a constant source of advice and encouragement.

Finally, the unfailing support of my wife Gwyn, the long hours she has put in typing manuscripts, and her tolerance of the time the book has taken up at home are all gratefully appreciated.

Contents

Chapter 15

Chapter 16

Chapter 17

Chapter 18

Chapter 19

Chapter 20

Chapter 21

Contributors

Professor Paul J. Abbas, PhD, Department of Speech Pathology and Audiology, and Department of Otolaryngology – Head and Neck Surgery, University of Iowa, Iowa City, USA

Anne L. Beiter, MS, Cochlear Corporation, Englewood, Colorado, USA

Karen Berliner, PhD, House Ear Institute, Los Angeles, California, USA

Judith A. Brimacombe, MA, Cochlear Corporation, Englewood, Colorado, USA

Carolyn J. Brown, PhD, Department of Otolaryngology – Head and Neck Surgery, University of Iowa, Iowa City, USA

Professor Graeme M. Clark, Department of Otolaryngology, University of Melbourne, The Royal Victorian Eye and Ear Hospital, East Melbourne, Victoria, Australia

Birgit Cook, MA, Department of Audiology, Södersjukhuset, Stockholm, Sweden

Huw Cooper, MSc, formerly of Royal Ear Hospital, London; now at Audiology Department, Queen Elizabeth Hospital, Birmingham, UK

Andrew Faulkner, DPhil, Department of Phonetics and Linguistics, University College London, London, UK

Dr B. K-H. G. Franz, Department of Otolaryngology, University of Melbourne and The Royal Victorian Eye and Ear Hospital, East Melbourne, Victoria, Australia

Graham Fraser, FRCS, Royal Ear Hospital, London, UK

John M. Graham, FRCS, Royal Ear Hospital, London, UK

Roger Gray, FRCS, Addenbrookes Hospital, Cambridge, UK

Professor Mark Haggard, Director, MRC Institute of Hearing Research, University of Nottingham, Nottingham, UK

Jonathan W.P. Hazell, FRCS, Royal National Institute for the Deaf, and University College and Middlesex Hospital Medical School, London, UK

Alison Heath, MA, ALA, High Wycombe, Bucks, UK

William House, MD, Hearing Associates, Newpont Beach, California, USA

Angela B. King, Royal National Institute for the Deaf, London, UK

Professor Dr Ernst Lehnhardt, Medizinische Hochschule, Hannover, Germany

Laurence McKenna, M Clin Psychol, Audiology Centre, Royal National Throat Nose and Ear Hospital, London, UK

Dianne J. Mecklenburg, PhD, Cavale International, Basel, Switzerland and Boulder, Colorado, USA

Dr B.C. Pyman, Department of Otolaryngology, University of Melbourne and The Royal Victorian Eye and Ear Hospital, East Melbourne, Victoria, Australia

Theodora Read, MCST, Royal Ear Hospital, London, UK

Sue Roberts, MA, Cochlear AG, London, UK

Margery N. Somers, PhD, House Ear Institute, Los Angeles, California, USA

Steven J. Staller, PhD, Cochlear Corporation, Englewood, Colorado, USA

Nancy Tye-Murray, PhD, Department of Otolaryngology – Head and Neck Surgery, University of Iowa, Iowa City, USA

Professor Richard S. Tyler, PhD, Department of Otolaryngology – Head and Neck Surgery, and Department of Speech Pathology and Audiology, University of Iowa, Iowa City, USA

Dr R.L. Webb, Department of Otolaryngology, University of Melbourne and The Royal Victorian Eye and Ear Hospital, East Melbourne, Victoria, Australia

Conferences and Symposia

The following list inlcudes the *major* meetings of the decade 1980–1990 and is not fully comprehensive. Note that the years shown refer to the year in which the meeting occurred, not to the year of publication of proceedings.

1982   New York   Cochlear Prostheses: An International Symposium
Publication: *Annals of the New York Academy of Sciences,*
405, 1–532
Editors: C.W. Parkins and S.W. Anderson

1982   Erlangen   Discussions on artificial auditory stimulation
Editors: W.D. Keidel and P. Finkezeller
Publishers: Commission of the European Communities

1983   San Francisco   Tenth Anniversary Conference on Cochlear Implants: An International Symposium
Publication: *Cochlear Implants*
Editors: R.A. Schindler and M.M. Merzenich
Publishers: Raven Press, New York

1983   Paris   Second International Symposium on Cochlear Implants
Publication: *Acta Oto-Laryngologica Supplementum*, 411

1985   Melbourne   International Cochlear Implant Symposium and Workshop
Editors: G.M. Clark and P.A. Busby
Publication: *Annals of Otology, Rhinology and Laryngology*
Suppl. 128, **96**(1), part 2

1985   Stockholm   Proceedings of the Nordic Workshop on Cochlear Implant, December
Editors: G. Bredberg and B. Lindstrom

1986   Colorado   Cochlear Implants in Children: Workshop Proceedings
Editor: D.J. Mecklenburg
Publication: *Seminars in Hearing* 7(4)

1986   New York   Speech recognition with cochlear implants issues, progress and trends
Abstracts: NYV Medical Center

1987	Düren	International Cochlear Implant Symposium, September Editor: P. Banfai
1989	Toulouse	Cochlear Implant: Acquisitions and Controversies, June Editors: B. Fraysse and N. Cochard
1990	Indianapolis	Third Symposium on Cochlear Implant in Children, January Publication: *American Journal of Otology* in press
1990	Iowa City	Second International Cochlear Implant Symposium, June Proceedings not published, but selected papers in press

Glossary

Apex of cochlea: that part of the cochlear duct furthest from the round and oval windows. In the tonotopical arrangement of the cochlea, the lowest pitch sensations are elicited here.

Basal turn (of the cochlea): the first turn of the cochlea, closest to the round and oval windows.

Bipolar electrodes: adjacent electrodes, arranged so that electrical current passes from one (active) to the other (return or ground), stimulating a relatively small area of surrounding tissue.

Dynamic range: the range, measured in either units of electrical current, stimulus units, or decibels, between the threshold for elicitation of the auditory sensation and the upper limit of comfort (the uncomfortable loudness level).

Extracochlear stimulation or electrodes: electrical stimulation of the auditory nerve by electrode(s) placed external to the cochlea itself, most commonly in the round window niche or on the promontory.

Feature extraction: extraction from the speech signal of those features thought to be most important for speech perception (as opposed to analogue or wideband speech processing, in which information about the entire speech signal is delivered to the electrode(s)).

Formants: resonances in the vocal tract giving rise to dominant spectral components in speech sounds. Spacing and frequencies of the formants are responsible for the timbre of speech sounds and the differences between vowels (see page 255 for full explanation).

Fundamental frequency: the rate of vocal fold closure, responsible for the pitch of a speaker's voice (see page 255).

Intracochlear stimulation or electrodes: electrical stimulation of the auditory nerve by an electrode(s) placed within the cochlea, most commonly within the scala tympani.

Mastoidectomy: surgical removal of the bone between the middle-ear cavity and the mastoid air cells, giving access to the round window via a posterior tympanotomy.

Monopolar stimulation: stimulation between an active electrode placed near to or in the cochlea and a return electrode at a relatively remote site (e.g. the temporal muscle). Stimulation of tissues is much less discrete and specified than with bipolar stimulation, but less current is normally required because current spread is greater, allowing a greater number of auditory neural elements to be stimulated.

Multichannel implants: devices in which each of an array of electrodes receives a different stimulus, thereby exciting different populations of auditory neurons with different signals.

Open-set speech recognition or discrimination: discrimination of speech (words or sentences) presented open set, i.e. without any closed response set being provided. Most commonly, this term is used to refer to the discrimination of speech without the aid of lipreading, through sound alone.

Oral methods of communication or education: approaches to education emphasising auditory reception of speech as opposed to the use of manual communication (sign).

Percutaneous connection: connection of the external part of the implant (speech processor) to the internal electrode array by wires passing through the skin, via a plug fixed to the bone under the skin.

Posterior tympanotomy: surgical access to the middle-ear cavity, giving a view of the round window, via an opening drilled through, following a cortical mastoidectomy (see page 159 for illustration).

Postlingual deafness: deafness acquired after the acquisition of normal speech and language. The definition of this term is intrinsically problematic because the process of acquisition of language continues over many years.

Prelingual deafness: deafness acquired before the acquisition of speech and spoken language (see proviso in definition of postlingual – above).

Promontory stimulation: experimental or acute (short-term) electrical stimulation of the cochlea via an electrode(s) placed on the promontory (the bony surface of the cochlea in the middle-ear cavity).

Single-channel implants: devices in which a single active electrode or electrode pair stimulates the auditory nerve. In some cases, e.g. the Vienna system, there is a choice of possible electrodes which can be activated and only one, or one pair, is selected to convey the electrical stimulus.

Transcutaneous signal transmission: transfer of signals across the skin from the external part of the implant (the speech processor) to the internal electrode(s) via an inductive or radio frequency link comprising a transmitter (external) and receiver (internal) coil.

Chapter 1
Introduction: Implants in Perspective

MARK HAGGARD

Cochlear implants have not merely become an accepted treatment for sensory deafness, they have come of age, and this book signals that fact. In their maturation, they have influenced the way in which requirements in services for the hearing impaired are construed, and they can be expected to contribute two other developments. The first, already becoming a reality, is an enhanced cooperation and mutual respect between otological surgeons and other professionals in the field of deafness, particularly audiologists. The other trend involves a more comprehensive assessment, and provision for the rehabilitation needs, of the severely and profoundly deaf (including non-candidates for implants), in respect of those problems that the implant alone does not automatically solve. In addition, the availability of implants as radical effective treatment for the needs of at least some deaf children may help to focus the need for screening and assessment of children more sharply, leading to more effective programmes. In the full realisation of these possible consequences of introducing cochlear implants, much will still depend upon actual adherence to explicit statements of policy. There remains some risk that the finite resources, attention and skills will be siphoned off from a direct assault on other important problems in hearing impairment, especially from the research, development and service provision needed for the larger numbers requiring hearing aids and other rehabilitation. However, there is no guarantee that such an assault would have occurred in isolation and, with vigilance and dedication, the risk may perhaps be avoided. Many working in the field of cochlear implantation believe that the new and exciting developments which they are pioneering will bring more resources into the whole field of hearing impairment, as well as diffusing benefits more directly to the profoundly deaf who are considered for, but do not receive, implants.

A Historical Viewpoint

It is fitting that the book starts in Chapter 2 with a historical chapter jointly authored by K. Berliner and W. House, among the main 'movers and shakers' of the field. Such historical accounts thrive on the stock-taking comments made in reviews of progress and in the introductions to books, so I am choosing my own words guardedly! The House–Berliner citation of the great originator – Blair Simmons – is also fitting. I recognise in myself the portrait of scientific caution in Simmons' account of the scientists in the 1970s; the scientists argued against a direct clinical approach to implantation. It may have been principled to raise such points of caution and to state the need for more basic research, but I think most of us also now readily acknowledge the vital contribution of the surgeons' direct approach. It is tempting to try to draw historical lessons to help following generations working on analogous problems to avoid unproductive delays. Possibly the American scientific and clinical environments were both overly competitive. If the National Institutes of Health in the USA had been prepared to take a more directive approach, the competitive element could have been restricted to tendering for subprojects within an overall agreed framework – as with the moon landings. However, it is very understandable that the NIH did not engage on the required scale, in that the evidence available (Bilger et al., 1977) was only mildly encouraging, and the scientific arguments for the benefits, being rather restricted, were also strong at the time. However, sequential decision strategy requires that when data are ambiguous but not outright negative, more data should be gathered. Agreement at any stage to proceed one stage further need not presuppose ideological commitment to the idea that a succesful outcome is inevitable. It is possible for sceptics and believers to agree in advance on the proper sequence of questions and interpretation of answers, whatever they may feel privately. Stringent criteria of evidence justifying continuation may be needed and sceptical scientists can be useful in formulating these. This stage-by-stage approach is as valuable in guiding technological development as it is in controlled clinical trials, and it is the most fundamentally scientific way to proceed in most human enterprises.

Now that we have seen the crumbling of the political and economic system of almost half of the world – the one built on centrally planned economies – it may seem anomalous to give (qualified) approval to the ability of central planning to deliver the goods and services that people require. However, the Australian experience allows the argument to be seriously put. About 10 years ago (Haggard, 1980), I wrote an article highly sceptical of the Australian Government ever seeing back the many millions of dollars it invested in the project that became the Cochlear Corporation (Nucleus) implant. The Australians had a hidden agenda: helping to spearhead the transition of their economy from one of primary production of raw materials to a high-technology manufacturing economy. In-company development has to be regarded as a returnable investment, but public sector research can probably never be, so perhaps my remarks missed the most relevant point. The difficulty lies not in accepting the truism about investment, but in defining the appropriate boundary between the sectors. The Australian Government was sufficiently pleased with its investment in the 'hi-tech' and high-prestige implant project to put the 'bionic ear' on a postage stamp recently. This particular product may be over-engineered for the requirements of many patients and hence may now appear over-priced. However, nobody was in a position to judge the general requirements in the early 1980s, and it is not certain that we will acquire the predictive ability to judge the issue in individual patients. The good reliability of the Cochlear Corporation implant, which is directly reflected in its cost, has made a material contribution to the widespread acceptance of implantation in general in the mid-1980s. Now that there is a competitor in the shape of the American (Ineraid – formerly Symbion) device produced by the Richards Company, and others are rumoured, it remains possible that these companies might not operate their implant business recurrently at a profit. We must hope, for the sake of long-term service to the many patients implanted, that these enterprises do show profit.

Implant work in the United Kingdom has so far experienced neither central planning nor large funding. British failures to develop successfully and exploit commercially the good and original fundamental UK research base are almost a cliché, more honoured and noteworthy in the exception than in the instance. The research of the late 1970s and early 1980s, particularly by the UCL–Guy's–Cambridge group, has not led to a substantial clinical or exploited development in implants, although its research findings have been of great value and the spin-off towards the production of signal-recoding acoustic aids has been significant. Clinical initiatives, coupled with the problems of high costs and supply of commercial implants, led the University College Hospital and RNID team, in the mid-1980s, to collaborate with the MRC Neurological Prostheses Unit to produce an affordable extracochlear implant. Not until this point were significant numbers of individuals implanted in the UK and a repeatable and reliable production technology developed. The team concentrated their efforts on a single aim in the development of a service and its essential technology. This was undertaken largely on charitable funding. In the remaining groups in the UK who have worked on implantation, the principal investigators have all had other major concerns or only marginal funding for implantation work. The overall picture indicates too little investment, too late and too thinly spread for a successfully exploitable development. Here we see a specific instance of the generalisation that most research and development (R & D) portfolios are too wide, because their planners are too risk averse.

Current Dilemmas

For some 5 years, developments in the UK were restricted in the way just described until, in 1988–89, three new teams began implantation on a small scale, also on charitable funding. These hard-won extensions to the nascent clinical service came together with mounting evidence from Australia and the USA of the very great benefit from implants and brought events to a head. Before 1989, the Department of Health had been inclined to view implantation as still 'at the research stage', and then latterly as either not of sufficiently high cost or not applying to cases of sufficiently low prevalence, to qualify under the rules obtaining for supraregional services (as apply for example to heart/lung transplants). In frustration at the difficulties in obtaining funding, the Royal National Institute for the Deaf and the British Cochlear Implant Group (an informal discussion forum and lobby for those professionally involved) made a concerted representation to the Minister of Health of the UK Government in 1989. Considering the many pressures on funding, and the political and organisational problems facing the Health Service at the time, the response was very pleasing. In January 1990, the Government announced an initial programme that would enable six English centres to build up publicly funded programmes for cochlear implantation and related rehabilitation, and Scotland and Wales have followed suite.

There are two consolations in the fact that cochlear implants have taken more time than originally anticipated to become established internationally, not merely in the UK. First, virtually all new developments see initial over-optimism, consolidation and then a second growth phase. Secondly, gradual development will have helped to minimise some of the considerable possibilities for misunderstanding by the public and the media, some of which remain. Until parents of deaf children have been carefully briefed, they are particularly vulnerable to simplifications by some types of newspaper and television programme. They need constructive encouragement from professionals and from other patients via self-help groups, but this must be tempered with realism concerning candidature and possible limits to benefit. Voluntary associations have an important role to play here and it was particularly pleasing at a recent implants conference in the UK (Haggard and Page, 1990) to see the past gaps bridged and disagreements overcome in the convergence of views from professionals and the National Deaf Children's Society on how to proceed in the implantation of children. A general pitfall is the tendency for the most widely seen media (television and popular newspapers) to over-simplify the description of implants as miracle gadgets that restore full hearing, and to fail to emphasise the need for some (re-)learning. Part of the difficulty arises in the statistical complexities of multiple criteria for candidature and the variability of the benefit displayed by patients; actual benefit is not yet predictable with high accuracy among those qualifying as candidates. The evidence on prediction of benefit need not be repeated here, but Chapter 6 by Huw Cooper can be conveniently cited to anyone doubting the appropriateness of caution in public statements.

Even with accurate information, conflicts and misunderstandings cannot be avoided. Hearing parents of deaf children place high value on a 'cure' that will make their children 'normal', sometimes clinging to this hope to an extent beyond that which the evidence reasonably permits. However, some activists among the signing deaf community still have a perspective completely opposed to implants, closely related to their assertion of the positive deaf identity; not merely is implantation thought unnecessary, it is to them a threat − at best paternalistic, but at worst sinister and bordering on genocide. This position is irreconcilable with that of the majority of parents prepared to do virtually anything that will enable their child to lead a normal life and to communicate with them. The professional is well advised to confront neither position, but to ensure that he or she fully understands these points of view, so as to be able to provide information that may correct the respective misunderstandings. This requires an awareness of those media that are informative and balanced, to counter those that are not, so as to point the patient/client towards the former. It can be helpful to refer to the existence of the extreme opinion which is the opposite of that being expressed.

The Future

The problem (perhaps somewhat delicate) of the attitudes of the activists among the signing deaf community has been worth raising here, because the problem of candidature among children is by no means resolved in detail. Among cooperating adults, many of the factors relevant to candidature can, in principle, be established by tests and worthwhile predictions of benefit can be made on that basis. In children, this picture breaks down; we need to consider freedom of the scalae of the cochlea from bony growth, absolute age, degree of present and past hearing loss plus the prognosis for deterioration, parental realism and support. Of great importance is the capacity and reliability of the rehabilitative context, i.e. the 'strong oral programme' in the criteria recommended by the Cochlear Corporation. But for children, the methods of measurement and the detailed criterion values for many of these quantities remain unclear. The polarised reactions to profound childhood deafness mentioned above only serve to complicate the parental and professional dilemmas, and do not assist the conduct of the difficult research necessary to establish knowledge from which authoritative recommendations can be made. Yet, both progress in establishing a clinical service and further research with children have high priority. After clearance of the adult prevalence backlog in 5–10 years' time, children will probably provide the majority of candidates on an incidence basis. On physiological grounds, the potential value of implants to certain subgroups is probably very high indeed. In addition, the number of years of life subsequent to implantation, plus the developmental influence of hearing on cognitive capacity, underline unambiguously the priority that those children who are suitable must be able to obtain implants.

At present, UK criteria for candidature embrace only post- and perilingually deafened children, but the larger group of prelingually deaf will probably in due course be considered appropriate. A further level of the candidature problem will then be met. Great demands will be made upon facilities for early detection, accurate assessment and, increasingly, for true aetiological diagnosis. Differential diagnosis has been neglected on the grounds that no differential action (bar counselling in dominant genetic deafness) would follow from the result. Diagnosis of pathology could eventually carry strong indications for or against candidature in children, although it barely does so currently in adults. True diagnostic facilities really only exist in a number of specialist centres (the word 'diagnosis' is often misused to refer to the confirmation of a suspected or detected case of deafness). It is disturbing that, in many countries becoming capable of delivering implant services, the cause of many children's deafness remains totally unknown, and that in many others the presumptive aetiology is not sufficiently certain to justify using it as a basis of candidature. An initiative is necessary to standardise and improve early detection plus true aetiological diagnosis. New diagnostic techniques, such as gene probes for various forms of recessive genetic deafness, will eventually have a role to play here. They may be 10 years in arriving, but so may be the knowledge linking diagnosis to prognosis for benefit. An alternative to the predictive approach might be the development of some more sensitive form of trial electrical stimulation on which a negative result would virtually rule out (unlike the present position) the possibility of material benefit from an implant. Techniques for gathering and analysing electrical responses in the nervous system, as well as stimulation techniques, would need to undergo considerable advances before the desired position can be reached.

Important issues in cochlear implantation for the future include the development and individual tailoring of signal-processing schemes to condition the audio signal and drive the electrodes. There is general equivalence of performance with the Cochlear (Nucleus) and Richards (Symbion/Ineraid) devices, despite very different amounts of analytical signal coding in the respective designs (see Chapter 4). This finding does not close the issue concerning further speech processing. Many interesting possibilities for recoding have yet to be tried, although there is a hint in the results that too much processing is not conducive to good performance in noise, a theoretically expected finding. M. Weiss (personal communication, 1989) has obtained suggestive evidence that a noise-reduction algorithm can improve intelligibility for an implantee. (In acoustic aiding systems for the moderately impaired, such algorithms currently assist quality and tolerance, but only assist intelligibility under highly constrained conditions.) I do not think that *the range of candidates* will be greatly widened overall by such means. However, I have little doubt that steady improvements in the computing power of microcircuitry will eventually lead to such algorithms giving materially greater average benefit scores for current candidates and a greater *range of circumstances* in which implants can be used effectively. It will take some time to delimit the signal-processing algorithms that are both effective and simple enough to implement in a miniaturised processor. For the same reasons of cosmetics and convenience as prevail in conventional hearing aids, the development of signal processing for implants is likely to be held back by pressures for small ear-level instruments. The advent of the percutaneous titanium plug may both assist developments at ear level and assist the development of signal-processing capacity, both because it offers a simple interface for experimentation and a high weight-carrying capacity. Problems of infection first need to be overcome, but this now seems very likely. Interesting issues are raised by the problems of defining the degree of auditory impairment at which an implant becomes a better option than a hearing aid, and of developing strategies whereby an aid and an implant can be constructively deployed on opposite ears.

Some desirable developments do not relate to the realm of technological research and development at all. An agenda has been set for service provision in the UK by the British Cochlear Implant Group. Based on epidemiological research by Dr A.R.D. Thornton (1986), it has recommended that provision in the UK should build up to about eight or nine implanting centres in all for the 56 million population of the UK, six of these in England; only one or two of these would take children initially. It is stipulated that each should be adequately staffed, including appropriate provision for rehabilitation. The virtue of this should be the avoidance of operations that have poor selection and follow-up, or undertaken in isolation (i.e. on very small caseloads) in the way that has occurred in some states of the USA. Local rehabilitation personnel will be required for any children not living within, say, a couple of hours' drive of the implanting centre. These professionals will, in most instances, not be adequately supplied from existing local services, but will need special training and possibly selection. They will need to continue the work started by the core team at the implantation centre, with continuity of methods. The selection criteria for these personnel and for robust exportable rehabilitation methods currently require to be clarified. The understandable tendency to involve whoever may be available has to be balanced by an ultimate responsibility to train, and to 'licence', on the part of those leading centres having expert knowledge of the relevant rehabilitative procedures. In the early years of paediatric cochlear implant programmes, the availability of the personnel and procedures will bear upon candidature; if rehabilitation is patchy the selection criteria must be stringent.

Virtually every new treatment introduced in medicine has had limitations and side effects – often unforeseen. So it may turn out with cochlear implants. At present, however, it is more important to emphasise their singular success, relative to what could have been scientifically hoped for 15 years ago. A realistic overall cost for selection, provision and intensive rehabilitative follow-up in the first year, using the more expensive technology available today is around £20 000 (US$40 000) per patient implanted, but elements of this cost will probably reduce as procedures become more standard. This is the same as the capital cost of a comfortable performance saloon car verging on the luxury bracket, or of 1 year's salary plus overheads for a low-to-middle grade public servant or junior executive. Provided that criteria are consistently applied which give a good chance of benefit according to what is known at the time, and provided that the contextual selection and rehabilitation maximise the benefit from the surgical implantation and hardware, this does not seem very much to pay for transforming a person's life. Formal measures of utility for everyday life which transcend particular domains of functioning or transcend medical specialities are, of course, still in their infancy and remain somewhat problematic. However, the strength of the statements of benefit received from patients – not just 'star' patients – suggests that the human benefit per pound invested will compare very favourably with that for the accepted treatments in many areas of hospital medicine.

References

BILGER, R.C., BLACK, F.O., HOPKINSON, N.T., MYERS, E.N., PAYNE, J.L., STENSON, N.R., VEGA, A. and WOLF, R.V. (1977). Evaluation of subjects presently fitted with implanted auditory prostheses. *Ann. Otol. Rhinol. Laryngol.* **86** (suppl. 38).

HAGGARD, M.P. (1980). Which baskets for our research eggs? *Hearing* **35**(4).

HAGGARD, M.P. and PAGE, M. (1990). Current approaches to cochlear implants. *Proceedings of the 1989 Conference.* Southampton: Duphar Laboratories.

THORNTON, A.R.D. (1986). Estimation of the numbers of patients who might be suitable for cochlear implants and similar procedures. *Br. J. Audiol.* **20**, 221–226.

Chapter 2
Cochlear Implants: From Idea to Clinical Practice

WILLIAM F. HOUSE and KAREN I. BERLINER

> If you're not up on something, you're down on it.
> Milus House, DDS (father of Drs William and Howard House)

Cochlear implants, not long ago a highly controversial topic, are now an accepted form of rehabilitation for selected deaf individuals. Controversy still exists, of course, but it centres not on whether cochlear implants should be performed in humans but rather on what type of device and in what patients. The road from idea to practical clinical application was, as they say, 'rocky'. As with many new ideas introduced into the practice of medicine, getting to the present state of acceptance required perseverance in the face of considerable criticism from the professional and scientific communities.

Although the printed literature never quite tells the whole story, we would like to take a look at the history of cochlear implants as perceived by those of us who were often at the centre of the controversy. It is most certainly not a literature review on the topic, and many fine publications and researchers are never mentioned. Most of that will be found elsewhere in this book. This is a history of the *idea*.

Cochlear Implants: Basic Principles

The cochlear implant is an electronic device, part of which is surgically implanted in the ear and part of which is worn externally like a hearing aid. It produces an electrical stimulus that bypasses the damaged or missing hair cells in profound sensorineural hearing loss and directly stimulates the remaining auditory neural elements.

Although there are presently a variety of cochlear implant devices in use around the world, they all have certain basic components in common. A microphone picks up sound and sends it as an electrical signal to a signal processor, where it is modified depending on the particular processing

9

scheme in use. The modified/processed signal is sent to an external transmitter where it is transferred through or across the skin to an implanted electrode or electrodes. This transmission may take place by use of electromagnetic induction or radiofrequency transmission to an internal receiver, or by direct connection via a percutaneous plug. Electrical current flows between one or more active electrodes and return electrodes, stimulating the auditory nerve to produce a sensation of sound. The devices differ with respect to processing schemes (e.g. analogue, feature extraction; single or multichannel), number (single or multi-) and placement (intra- or extracochlear) of electrodes, method of transmission through the skin (transcutaneous or percutaneous) and stimulation configuration (e.g. monopolar, bipolar).

The Modern History of Electrical Stimulation as a Treatment for Profound Sensorineural Hearing Loss

Auditory sensation as a result of electrical stimulation dates back at least as far as 1800, when Volta (1800) inserted metal rods in each of his ears and attached them to a circuit containing 30 or 40 of his newly developed electrolytic cells. Volta did not repeat that experiment. In the last half of the nineteenth century, there were numerous investigations of the phenomenon. By the late nineteenth century, a new field referred to as 'electro-otiatrics' had been developed, but by the turn of the century it died out. The modern history of electrical stimulation of the auditory nerve is generally acknowledged as beginning with the reports of Djourno and Eyries (1957) in France.

Several detailed histories and reviews of electrical stimulation of hearing have been written, and we do not wish to repeat those here (e.g. Simmons, 1966; Berliner, Luxford and House, 1985; Luxford and Brackmann, 1985). However, over the 30-year history of cochlear implants, a number of themes developed that had great impact on the directions of the work and the current attitudes. Each decade brought its own set of issues, concerns and advances, and it is these that we will try to present, using the printed literature to illustrate our interpretation of each era.

The 1960s

During the 1960s, cochlear implant activity was highly localised to the West Coast of the USA, in particular California. Several problems plagued this early work. The technology of implantable materials was not yet ready, and also the scientific community was not ready to accept this new challenge.

In Los Angeles, House began with studies of electrical stimulation in patients undergoing middle-ear surgery, followed by implantation of several deaf patients in 1961, one of whom received a multielectrode device. However, this latter device was removed when redness and swelling developed. Unfortunately, the engineer involved at the time had encouraged newspaper articles about the work, leading to a deluge of calls from people who had heard about the implant and its possibilities. The premature publicity and the lack of appropriate insulation materials brought this first phase of implant research to a halt. House later teamed up with engineer Jack Urban and implanted three patients in 1969–1970 with a multielectrode 'hard-wired' device. By then, pacemakers were being implanted and improved materials had been developed. Considerable testing was performed using laboratory equipment developed for the purpose (Figure 2.1).

In addition to Los Angeles, Robin Michelson at the University of California, San Francisco and Blair Simmons at Stanford were actively pursuing both animal and human research. At a later time, Simmons shared some personal perspectives on the early history of implants:

> While skepticism engendered by claimed miracles is healthy, outright denial that a genuine research problem exists is not. While my 1964–65 experiments were in progress I contacted at least six of the most prominent researchers in speech coding and others in auditory psychophysics. None of these persons were willing or interested in suggesting experiments which might have helped define speech coding strategies for the future. I got a distinct impression, perhaps colored by a little personal paranoia after the first few rejections, that most everyone was either incapable of thinking about the many problems involved or would rather not risk tainting their scientific careers. I do not believe this problem has disappeared completely in the subsequent 20 years.
>
> (Simmons, 1985, p. 4)

It took House, Michelson and Simmons a decade to get others interested in the concept of cochlear implantation. The interest, when it did emerge, spanned the entire range from enthusiasm to outrage.

The 1970s

The 1970s were a provocative era in the history of cochlear implants. Themes endemic to this decade included feelings like: 'It won't work'; 'It's not perfect so we shouldn't use it'; 'We don't know why it works, but are going to use it anyway'; 'It will destroy the auditory system and won't continue to work in the long run'; and so on. In general, these themes pitted the clinical community against the scientific community. Also, during this era, we saw the development of complete clinical programmes for implantation, including development of materials and methods for device fitting, rehabilitation and assessment.

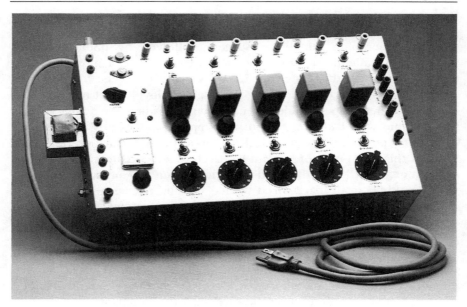

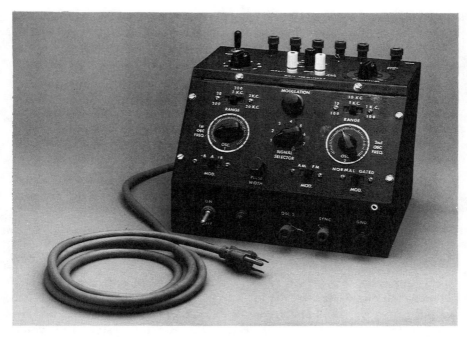

Figure 2.1. Signal processing equipment used to test subjects with multielectrode cochlear implants (about 1969). Different stimuli could be presented to each electrode, with a time delay incorporated to simulate the lag which occurs when the vibrations travel through the fluids in a normal cochlea. Sine, square or triangle waves could be generated. The signal could be divided by bandwidths, 'counted down/transposed', carried by frequency or amplitude modulation and otherwise altered.

The 1970s began with the first wearable devices and long-term human implantations (Michelson, 1971; House and Urban, 1973). House and Urban reported that:

> During the next year and a half [1971–1972] we constructed and tested many devices giving variations in signals ... Many of these devices took months to construct and proved worthless after a few hours of testing. We finally put the most worthy features into one unit and allowed C.G. to vary the signal to suit himself ... He settled on a rather simple circuit ... Because of its simplicity, this circuit was miniaturized and given to C.G. as a wearable aid. For the first time [May, 1972] he was able to walk out of the laboratory and perceive the sensation of sound.
>
> (House and Urban, 1973, pp. 5–6)

They concluded:

> We feel that the electronic cochlea is now ready for more widespread testing and development; this does not mean its uncontrolled implantation and use, but careful investigation by teams of surgeons, electronics experts and rehabilitation personnel.
>
> (House and Urban, 1973, p. 7)

In 1973, the American Otological Society meeting held a session on cochlear implants. The journal printed, as an attachment to the House and Urban (1973) paper, discussion comments by others present at the meeting. Many of these comments suggested that cochlear implants could not work, that we should not use them because they cannot restore normal hearing or that we should use them regardless of our understanding of the mechanism by which they might work.

Dr Merzenich of the San Francisco group commented:

> Dr. Kiang's remarks suggest little or no discriminative hearing can be generated from a single electrode pair. However, it should be pointed out that these subjects do have some discriminative hearing in the sense that small differences in stimulus frequency can be detected. And subjects describe sounds which they hear as 'tones'. This must be faced up to and explained. These and other qualitative observations on hearing in these subjects have also been made by Dr. Simmons and others. They are bonafide, as you will appreciate the first time that you see a patient. They simply must be explained in terms of neural mechanisms.
>
> (House and Urban, 1973, p. 13)

Dr House said:

> Now, what are our goals? ... Well, let us take the example of a patient who has no leg. Shall I wait until our tissue transplantation has progressed far enough that I can transplant a leg on him that will work as well as yours and mine or shall I offer him a peg or a wooden leg? I shall offer him a peg or wooden leg and that is where we are at this point in our cochlear implant work.
>
> We are entering a new era of otology. For the past thirty years we have been in the conductive hearing loss era ... but we are now entering the era of the sensory hearing loss. ...
>
> I believe we, as doctors, should meet this challenge and form groups all around the world, groups of engineers, otologists, rehabilitation experts and anybody who

has anything to offer, who will study this problem intensively. In three years we should know the best electrode system, the best methods of stimulating these inner ears and what the risks involved are. If we do not do this, we shall have been remiss in our efforts as otologists.

(House and Urban, 1973, p. 14)

Finally, the last discussant, Dr Dobelle:

I cheerfully confess that I do not know why stimulation of the auditory cortex results in subjective sensations of sound, Dr. Kiang. However, I agree with Dr. William House's approach. If such stimulation results in the sensation of sound — and it certainly does — I will be delighted to take advantage of the phenomenon even if I do not understand the underlying physiological mechanisms.

By analogy, I think a recent remark made in my presence by 'Pim' Kolff, inventor of the artificial kidney, is very important and bears repeating. When asked about the fact that, after 30 years, the artificial kidney was still not fully understood, he replied, 'If I really worried how it worked, I would still be studying membrane transport in cellophane, instead of building the first artificial kidney; I feel the same way about the auditory prosthesis. If it works, I will take it. Auditory physiologists. . . can then try to explain why.'

(House and Urban, 1973, p. 14)

Already the attitude differences between the scientific community and the clinical community were apparent.

A few months after the American Otologic meeting, a conference entitled 'The First International Conference on Electrical Stimulation of the Acoustic Nerve as a Treatment for Profound Sensorineural Deafness in Man' was held. In the foreword to the printed proceedings, it states that the purpose of the conference was 'To demonstrate to the scientific and otolaryngologic community the very marked limitations of the present devices (essentially only sound perception)' (Merzenich, Schindler and Sooy, 1974, p. vii). The foreword further says: 'Their [Michelson and Merzenich's] work also suggested that the remaining obstacles to a practical implant, namely; multiple electrodes, multi-channel receivers, etc. could be solved in a relatively short time using standard neurophysiologic techniques and laboratory animals' (p. vii).

The thoughts contained in the foreword to the proceedings of the first major meeting on cochlear implants represent attitudes that carried throughout the 1970s. One consequence of the meeting was a view that multichannel devices were 'just around the corner' and that implantation of single-channel cochlear implants should be curtailed because they would never provide full speech discrimination. In fact, many seemed to believe that it had already been demonstrated that multielectrode implants were the only practical approach. It must be borne in mind that at that time there were only a few patients using single-channel implants and *none* using multichannel stimulation.

The second attitude represented was that only animal work was needed to solve the major problems. This perspective fuelled the controversy over human implantation. Thirdly, a judgement was made by normally hearing individuals that the benefits demonstrated at that time were of little value, i.e. 'only sound perception'. This theme recurs frequently – that anything less than provision of true speech discrimination is not worth while.

The apparent conflict between the basic scientists and the clinicians continued to be a prominent theme. Blair Simmons addressed this issue:

> Much of what I hear coming from the scientists and aimed at the clinician says, 'keep your hands out of our Cochlea.' The scientist have (sic) a legitimate complaint. For many years clinicians have cared little for what goes on in there, just as long as the ear works. The scientist, on the other hand is far more interested in knowing about the normal cochlea and has a heavy commitment to finding out. Now, all of a sudden the cochlea seems to be going clinical. Giving up even a piece of one's territorial prerogative is difficult.
>
> Clinicians, on the other hand, are distinctly guilty of down-playing the tremendous wealth of information available from the basic scientist of hearing.
>
> (Merzenich, Schindler and Sooy, 1974, p. 211)

One important stated goal of this 1973 conference was to identify the most urgent unsolved problems and, in the interest of time, coordinate a cooperative international effort to solve these. It is likely that increased interest in cochlear implants did result from this meeting and others that followed. Many centres world wide began either animal or human research in cochlear implantation, although the degree of formal cooperation was minimal.

Not everyone attending the conference was in favour of the idea of cochlear implants at all. In one of the concluding statements from the proceedings of the 1973 meeting, one researcher/clinician said: 'I have the utmost admiration for the courage of those surgeons who have implanted humans, and I will admit that we need a new operation in otology but I am afraid this is not it' (Merzenich, Schindler and Sooy, 1974, p. 209).

In 1976, a monograph was published detailing the events and results of 15 years of work (House et al., 1976). In the last chapter ('Prospects'), we said:

> Our present view of cochlear implants is that we are only at an early stage in their development. This estimate may well be an overoptimistic evaluation of what the future holds. We are therefore committed to the primary task of trying to define the realistic limits of cochlear implants. Is an exciting vista opening before us, or have we reached the zenith of our expectations?.
>
> ... we have reached a stage in the development of implants in which observation and research on a large population is required for a substantive answer to the fundamental question, 'Do cochlear implants make a significant difference to individuals with a profound sensory hearing loss?'
>
> (House et al., 1976, pp. 51–52)

During this period, the National Institutes of Health (NIH) in the USA sponsored an independent evaluation of the patients then implanted with single-channel implants. The results of this study of 13 subjects, using either the House–Urban implant or the Michelson device, were published in 1977 (Bilger et al., 1977) and generally confirmed the clinical findings that had been reported by the implanting clinics: the implant provided detection of sound over the entire frequency range, patients could identify environmental sounds, speech reading was improved with the implant on, patients could better monitor their own speech production and patients felt that their quality of life was improved.

From the perspective of history, what is interesting about this study is that these positive findings tended to take a backseat publicly to two 'negative' findings, which were widely cited. First, implant patients were bothered by noise. In particular, they found traffic noise bothersome when in an automobile on the freeway (or motorway). This would not seem to be a surprising finding for a hearing-impaired listener. However, in this case, some professionals interpreted the noise problem as a function of 'one-channel' listening. Secondly, increased postural instability on one or more measures, as measured by a posturography platform, was reported to occur with stimulation from the implant. This was interesting in light of the fact that none of the patients noted any clinical vestibular symptoms upon implant use. Later studies (e.g. Eisenberg, Nelson and House, 1982) found no evidence for increased postural instability, and this issue has long since disappeared.

Even this first independent study of implanted subjects was influenced by the attitude of the times. In an overview of the study, the authors discuss the study design:

> The psychoacoustic protocol was designed primarily to specify the nature of auditory discriminations possible with present-day auditory prostheses and did not stress tasks that would require the subjects to provide an absolute identification of the stimulus (e.g. repeat the word), since it is well-accepted that subjects using auditory prostheses cannot understand speech with them.
>
> (Bilger and Black, 1977, p. 4)

They go on to say, 'Above all, a single channel auditory input will not provide a speech input that either sounds speech-like or is understandable' (p. 4). Although the number of subjects who had cochlear implants at the time was small, and speech recognition was not thoroughly tested, this study continued to fuel the existing *assumption* that no speech understanding was possible with any single-channel device. Since then, work with more patients and a variety of single-channel devices has shown that this assumption is not entirely accurate (e.g. Hochmair-Desoyer, Hochmair and Stiglbrunner, 1985; Berliner et al., 1989). However, the belief that single-channel cochlear implants could not provide speech discrimination persisted throughout the 1970s and had lasting effects on device development. It greatly narrowed the perspective of workers in this field and excluded from pursuit many possible approaches to signal processing.

Probably the next major event in the 1970s was a meeting in 1977 sponsored by what is known now as the House Ear Institute. Since nearly all cochlear implant work in the USA at that time was taking place on the west coast, we felt that more interaction and cooperative effort was possible and desirable. That first meeting was called the 'Electroanatomy Conference', but it evolved into what became known as the 'West Coast Cochlear Prosthesis Workshop' which was held every 12–18 months. The idea was to rotate the meeting site so that laboratories and facilities of each group could be visited. Furthermore, strong effort was made to keep costs minimal so that laboratory personnel, graduate students and others who form the backbone of much of the work would be able to attend and share their information and experience. At the 1977 meeting, Dr House proposed that participants agree on a minimum test battery to be performed in common so that results could be more readily compared. But an attempt at agreement on a common test battery did not occur until almost 10 years later.

Given a continuing level of controversy and the consequent uncertainty regarding the future of cochlear implants in the USA, Dr House decided in 1977 to hold the First International Cochlear Implant Conference. This was a training course to which 10 teams of surgeons, audiologists and engineers from outside the USA were invited. Manuals and other training materials were provided. The intent was to assure that, if cochlear implants could not progress within the USA, perhaps they could flourish in other countries where barriers to new innovations in medicine were, possibly, lower.

Several of the barriers present in the USA in the mid-1970s are illustrated, at least indirectly, by the published literature, for example: 'An experimental neurophysiological study ... addressed itself specifically to the problem of the *handicap* [our italics] of patients with single-wire prostheses' (Tonndorf, 1977, p. 11).

In its complete context, the idea expressed here represents one common perspective at the time. Some, particularly the scientists, compared the less-than-perfect hearing provided by the implant to normal hearing, and perceived the 'handicap'. Others, particularly those clinicians working with the implant and profoundly deaf patients, compared implant performance to deafness, and perceived the benefits. These contrasting perspectives, we believe, acted as a barrier to understanding between these two communities.

About the same time, there were still some strong feelings regarding the propriety of implanting humans at all. The issue was animal vs human research. Simmons recalls: '. . . as late as 1978 our purpose to pursue human research was disapproved on "moral grounds" by the same peer review group that gave us high marks for the scientific quality of the proposal itself. That decision was subsequently reversed at a higher level of review at NIH' (Simmons, 1985, p. 5).

Others had a more positive attitude towards cochlear implantation:

> Once in a great while our surgical specialties can point to a single dramatic advance in surgical technique, outshining in importance all other developments in the area. Such a revolutionary advance is now taking place in otolaryngology, an advance offering for the first time a means of improving the communicative abilities of post-lingually profoundly deaf subjects.
>
> ... Present techniques must be regarded as only a simple beginning; much work remains to be done in all areas related to the use of electronic cochlear implants ... Nevertheless, a promising start has been made as it has been demonstrated that even with the severe limitations of present techniques – techniques that will undoubtedly be regarded in years to come as primitive – measurable benefits to hearing may be obtained. . .
>
> This surgical technique, the study [the Bilger et al. study], and its results constitute a spectacular advance in otolaryngology that may well prove to be the most significant development, not merely of the past year, but of the past decade or more.
>
> (Naunton, 1977, pp. 33, 35)

Although cochlear implants may have been controversial, those who were dealing with patients made concerted efforts during the 1970s to develop clinical programmes for the selection, assessment and rehabilitation of the patients. In 1979, an article was published on the present status and future directions of the authors' implant programme (House, Berliner and Eisenberg, 1979). As of August 1978, 33 adult patients had received the House single-electrode cochlear implant, and testing and rehabilitation programmes and materials had been developed. We concluded:

> Development of test and training methods and materials for use with profoundly deafened adults will continue, and a program for the prelingually deaf adult is being considered for the future [footnote: One pre-lingually deaf subject was recently selected and implanted to begin research on the usefulness of the prosthesis for that population].
>
> ... We feel that the single-electrode cochlear implant is an already available, surgically and electronically 'simple' device from which to gather baseline data on electrical stimulation, gain subject-hours of experience, and, at the same time, provide the deafened adult with auditory rehabilitation.
>
> (House, Berliner and Eisenberg, 1979, p. 183)

During this time period, work was progressing outside the USA, most notably in Australia where Clark and colleagues were developing a multichannel cochlear implant that was, in the last half of the 1980s, to become the single most used device in the world under the name 'Nucleus Multichannel Cochlear Implant' (Clark et al., 1977).

Finally for the 1970s, the authors' 1979 cochlear implant training course should be mentioned. A select group of otologists from within the USA were invited to consider becoming co-investigators in a multicentre study of the House cochlear implant in adults. They were required to bring to the training course a complete cochlear implant team, including an audiologist and a psychologist. The pattern set by this course and its requirement for a cochlear implant team has continued to dominate the clinical approach to cochlear implantation.

The 1980s

The 1980s brought with them US Food and Drug Administration (FDA) medical device regulations, large-scale clinical trials of several different cochlear implant devices in both adults and children, the introduction into the field of commercial manufacturers, and numerous national and international meetings on cochlear implants. Although there was continued controversy, vigorously renewed by the implantation of children, the latter part of the 1980s brought acceptance of cochlear implants as a form of rehabilitation for selected, profoundly deaf patients.

In a review of cochlear implant work through 1980, it was pointed out that about 50% of the 129 references had only been published since 1977 (Berliner and House, 1981). There was clearly a rapidly increasing interest in cochlear implants.

By August 1980, 110 patients had received the House device, 13 of them being prelingually deaf. Also the first implantation of the device in a child, a 9-year-old congenitally deaf boy, was reported (House et al., 1981):

> During the past few years, we have greatly refined the implant program for the postlingually deafened adult. We have streamlined the evaluation and rehabilitation procedures, written these procedures in step-by-step manuals that can be used by others, developed instrumentation for easy testing of electrical thresholds, and developed an efficient glasses coil holder for holding the external coil in place.
>
> We are now exploring means of coil placement without glasses, in particular, the use of implanted magnets. We have recently developed and used on one patient a method for replacing a malfunctioning internal coil without removing the implanted electrodes. Both of these represent necessary steps towards the future possibility of implanting deaf infants.
>
> Use of the implant by the prelingually deaf will continue to be explored, with emphasis over the next few years on developing a program to work with and study the deaf child.
>
> (House et al., 1981, p. 462)

By the end of 1981, the authors had implanted 12 children (under the age of 18 years), including two preschool-age children, with the House cochlear implant. Results were detailed in Eisenberg and House (1982). A new era of controversy had begun.

Two major meetings, specifically on cochlear implants, took place in the first half of the 1980s. The first conference was held in 1982 by the New York Academy of Sciences. The second, held in 1983, was the Tenth

Anniversary Conference on Cochlear Implants: An International Symposium. Proceedings of both of these meetings were published (Parkins and
Anderson, 1983; Schindler and Merzenich, 1985). The difference between
the preface to the book resulting from the Tenth Anniversary Conference
and that from the 1973 Proceedings (see above) illustrates the major
change in attitude towards cochlear implants that took place in the early
1980s. This preface (Schindler and Merzenich, 1985) says:

> Studies on the development and application of cochlear implants represent an
> exciting, unprecedented multidisciplinary endeavor in otolaryngology...
> The present volume provides hearing and speech scientists, engineers, and
> clinicians an opportunity to review reports from a distinguished group of cochlear
> implant researchers representing most of the major research and applications
> centers in the world...
> It is clear that the current generation of cochlear implants are of benefit to carefully
> selected deaf individuals. It is likely that future cochlear implant devices, particularly
> those that have multichannel capabilities, will provide substantially greater benefit.
> Cochlear implants are rapidly becoming a major treatment modality for the deaf...
> (Schindler and Merzenich, 1985, p. v)

One of the basic science participants of the 1983 conference pointed out:

> Over the past three decades, the notion of restoring hearing to patients with hair
> cell deafness has progressed from the realm of science fiction to a commercially
> viable industry. This might be attributed to advances in electronic technology and
> in our understanding of the normal function and pathology of the auditory system,
> but it is largely the result of determined, even dogged, trial-and-error experimenta-
> tion by a courageous group of pioneers scattered around the globe.
> (Loeb, 1985, p. 17)

On November 26, 1984, the US Food and Drug Administration formally
recognised the '3M Cochlear Implant System/House Design' as a safe and
effective treatment for profoundly deaf adults by granting marketing
approval to the manufacturer. In a press conference, the FDA spokesperson
noted that this was the first time that a medical device had been approved
which partially restored one of the five major senses.

Table 2.1 recaps some of the steps in arriving at that point. Of course,
considerable work by other implant researchers was ongoing during this
period. We wish simply to show the considerable time span required to
get 'from idea to clinical practice'. As we later commented:

> The House/3M cochlear implant has had a significant impact in the treatment of the
> profoundly deaf, even while in the investigational stage. First and foremost, patients
> who were previously turned away as 'untreatable' were provided with a new option.
> Furthermore, the professionals – otologists and audiologists – had a new set of tools,
> including assessment and rehabilitation materials, to use in dealing with the
> profoundly deaf patient. These patients can now be provided more effective care
> whether they obtain an implant or a hearing aid. Finally, the introduction of this

Table 2.1 The House Cochlear Implant: from idea to clinical practice

Year	Event
1957	Patient brings William F. House, MD news article of patient in France implanted for electrical stimulation of hearing
1961	House implants two patients with single gold electrodes for short-term stimulation of hearing. One patient receives a multiple-electrode implant
1965	House teams up with engineer Jack Urban to develop system for chronic use
1969–70	Multiple silver electrodes with percutaneous system implanted in three patients
1972	First 'take-home' wearable signal processor
1972	First single platinum electrode, induction coil system implanted. Prototype of present device
1973	Begin clinical trials – diagnostic, evaluative and training procedures initiated. Five patients implanted
1974–79	A total of 31 patients receive the cochlear implant
1979	'Co-investigator' programme initiated, with training course. A total of 41 patients implanted in this year alone
Jan. 1980	Federal medical device regulations published by FDA
June 1980	Use of magnets to hold external receiver in place
July 1980	First child (under 18 years of age) implanted
Nov. 1980	Investigational Device Exemption (IDE) application submitted to FDA by House Ear Institute
Dec. 1980	IDE conditionally approved by FDA
Mar. 1982	First Model 7700 ('Alpha') device implanted after development by 3M (smaller, lighter weight, new magnet system)
Aug. 1982	Co-investigator activity halted by FDA pending Institutional Review Board (IRB) approvals of device modifications
Oct. 1982	Clinical investigation continues
April 1983	Database close for Pre Market Approval (PMA) application for adult patients
Oct. 1983	PMA submitted to FDA by 3M Company
May 1984	Supplements to PMA submitted. Total database now includes 163 patients with Model 7700 device and 206 patients with prior devices, implanted by 36 different clinics
June 1984	Second FDA ENT Advisory Panel meeting – unanimous vote to recommend approval
Nov. 1984	FDA announces approval of 3M Cochlear Implant System/House Design for use in adults

device stimulated the development of better devices, better assessment tools, and other alternatives.

(House and Berliner, 1986, p. 284).

These statements are true for the entire field of cochlear implants. The impact of the introduction of these devices goes well beyond the patients who actually receive one of them.

By 1984, clinical trials of the 3M/House single-channel cochlear implant in children had also been ongoing for several years. Yet the controversy was still emotionally packed. In a 1984 news magazine article, a well-known paediatric otolaryngologist was interviewed on the topic of cochlear implants in children:

'There is no moral justification for an invasive electrode for children' ... Speaking for himself, he says he finds the cochlear implant a costly and 'cruel incentive', designed to appeal to conscientious parents who may seek any means that will enable their children to hear. 'It's a toboggan ride for those parents, and at the end of the ride is only a deep depression – and you may hurt the kid.'

(*Medical World News*, June 11, 1984, p. 34)

In 1985, we again reviewed the literature on cochlear implants:

During the years 1981 to 1985, more than 200 articles were published, approximately twice as many as in the previous four-year period... In 1981, approximately 200 patients worldwide had received cochlear implants. Patients now number more than 750.

(Berliner, Luxford and House, 1985, p. 173)

We went on to conclude:

There seems to be general agreement that cochlear implants are a feasible means of restoring at least some hearing to deaf humans. There is less agreement about which device is 'best', which patients should be considered appropriate candidates, and how to assess results of implantation.

(Berliner, Luxford and House, 1985, p. 179)

Also in 1985, a 69-page journal supplement was published detailing the authors' programme and results to date with the single-channel cochlear implant in children (Berliner, Eisenberg and House, 1985). In his Editorial comment, the journal Editor-in-Chief says:

With the publication of this supplement the HEI [House Ear Institute] has provided information on the development of the children's cochlear implant program, and submitted their early results for your scrutiny. It is hoped that the publication of these preliminary data will allow the reader to begin to develop an informed opinion about this procedure.

(Keith, 1985, p. 1S)

By 1986, the authors were beginning to notice an interesting phenom-enon. Children were showing signs of the kind of auditory performance that theorists had proclaimed was not possible with a single-channel cochlear implant – open-set auditory-only speech recognition. Had we erred in our expectations? This issue was addressed by Berliner and Eisenberg (1987) who concluded:

> As professionals, we may be doing our patients a disservice to limit our expectations for their success with a cochlear implant – any cochlear implant. We should be more open to possibility and less tied to theory, at least until we have an objective basis for defining our expectations.
>
> (Berliner and Eisenberg, 1987, p. 229)

Unfortunately, the historical prejudice about this topic (open-set speech recognition with single-channel implants) is so strong that there has been little acknowledgement or utilisation of this finding. This is truly lamentable, since scientific curiosity should, at the least, lead us to wonder how we can fit theory to the facts and explain the phenomenon.

It is difficult to pick the time in history when cochlear implants became 'respectable'. By 1986, however, the American Academy of Otolaryngology – Head and Neck Surgery decided to make some recommendations for standardising the reporting of results, since it was by then established that many centres were doing clinical research and/or clinical rehabilitation with a number of different cochlear implant devices. The number of papers submitted for publication was increasing rapidly and the professional public would need to be able to make comparisons. An ad hoc committee was appointed, which Dr Karen Berliner chaired, and standards were developed for reporting results of cochlear implantation in adults (Brackmann, 1987).

This brings us to the present – 1990. By this time, a second cochlear implant device, the Nucleus Multichannel Cochlear Implant, has long since been approved by FDA for marketing to postlingually deaf adults; a third device, the Symbion (now Richards') Ineraid artificial ear will probably have received marketing approval for use in deaf adults by the time of publication, a recommendation having recently been received for approval from the FDA Advisory Panel; a PreMarket Approval (PMA) Application for the 3M/House single-channel cochlear implant in children aged 2 through to 17 years has been submitted to the FDA, the FDA Advisory Panel has recommended approval and a final decision by the FDA is being awaited; by publication date, a PMA will probably have been approved for the Nucleus Multichannel Cochlear Implant in children.

Considerable chunks of the history of cochlear implants have been omitted from this chronology through lack of reference to the animal and basic science research that has occurred and the clinical research of many other cochlear implant teams world wide. Ours is only a history of the idea, and of the attitudes towards that idea. From our experience, which spans most of the modern history of cochlear implants, we can identify many issues that are important to understanding the milieu that surrounds this topic. Some of these are addressed in the following section.

Issues and Perspectives

Role of the FDA

In 1976, the Medical Device Amendments to the Food, Drug and Cosmetic Act in the USA gave the FDA authority to regulate new medical devices. The law basically requires that safety and effectiveness be adequately demonstrated through clinical investigations before a device such as the cochlear implant can be marketed. Specific regulations were published in January 1980 to go into effect near the end of that year. The FDA regulations had an impact that we believe many in the professional and scientific communities fail to appreciate.

First, to use a device at all in human subjects, even one subject, required submission of an Investigational Device Exemption (IDE) application for approval by the FDA. The purpose of an IDE study is to gather clinical data on safety and efficacy eventually to be submitted for review for marketing approval by the FDA, i.e. implicit in the process is the goal of large-scale clinical trials in human subjects to result eventually in commercial marketing. This added, perhaps, a different perspective from that held by the research community.

Secondly, an IDE had to include a detailed protocol for gathering the data on safety and efficacy. Although the protocol could be changed, to do so required formal submissions and the consequent time lags until approval. Further, once a study had been under way for some time, changing the protocol would produce a significant setback in compilation of consistent data to submit for required reports and for marketing approval, i.e. it became impractical to change the assessment measures used every time a new measure had become available and had garnered popular endorsement.

Thirdly, although use of an investigational device was limited to a small number of approved sites, use could not continue indefinitely on an investigational basis, i.e. the very nature of the regulations required an eventual move to make the device generally available for use by the professional public, something that did not go over well with many critics of cochlear implants.

Finally, large-scale clinical trials require staff such as regulatory personnel, clinical specialists to maintain data and assure adherence to protocol, and a team to train and support investigators. They further require extensive data handling and analysis, report writing and travel for meetings with investigators and the FDA. In other words, clinical trials are expensive. In addition, the more patients included in the clinical trials, the more patient needs become the time-consuming priority. Thus, performing appropriate FDA-approved clinical trials may deplete resources (both time and money) to the extent that other questions of mere scientific curiosity must go unexplored or must be delayed.

From the historical perspective, there are some very positive aspects to the implementation of the FDA regulations. Clinicians who are allowed to obtain the device and perform the procedure are limited during the investigational phases to only those who meet the study sponsor's qualifications. They are typically required to take an in-depth training course. They are also required to sign an investigator agreement indicating that they agree to follow the study protocol.

In addition, the IDE regulations encourage the use of multicentre clinical trials – a rather unique approach in otology. In the case of cochlear implants, this involvement of a number of different centres helped to lend considerable credibility to the claimed results. And, of course, it makes a new device more geographically accessible to patients than if only one investigational site was involved.

Role of commercial manufacturers

In the 1980s, commercial medical manufacturing companies began to play a larger role in the field of cochlear implants. This was a necessary step for the large-scale clinical application of these prostheses. The 3M Company was, to our knowledge, the first major commercial company to investigate the possibility of getting into cochlear implants as a future product. In 1978, they began reviewing the field on a world-wide basis, making visits to some of the active implant research centres. In 1980, 3M became formally involved with the 'House' device and eventually developed some significant improvements in size and power requirements for successful transmission of the signal through the skin. Nucleus Limited, in Australia, became associated with the University of Melbourne implant project and later introduced its American subsidiary, Cochlear Corporation; Symbion (now Ineraid) became associated with the University of Utah implant, which has now been taken on by Richards Medical Company; and a variety of companies from 3M to Storz to MiniMed have collaborated with the University of California at San Francisco. For a brief period, a company named Biostim produced a single-channel cochlear implant in association with Stanford University's implant project personnel. In Europe, several devices were produced by commercial companies, and details of these are to be found in the next chapter.

The introduction of commercial companies to the field provided additional resources that were sorely needed to advance the clinical application of cochlear implants. In addition to rendering the devices, accessory equipment, printed literature and training courses to a 'professional' level, these companies provided much-needed support for repair and maintenance of patient equipment. They also provided the regulatory support that became necessary with the introduction of the FDA medical device regulations in the USA.

However, the presence of commercial companies took the cochlear implant out of the realm of academic and private non-profit institutions and placed it in the commercial marketplace where the objective is rapid development of profitable products. The accompanying aggressive marketing strategies and sometimes cut-throat competitive practices are foreign to the clinical and academic researchers involved in this field.

The concept of channels

Use of the term 'channel' was introduced to the cochlear implant field by those who made analogy to information processing theory. It was assumed that one electrode was analogous to one channel and that, therefore, performance expectations for a single-electrode device could be based on what was known about the capacity of one channel. Although the assumption may be correct, it is not self-evident that a single wire equates to a single channel in the same sense. In the normal ear, we have only one tympanic membrane, one set of ossicles, one oval window membrane. Yet each of these elements along the sound reception pathway is able to receive and pass on complex signals. Not until we begin to describe what happens inside the cochlea does the issue of channels arise, relating different bundles of nerve fibres to the concept of multiple channels. It may or may not be possible for an electrical stimulus presented on a single wire to maintain a significant level of complexity, but because of the assumption behind use of a specific term, 'single-channel', this possibility has gone unexplored.

Teamwork

One important general contribution of the cochlear implant to hearing healthcare was commented on in the preface to the 1985 supplement:

> Cochlear implants are clearly here to stay. They have introduced a unique concept into the treatment of profound sensorineural deafness – teamwork. This is not just a surgical treatment nor just an audiological treatment. It absolutely requires the cooperative efforts of both professions. For children, professionals from a variety of disciplines must work together to maximize the potential benefits for the child. An exciting challenge now exists for hearing-healthcare professionals to integrate this new alternative into their educational programs and their clinical practices.
>
> (Berliner, Eisenberg and House, 1985, p. 5S)

We truly believe that the cochlear implant has changed the practice of both otology and audiology. The interaction between these two professions, which developed for the purposes of providing a successful cochlear implant programme, has had lasting impact. It is interesting, too, that cochlear implants are one of the few topics on which papers are presented with equal frequency at both medical and speech and hearing meetings. Additionally, most of these papers are co-authored by an otologist and an audiologist. The introduction of new devices, such as partially implantable hearing aids, will benefit from these interactions as will the general quality of care for the hearing-impaired.

Other issues

There are any number of other issues that have been hotly debated in the history of cochlear implants or that have quietly played a role in shaping clinical application of these devices. There are just a few on which we wish to comment.

One area of controversy for many years dealt with placement of the electrode(s) inside the cochlea (intracochlear) or outside the cochlea (extracochlear). Devices of both types have been used. This issue was debated more strongly, perhaps, in Europe than in the USA. However, as time has yielded little evidence of significant clinical problems in patients with intracochlear implants, this issue has faded somewhat from the fore.

We have not discussed animal research or its role in the history of cochlear implants. However, there is one interesting historical trend that we would like to note. Early animal work was performed by some of the groups also interested in human studies and was directed towards issues of electrode placement, demonstration of in vivo electrode tolerance and so on. The 'middle' history of animal studies was highly oriented towards demonstrating the damage that cochlear implants might potentially cause. Results of some of these studies, using non-deafened animals and high levels of electrical stimulation, had a considerable negative impact on the attitudes towards human implantation, fuelling the controversy over this form of treatment for sensorineural deafness. Only in recent years has there been an interest in the possible beneficial effects of electrical stimulation on the auditory system. A number of animal studies are now being oriented in this direction.

Finally, we would like to comment on 'the little things' that make cochlear implants a clinically feasible rehabilitative tool. Too often, the clinical advances take a backseat in history. We have already mentioned the introduction of the magnet system for holding the external transmitter in place (see also Dormer et al., 1980) and the reconnect system for replacing an internal receiver without removing the intracochlear electrode. The magnet, in particular, was seen as a key step towards being able to use the device clinically in children. Prior to this, a variety of 'coil-holder' systems had been devised, including headbands, ear moulds and, finally, a fully adjustable system for fitting the transmitter coil to the temple

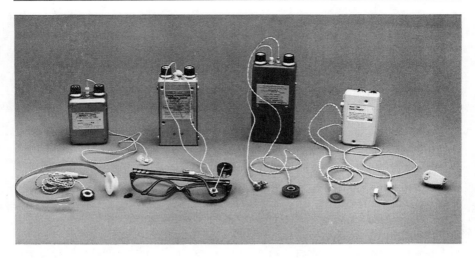

Figure 2.2. From left to right, chronological development of the House Cochlear Implant system, showing use of various methods for securing external transmitter in place (headband, spectacles, 'ring' magnet, 'centre' magnet) and various microphone placement techniques (ear mould, spectacles, tie tack, ear hook). At far right is the newest version – a miniaturised device in which microphone, transmitter and signal processor are all contained in an on-the-head case held in place by a magnet (thus, no cords or body-worn package is required).

piece of spectacles. None of these was totally satisfactory for the daily use of the device by patients. Figure 2.2 shows the transition over time to the present 3M/House device with magnetic attachment system. Similar evolutions have occurred with other cochlear implant devices.

In addition to patient hardware needs, development of written information materials for patients, rehabilitation techniques and materials, training manuals for co-investigators and patient assessment tools all played a significant role in making cochlear implants a clinically feasible prosthesis. Without some allotment of resources towards these clinical necessities, cochlear implants may well have disappeared from the scene. Each and every clinical implant programme around the world has had to deal with this issue, and many have made contributions to the field in the form of patient fitting techniques, rehabilitation materials, test procedures and information booklets.

A major contributor

In 1981, Mr Jack Urban died. Jack had devoted his time and the facilities of his company to the development of the 'House' cochlear implant at no charge. He is perhaps the single most unacknowledged figure in the history of cochlear implants. Apparently because this engineer, whose basic

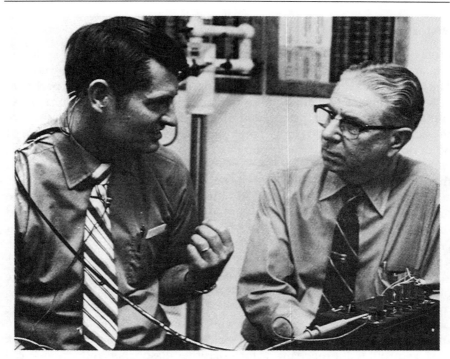

Figure 2.3.   Engineer Jack Urban testing patient who has multiple electrodes and percutaneous plug.

cochlear implant design is even today in use in large numbers of profoundly deaf adults and children, was not in an academic setting and/ or because he was an unknown to the basic hearing science community, he was never credited with the expertise and intellect that he possessed. Jack had a long and admirable history in engineering, but it was in the field of optics that he performed work for many years for NASA.

It was said on more than one occasion by members of the scientific community that the House cochlear implant which he designed was not 'engineered' but rather was 'gadgeteered'. This judgement was based on no knowledge of the research that Jack Urban performed, since it was not his highest priority to publish his work. The multichannel cochlear implant and the laboratory-based stimulation equipment that he developed in 1969 (see Figure 2.1) performed most of the processing tasks that even today are discussed in relation to multichannel stimulation (Figure 2.3). Also, it was Jack's multichannel electrode and percutaneous plug system that was first used in the University of Utah programme. No history of cochlear implants is truly complete without some acknowledgement of the role that this man played.

Historical cycles

Probably typical of most new innovations in medicine, the cochlear implant has passed through several stages regarding attitudes towards it. The cycle is repeated with each foray into a new dimension of the problem.

When cochlear implantation in human adult subjects first began at the authors' clinic, it was considered highly unacceptable by large numbers of the scientific and professional communities. 'More animal studies should be done first; benefits aren't enough to warrant an "invasive" procedure; we can do just as well with hearing aids; something better is just around the corner so stop using those primitive single-electrode devices' etc., etc. When it became clear that cochlear implants were not going to simply fade out of the picture, that some patients were undoubtedly benefiting and that newer devices would become available, the attitude changed, albeit gradually, to one of acceptance. This whole cycle started again with the first implantation of children.

As active members of a professional or scientific community, we are often called upon to voice our opinions on new ideas or practices in medicine. Our frailty is that once we have taken a highly visible public position on an issue, we are hesitant to concede a change in opinion. In the arena of cochlear implants, the introduction of newer, more complex devices provided a mechanism for cognitive dissonance reduction and a public rationale for a change in perspective. Thus, although most of the original concerns regarding damage to the auditory system, long-term effectiveness, growth and development in children etc. were at least as relevant for new devices as for the 'old' devices, these concerns were suddenly pushed aside in a new wave of acceptance.

In this cycle, we tend to forget that innovation does not often leapfrog directly to the ultimate answer. Without the steady, daily work of starting with the first step, in this case the single-electrode cochlear implant, and developing the clinical application (e.g. selection criteria, equipment and procedures for fitting and adjusting the device, rehabilitation techniques, patient information brochures, professional training materials and courses), we would not have the present 'state-of-the-art' cochlear implant. Furthermore, because of the mechanism of change in attitude, there is often little acknowledgement of the possible need for a variety of options. The 'old' need not be thrown out when the 'new' becomes available if there is still a useful role for it. We believe that there is, at the present time, still an important niche for every cochlear implant device currently available, including both single-channel and multichannel devices.

The Future of Cochlear Implants

There is now no question that electrical stimulation of the auditory system is an effective treatment for profound sensorineural deafness. We have not yet reached, and may never reach, the ultimate goal of restoring normal hearing to all patients who undergo this form of treatment. Yet it is clear that even were no further advances to be made, cochlear implants would continue to be viewed as an appropriate form of rehabilitation.

It is important to acknowledge that progress in this field has been, and will probably continue to be, slow. Present cochlear implant devices, both commercially available and investigational, are essentially the same devices that have been around for the last 5–10 years.

The number of patients seeking cochlear implants has been disappointingly small. All of the commercial manufacturers presently involved in this type of product performed marketing studies. Their projected number of consumers has failed to materialise. This is a significant problem. If commercial companies cannot make a profit or, at the very least, break even, the future of these devices may be unclear.

We are seriously concerned that cochlear implants may be an 'orphan product', i.e. there may not be a large enough market to induce manufacturers to go through the considerable expense of performing clinical trials. Under such circumstances, even if a company has a large enough share of the limited market to continue providing some of the current products, it is doubtful whether any significant amount of commercial resources will be expended towards future improvements. The next few years will tell.

Just since this chapter was first drafted, 3M Company has dropped out of the cochlear implant market, transferring rights to its products and developments to Cochlear Corporation. The 3M/House single-channel cochlear implant will probably no longer be commercially available. However, Cochlear Corporation has recently introduced a modification of the signal processing scheme for the Nucleus multichannel implant, and MiniMed is about to begin trials of a new device developed out of their collaboration with the University of California at San Francisco. We hope that progress such as that represented in these new device introductions will continue.

It is extremely disconcerting to feel so pessimistic just at the time when we have witnessed the outstanding benefits that the implant can provide to children. The future prospects for children implanted at a young age are extremely bright. The question is whether the cochlear implant will continue to be available for those children.

We would like to end by repeating what Dr Bill House said in 1986:

I am not discouraged. I am simply much wiser about cochlear implants. Twenty years ago I thought implants could be developed and widely applied in 4 to 5 years. Let us all recognize that we have at least another 20 years of painful, step-by-small-step development if we are to continue to improve the cochlear implant.

(House, 1986, p. 218)

References

BERLINER, K.I. and EISENBERG, L.S. (1987). Our experience with cochlear implants: Have we erred in our expectations? *Am. J. Otol.* **8**, 222–229.

BERLINER, K.I., EISENBERG, L.S. and HOUSE, W.F. (Eds) (1985). The cochlear implant: An auditory prosthesis for the profoundly deaf child. *Ear Hear.* **6**(suppl.), 1S–69S.

BERLINER, K.I. and HOUSE, W.F. (1981). Cochlear implants: An overview and bibliography. *Am. J. Otol.* **2**, 277–282.

BERLINER, K.I., LUXFORD, W.M. and HOUSE, W.F. (1985). Cochlear implants: 1981 to 1985. *Am. J. Otol.* **6**, 173–186.

BERLINER, K.I., TONOKAWA, L.L., DYE, L.M. and HOUSE, W.F. (1989). Open-set speech recognition in children with a single-channel cochlear implant. *Ear Hear.* **10**, 237–242.

BILGER, R.F. and BLACK, F.O. (1977). Auditory prostheses in perspective. Evaluation of subjects presently fitted with implanted auditory prostheses. *Ann. Otol. Rhinol. Laryngol.* **86**(suppl. 38), 3–10.

BILGER, R.C., BLACK, F.O., HOPKINSON, N.T., MYERS, E.N., PAYNE, J.L., STENSON, N.R., VEGA, A. and WOLF, R.V. (1977). Evaluation of subjects presently fitted with implanted auditory prostheses. *Ann. Otol. Rhinol. Laryngol.* **86**(suppl. 38).

BRACKMANN, D.E. (1987). Recommendations for the reporting of preoperative testing and postoperative results in cochlear implantation. *Otolaryngol. Head Neck Surg.* **97**, 519–521.

CLARK, G.M., TONG, Y.C., BLACK, R., FORSTER, I.C., PATRICK, J.F. and DEWHURST, D.J. (1977). A multiple electrode cochlear implant. *J. Laryngol. Otol.* **91**, 935–945.

DJOURNO, A. and EYRIES, C. (1957). Prosthese auditive par excitation electrique a distance du nerf sensoriel a l'aide d'un bobinage inclus a demeure. *Presse Med.* **35**, 14–17.

DORMER, K.J., RICHARD, G., HOUGH, J.V.D. and HEWETT, T. (1980). The cochlear implant (auditory prosthesis) utilizing rare earth magnets. *Am. J. Otol.* **2**, 22–27.

EISENBERG, L.S. and HOUSE, W.F. (1982). Initial experience with the cochlear implant in children. Cochlear implants: progress and perspectives. *Ann. Otol. Rhinol. Laryngol.* **91**(suppl. 91), 67–73.

EISENBERG, L.S., NELSON, J.R. and HOUSE, W.F. (1982). Effects of the single-electrode cochlear implant on the vestibular system of the profoundly deaf adult. Cochlear implants: progress and perspectives. *Ann. Otol. Rhinol. Laryngol.* **91**(suppl. 91), 47–54.

HOCHMAIR-DESOYER, I.J., HOCHMAIR, E.S. and STIGLBRUNNER, H.K. (1985). Psychoacoustic temporal processing and speech understanding in cochlear implant patients. In: Schindler, R.A. and Merzenich, M.M. (eds) *Cochlear Implants*, pp. 291–304. New York: Raven Press.

HOUSE, W.F. (1986). Cochlear implants present and future. *Otolaryngol. Clin. North Am.* **19**, 217–218.

HOUSE, W.F., BERLINER, K.I., CRARY, W.G., GRAHAM, M., LUCKEY, R., NORTON, N., SELTERS, W., TOBIN, H., URBAN, J. and WEXLER, M. (1976). Cochlear implants. *Ann. Otol. Rhinol. Laryngol.* **85**(suppl. 27).

HOUSE, W.F. and BERLINER, K.I. (1986). Safety and efficacy of the House/3M cochlear implant in profoundly deaf adults. *Otolaryngol. Clin. North Am.* **19**, 275–286.

HOUSE, W.F., BERLINER, K.I. and EISENBERG, L.S. (1979). Present status and future directions of the Ear Research Institute cochlear implant program. *Acta Oto-Laryngol.* **87**, 176–184.

HOUSE, W.F., BERLINER, K.I., EISENBERG, L.S., EDGERTON, B.J. and THIELEMEIR, M.A. (1981). The cochlear implant: 1980 update. *Acta Oto-Laryngol.* **91**, 457–462.

HOUSE, W.F. and URBAN, J. (1973). Long term results of electrode implantation and electronic stimulation of the cochlea in man. *Ann. Otol. Rhinol. Laryngol.* **82**, 504–514.

KEITH, R.W. (1985). Editorial comment. In: Berliner, K.I., Eisenberg, L.S. and House, W.F. (eds) The cochlear implant: An auditory prosthesis for the profoundly deaf child. *Ear Hear.* **6**(suppl.), 1S.

LOEB, G.E. (1985). Single and multichannel cochlear prostheses: Rationale, strategies, and potential. In: Schindler, R.A. and Merzenich, M.M. (eds) *Cochlear Implants*, pp. 17–28. New York: Raven Press.

LUXFORD, W.M. and BRACKMANN, D.E. (1985). The history of cochlear implants. In: Gray, R.F. (ed.) *Cochlear Implants*, pp. 1–26. London: Croom Helm.

Medical World News June 11, 1984, p. 34.

MERZENICH, M.M., SCHINDLER, R.A. and SOOY, F. (eds) (1974). *Proceedings of the First International Conference on Electrical Stimulation of the Acoustic Nerve as a Treatment for Profound Sensorineural Deafness in Man.* San Francisco: University of California.

MICHELSON, R.P. (1971). Electrical stimulation of the human cochlea. *Arch. Otolaryngol.* **93**, 317–323.

NAUNTON, R.F. (1977). Otolaryngology. *Bull. Am. Coll. Surg.* **62**, 33–35.

PARKINS, C.W. and ANDERSON, S.W. (eds) (1983). Cochlear prostheses: An international symposium. *Ann. N.Y. Acad. Sci.* **405**, 1–532.

SCHINDLER, R.A. and MERZENICH, M.M. (eds) (1985). *Cochlear Implants.* New York: Raven Press.

SIMMONS, F.B. (1966). Electrical stimulation of the auditory nerve in man. *Arch. Otolaryngol.* **84**, 24–76.

SIMMONS, F.B. (1985). History of cochlear implants in the United States: A personal perspective. In: Schindler, R.A. and Merzenich, M.M. (eds) *Cochlear Implants*, pp. 1–7. New York: Raven Press.

TONNDORF, J. (1977). Cochlear prostheses: A state-of-the-art review. *Ann. Otol. Rhinol. Laryngol.* **86**(suppl. 44).

VOLTA, A. (1800). On the electricity excited by mere contact of conducting substances of different kinds. *Trans. R. Soc. Phil.* **90**, 403–431.

Chapter 3
The Development of Cochlear Implants in Europe, Asia and Australia

DIANNE MECKLENBURG and ERNST LEHNHARDT

A History of Cochlear Implants outside the Americas

The history of electrical stimulation of the auditory system in Europe spans 200 years, beginning in 1800 when Count Alessandro Volta first applied a rather large voltage (50 V) via two metal rods inserted into his ear canals that produced a sensation of sound described as the 'boiling of viscous fluid' (Luxford and Brackmann, 1985). More directly related to cochlear implants was the work carried out by two Frenchmen, Djourno and Eyries (1957). They placed wire electrodes into the cochlea of two deaf patients who subsequently reported being able to differentiate several frequencies and also a few words without lipreading. The European news spread to the USA and three pioneer researchers – House, Michelson and Simmons – began independent studies in the 1960s, bringing further credibility to auditory prostheses.

Outside the USA, the earliest reported interest in cochlear implantation was by Graeme Clark in Australia and Claude Chouard in France. These pioneers, and numerous other researchers, contributed new knowledge in the areas of microsurgical techniques, electrode design, cochlear anatomy, histological findings relating to electrical stimulation and acoustic deprivation, psychophysics, speech coding, electrophysiology and evaluation techniques. The Clark team approached the subject of cochlear implants using scientific stratagem whilst Chouard approached the subject from a more clinically based philosophy. It is not surprising, then, that Chouard was the first surgeon outside of the USA to place a cochlear implant in a human being.

Professor Graeme Clark's early interest stemmed from the work of Simmons (1967) and the belief that a multichannel approach to stimulating the cochlea in a meaningful fashion would be essential. To this end, he left his surgical practice in 1967 and began research on animals to investigate auditory neural mechanisms and the application of electrical stimulation for the management of deafness (Epstein, 1989). Professor Claude Chouard, however, was guided by the desire to provide more information to implant subjects than that which had been available through single-channel devices. He, as a young intern working under Dr Eyries in the late 1960s, learned about the details of the earliest single-wire-electrode implant and became convinced that the most effective regime for cochlear stimulation would be multichannel (Chouard, 1978). Although it was several years before these men implanted their first patients, both aspired to provide deaf individuals with more than just 'contact' with an acoustic environment, but rather electrical signals that would supply adequate information for speech understanding. During the following decades, at least 38 different cochlear implant configurations from 12 different countries were developed by 22 investigating teams. Table 3.1 provides an overview of the multinational activity. It must be noted that 'subjects implanted' reflects only recipients outside North and South America. The greatest number of implanted subjects have emanated from ideas originating in France, Australia, Austria and Germany. As of November 1990, world wide, including all cochlear implant variations, nearly 5000 individuals (adults and children) have received some type of cochlear implant system.

Early Investigators

France: Paris

Chouard and Macleod developed a bundle of electrodes, each of which could be inserted into the cochlea independently, coupled with a digital speech processing strategy, and implanted Europe's first patients in 1973 (MacLeod, Chouard and Weber, 1985); by 1975 they had implanted 20 subjects (Luxford and Brackmann, 1985). These first patients had five to seven monopolar, individual electrodes placed into the cochlea through holes drilled in the promontory. Each electrode was separated by several millimetres and isolated with a Silastic sleeve. The transmission link was percutaneous, with a large, but wearable, processing unit. A second-generation electrode and speech processor was designed by 1976 and, in the following years, underwent several iterations. The first new electrode was expanded to 12 channels using the same bundle design as the previous version. Later, an intracochlear carrier was developed and 12 electrodes placed along the array in Silastic depressions. The coding for the speech processor used a filter-bank approach for signals between 100 and 3000 Hz. It drove the electrodes with square waves at a rate equal to or less than 300 pulses per second. Both amplitude and pulse duration were varied to increase or decrease loudness (MacLeod, Chouard and Weber, 1985). In 1982, the results of comparative studies brought to question

Table 3.1 Description of 38 cochlear implant configurations developed, excluding those developed in the Americas

Primary investigator	Country	City	Year of first interest	Year of first implant	Channels	Electrodes	Location	Subjects* implanted	Comments
Hochmair-Desoyer/ Hochmair	Austria	Vienna/ Innsbruck	1975	1977	1	Single	Extra-	125	Round window
					1	Multi-	Intra-	72	Two bipolar pairs but chooses only one pair
						Multi-	Intra-	5	Combines analogue and digital stimulation
Graeme Clark	Australia	Melbourne	1967	1978	22	Multi-	Intra-	691	Programmable, bipolar or common ground
Nucleus	Australia	Sydney	1986	1988	1	Single	Intra-	0	Driven by a multichannel processor
					5	Multi-	Extra-	5	Promontory placement
Marquet/Peeters LAURA	Belgium	Antwerp	1978	1986	8	Multi-	Intra-	2	Internal canal antenna; all-in-ear mic/ pre-amp/antenna/data control circuit
					6	Multi-	Extra-	?	
Gersdorff/Schneppe	Belgium	Brussels	1984	1985	1	Single	Intra-	5	Initially, extracochlear
Goa	China	Shanghai	?	?	1	Single	Intra-	1	
					3	Multi-	Intra-	1	
Chen	China	Guangzhoi	1983	1984	4	Multi-	Both	20	
Valvoda	Czechoslovakia	Prague	1982	1987	1	Single	Extra-	3	Round window
Tichy	Czechoslovakia	Prague	1979	1982	1	Single	Intra-	1	
Bonding/Lauridsen	Denmark	Copenhagen	1980	1983	?	Multi-	Intra-	2	Expanding array
Gerhardt	East Germany	East Berlin	1985	1986	1	Single	Extra-	5	
Chouard	France	Paris	1968	1974	12	Both	Intra-	170	Monopolar stimulation, programmable
				1985	1	Single	Both		
				1989	15	Multi-	Intra-		
Frachet	France	Bobigny	1986	1987	1	Single	Extra-	1	Oval window placement
Fraysse	France	Toulouse	1980	1981	1	Single	Extra-	22	Receiver implanted in chest

37

Name	Country	City								Description
Portmann	France	Bordeaux	1978	1980	1	Single	Extra-	30		Multiple subcutaneous receivers
Morrison/Evans	UK	London	1981	1984	5	Both	Both	5		Implanted lower rib cage
Douek/Fourcin/ Moore	UK	London	1975	1978	1	Single	Extra-	14		(Original) retractable electrode
				1990	3	Multi-	Extra-	3		Promontory grooves for electrode Bioglass, neural network programming Round window and promontory stimulation
Fraser	UK	London	1983	1983	1	Single	Extra-	56		Round window
Bosch/Colomina	Spain	Barcelona	1976	–	6	(Multi-)	(Intra-)	0		Multiple subcutaneous receivers Six bipolar electrode pairs
Dillier/Fisch/ Spillmann	Switzerland	Zürich	1974	1979	1	Single	Extra-	12		Vienna implant used with their own processor
Kanchanarak	Thailand	Chaing Mai	1989	?	1	Single	Intra-	?		
Banfai	West Germany	Cologne-Düren	1976	1977	8/14	Multi-	Extra-	208		Promontory stimulation
					16	Multi-	Both	?		Analogue/digital, transcutaneous, programmable
Hortmann	West Germany	Neckartanzlingen	1977	1984	8	Multi-	Both	120		Promontory or scala stimulation
					1	Single	Intra-			Driven by a multichannel processor

*Implant numbers (adults and children) not including the Americas as of February 1990.

the efficacy of implanting multichannel devices in subjects who may have severely compromised auditory systems. Consideration was also given to the large expense surrounding multichannel equipment. To this end, a single-channel electrode and processing unit was developed. The electrode was a simple ball electrode which could be placed either in an extra- or intracochlear position. The processing unit used a feature extraction method for the pitch of the signal – voicing pitch – and presented a square wave at the rate of that frequency (Chouard et al., 1987).

Improvements to the multichannel system led to more efficient coding, flexible programmable memory and increased channels used for transmission in a device described as a 'multifunctional, programmable, physiological stimulator' (Chouard, C.H. 1990, personal communication). This newest system uses advanced digital signal processing. The acoustic signals are fast Fourier transformed into 15 channels lying between 100 and 4000 Hz. Each channel is assigned to a specific electrode located on a 17-mm electrode array. The electrodes are always stimulated sequentially, in numerical order along the array, at 300 pulses per second. The transmission link is transcutaneous to a hermetically sealed ceramic receiver/stimulator. There are two electrode-array designs: one each for the right and left cochlea. However, the single-channel system continues to be the device of choice for elderly patients and young children. By 1984, 91 pre- and postlinguistically deafened adults, and 9 children had been implanted; a total of 126 by 1988; and at the time of writing, 170 subjects had received implants derived from concepts associated with Chouard.

Australia: Melbourne/Sydney

A more complex feature extraction system was developed by the work of Clark and his team at the University of Melbourne. Three subjects were implanted with a 20-electrode, 10-channel, bipolar electrode array in 1978 (Clark, 1987). Extensive psychophysical experimentation took place, resulting in the selection of more definitive coding parameters for their feature extraction coding strategy. The earliest, small, wearable, processing units, available in 1982 through Nucleus, used a digitally controlled stimulation regime. It transmitted the voicing feature, F_0, as the rate of stimulation; the frequency feature of the second formant (F_2) as place of stimulation corresponding to electrode location and the amplitude feature of the speech waveform as the level of applied current. After having gathered data from about 100 adult, postlinguistically deafened, implanted subjects, the feature extraction strategy was expanded to include another frequency feature – the first formant F_1 (Clark, 1987) and its corresponding amplitude. Thus, two features activated electrodes located along the array tonotopically. This was accomplished sequentially, although the electrodes were not stimulated in order, e.g. 1 – 22, but determined by the occurrence of frequency-band-to-electrode location determined by the maxima for F_1 and F_2. The new wearable processor then extracted five speech features: F_0, F_1, F_2 and the two-formant amplitudes. A new strategy called MULTIPEAK, released by Nucleus in 1989, now provides an additional three bandpass filters for formant extraction, emphasising high-frequency information. They range from 2000 to 7000 Hz. The amplitude of the three filter bands is also estimated and mapped to current. The new coding scheme stimulates four electrodes in rapid succession for each F_0 period. Special algorithms have been incorporated which alter the relationship between pulse amplitude and pulse duration in order to allow the four pulses to occur within each frame (Lehnhardt, von Wallenberg and Battmer, 1990).

To date, more than 4000 deaf individuals have received some type of Nucleus system world wide; nearly 700 of these have been implanted outside of North America. The Nucleus MiniSystem 22 is currently the only cochlear implant system satisfying the safety and effectiveness require-ments of the US Food and Drug Administration (FDA) for implanting both adults and children. The youngest recipient has been a 2;3 year old and the oldest recipient was 87 years old. Continued work from the Department of Otolaryngology at Melbourne University has resulted in a novel time-division current multiplexing technique called 'quasi-simultaneous stimulation' (McDermott, 1987). Along with the desire to provide better speech perception, it has been developed to minimise potential electrical interactions at the active electrodes. The stimuli are independently controllable in current amplitude, duration and onset time; groups of three stimuli can be generated typically at a rate of 500 Hz. The device also incorporates an outward telemetry system that enables electrode voltage waveforms to be monitored externally any time after implantation (McDermott, 1989). This facility permits the electrical performance of the stimulator and electrode array to be checked in vivo and reportedly is proving useful in long-term studies aimed at characteris-ing the electrical properties of the electrodes and their environment. To date, three totally deaf individuals have received the advanced implant (H.J. McDermott, 1990, personal communication).

Belgium: Antwerp

In 1978, a team of researchers in Belgium, represented in the acronym 'LAURA', began development of a multichannel, programmable device that could stimulate both 'simultaneously or sequentially with analog or pulse-type stimuli' (Peeters et al., 1987). Encouraged by the work of Merzenich in the USA and Clark in Australia, they focused on designing a multichannel system that had effective channel separation and used a feature extraction approach to coding. The 21-mm electrode array had 16 ball electrodes placed in preformed cups along a silicon carrier. Many changes to the implanted electronics and the electrode design and fabrication have occurred. The feature extraction processing had strong similarities to the Clark coding scheme. The fundamental frequency controlled the rate of stimulation, and maxima from four frequency bands were estimated and translated to electrode place and signal amplitude. All eight electrodes would be stimulated when voiced sounds were detected and only four electrodes would be activated when unvoiced sounds were detected (Peeters et al., 1990). The externally worn ear mould contained a transmitting antenna, a microphone/preamplifier and a data modulation circuit. The internal, receiving antenna was placed around the external ear canal. A unique feature of the receiver/stimulator was, at that time, a feedback control system that allowed the status of the internal elements to be monitored, e.g. voltage measurements at the tip of each electrode. Future developments will be improved speech algorithms and size reduction of the external equipment.

Controversy Develops

A great deal of publicity surrounded the first implantations, both by Chouard in France and by House in the USA. It appeared to the medical and scientific communities that, perhaps, events were unfolding too rapidly for human subjects without enough supporting basic research. There was a strong need to understand better what the mechanisms for direct electrical stimulation of the eighth nerve were and how it might affect long-term safety and perceptual performance.

England: London (EPI)

In this atmosphere, the United Kingdom's External Pattern Input (EPI) Group was formed in 1975 with the triad of Douek, Fourcin and Moore as the primary investigators. Their stated purpose was to learn whether electrical stimulation of the eighth nerve was a viable means of transmitting information if the stimulation were presented external to the scala tympani, i.e. without invasion of the cochlea. They were also seeking to learn what types of acoustic patterns could be used to transmit speech most effectively to the eighth nerve. Their earliest work concentrated on demonstrating that round window stimulation could provide equivalent results to that of single-channel, intracochlear electrodes (Moore et al., 1984). A most creative method was used not only to devise an 'implant' that was not implanted (Walliker et al., 1985), but also, eventually, to devise a surgical technique (no longer in use) called a 'tympanopexy' (Douek and Faulkner, 1987). The active electrode was located on a stiff wire protruding from the end of the distal portion of an ear mould. When the ear mould was placed in the ear canal, the tip of electrode would rest on the promontory, providing extracochlear stimulation. The stimuli presented were charge-balanced square waves which varied in amplitude and rate with the changing fundamental frequency (F_0) of a speaker's voice. The EPI group were the first to develop an efficient F_0 extractor. The first subjects received this extracochlear, removable electrode in 1978.

Since that time, the EPI group has been experimenting with permanently implanted electrodes. In order to evaluate the fixing of an electrode to the promontory, they conducted animal experiments using Bioglass, a material that completely integrates with bone. The first patient to receive the new single extracochlear electrode was in 1987. It consisted of a 5-mm disc of Bioglass with a concave platinum contact pad. The pad was welded to a PT foil electrode which passed through Bioglass and was embedded in the promontory. The pad was contacted by the ear mould electrode. This method provided improved dynamic range and ensured that the electrode placement was constant (A. Faulkner, 1990, personal communication). Having found these improvements, they next implanted two subjects in 1990 with multiple electrodes. The array of electrodes consisted of one indifferent electrode and three active, the latter three being placed independently at the round window, the second turn of the cochlea and the apex of the cochlea. In keeping with the philosophy, and the name of the group, the electrodes were placed outside of the cochlea. Those placed in grooves made in the promontory were fixed with Bioglass. The array was implanted using a meatal approach and the connector embedded in the external auditory canal, thus providing a percutaneous connection. The first two patients with the new array are undergoing psychophysical testing to determine whether channel separation can be obtained using this type of electrode placement, and what the best types of stimuli might be. Currently, the patients receive sound sensations from laboratory clinical stimulators but will obtain wearable stimulating units in the future. Because the connector sits outside the otic capsule, eventually the externally worn stimulator would be attached directly to it and worn in the pocket or on a belt. A more conventional postauricular placement of the microphone should also be possible.

Another innovation from this group is the use of neural-network classifiers for real-time speech processing. Three complex algorithms depend upon a training phase during which the network 'learns' which features of the speech waveform reliably indicate the pattern to be extracted. The first application has been for voice fundamental period estimation, in which the period of each successive cycle of vocal fold closure, measured by an electrolaryngograph, provides an ideal reference for training the network to provide a period-by-period estimate of

fundamental frequency. Classifiers can be trained in noise and reverberation, so as to be more robust in such conditions (Howard and Huckvale,
1988). A wearable speech processor which runs this neural-network F_0
extraction algorithm on a TMS320C25 chip is currently under development (Walliker and Howard, 1990).

Austria: Vienna/Innsbruck

Austrian interests were proceeding through the Cochlear Implant Project
in Vienna under the guidance of Burian, Hochmair-Desoyer and Hochmair.
Their first approach was to utilise a hermetically sealed electronics
package attached to an intracochlear, eight-electrode array. Two patients
were implanted with this system that presented pulsatile stimuli delivered
from a transcutaneously linked external processor (Hochmair-Desoyer et
al., 1981). Later, the goal of the team was to make the internal implant
signal transparent, i.e. so that it could be driven by any external processor.
They also changed the configuration of the stimulus presentation to a
single, bipolar pair of intracochlear electrodes and developed a single-
channel extracochlear ball electrode. The transparency of the receiver/
stimulator added flexibility to the use of the implants as they could be
interfaced with other research devices. The multielectrode array had two
implanted receivers (Burian et al., 1984). For their designs, they always
selected one pair of electrodes for broad-band analogue stimulation: in the
case of the intracochlear device one pair of the available four was chosen.
A technique of equalising the loudness of different frequency bands was
utilised with a method they called 'multifrequency coding', i.e. four
separate bands which could be adjusted until the entire frequency range
sounded equally loud. These adjustments were carried out through a
computer-controlled fitting system. Once the amplitude of the frequency
bands was equalised, they were recombined and transmitted as one
channel of information (Hochmair-Desoyer et al., 1989). The most recent
research efforts have re-examined the use of multichannel stimulation. A
method of simultaneously transmitting pulsatile and analogue signals has
been developed (von Wallenberg, Hochmair and Hochmair-Desoyer,
1990). The second formant frequency, F_2, is coded to electrode place
(place-pitch) and presented as pulsatile signals, whilst one other channel
receives the analogue signal (rate-pitch). In this way, the designers
speculate that both pitch and timing characteristics of a speech signal will
be preserved. Five patients have been evaluated with this new technique.

Switzerland: Zürich

In Switzerland, research into coding first began in 1974 by Dillier, Leifer
and Fisch. Their main interest was to evaluate electrical auditory responses
to simply coded data which could eventually lead to an understanding of
the parameters needed for an efficient and effective multichannel

prosthesis (Dillier, Leifer and Fisch, 1976). The first implanted patients, in 1977, received a hard-wired, two-channel bipolar implant with the electrodes placed in the modiolus (Dillier, Spillmann and De Min, 1987). Each electrode was stimulated independently. A percutaneous connection was chosen only for these early experiments in order to access the implanted electrodes directly. The aim, however, was to implement a transcutaneous system thereafter (Dillier and Spillmann, 1978). It is not clear why the team abandoned the modiolar placement, but they did report difficulties with the percutaneous connection.

Their next experiments were with electrodes placed at the round window. They directed attention to speech processing and interfaced their external system(s) with the transparent, single-channel, monopolar, round window electrode produced by the Vienna team. The Zürich team was the first outside the USA to use pulsatile stimulation regimes. Their single-channel pulsatile stimulator employed a number of variable parameters which allowed them to evaluate subjects in different coding conditions (Dillier and Spillmann, 1984). Ten such systems have been implanted. The results of their studies demonstrated, like the EPI group in London, that auditory perceptual performance similar to that obtained by investigators implanting intracochlear single-channel electrodes could be obtained with extracochlear stimulation. Later, computer-controlled fitting software was designed for the implementation of pulsatile and analogue coding strategies. Their future aim is to develop a portable TMS320 system, through which flexible, experimental coding strategies can be applied to subjects already using implanted electrode(s). This approach would allow subjects to have access to a variety of sophisticated laboratory coding approaches and, at the same time, have a take-home device from which more experience can be gained.

West Germany: Cologne-Düren/Neckartanzlingen

Paul Banfai developed an interest in cochlear implants in 1975 after travelling to the Los Angeles group where he learned first-hand about the device developed by William House and Jack Urban (1973). He brought the single-channel device to Germany and implanted his first patient shortly thereafter. However, he felt that the results were not satisfactory and decided to devise a system which would be more specialised in providing independent frequency information. He contacted Gunter Hortmann, an engineer, and together they revisited the LA team. There they observed the preoperative evaluation procedure of promontory stimulation and reasoned that the placement of multiple electrodes on the promontory would provide both a non-invasive placement and the potential for multichannel, frequency-specific stimulation (G. Hortmann, 1990, personal communication). The collaboration resulted in a device which employed a modified Vocoder principle to multiple electrodes placed in an extracochlear position. To gather psychoacoustic and electrophysiological data, in 1977, Banfai implanted a four-electrode array in two patients. The active, spiral-shaped electrodes were anchored in holes drilled at regular intervals in the promontory wall. The ground electrode was anchored in the mastoid cavity. The transmission link was percutaneous and stimulation was provided directly from a computer-based signal generator.

From these early studies, Hortmann developed a portable processing unit which consisted of four bandpass filters connected to four square-wave generators with a step-down (counter/divider) function. The square-wave pulse generators were automatically activated when the filter output exceeded 55dB. The stimulus source was a constant-current output whose stimulus amplitude was permanently set, i.e. each channel was set for equal loudness (Hortmann, 1990). This was accomplished by directly testing a patient. Banfai and Hortmann soon increased the number of channels from four to eight (in 1981) and used what they termed 'an anti-coincidence circuit' which allowed only one stimulus impulse at a time to act on one of the eight active electrodes. The electrodes protruded from a contact plate in an arrangement that would, theoretically, allow for tonotopic stimulation of the underlying cochlear region. The implant was termed a 'hedgehog' (Banfai et al., 1984). During 1984, Banfai and Hortmann began to develop their own separate units. The first patients implanted with the newly designed Hortmann implant were implanted in late 1984 by Morgenstern in Düsseldorf. It utilised the same electrode, but differed in that it was equipped with analogue high-frequency transmission, and the output signal was digitalised. Innovative placement of the receiving antenna was part of the system. It was located around the external auditory meatus, and an ear mould-type transducer was placed in the ear canal. In 1987, Hortmann introduced an intracochlear electrode array with eight active monopolar-stimulating electrodes. A single-channel monopolar electrode that was driven by the 12-channel processor became available in 1989.

To date, including all three implant systems, there are a total of 100 Hortmann implants in 12 different countries (Hortmann, 1990). The device utilised by Banfai became a 16-electrode array, could be used either percutaneously or transcutaneously and included digital transmission of the data (Banfai et al., 1987). Their most recent programmable speech processor has made it possible to select varying bipolar pairs for stimulation and to adjust stimulus intensities for each. They have applied their signal presentation in both a single-channel and a multichannel configuration, i.e. as with the multielectrode Vienna device, they might choose only one bipolar pair for stimulation. Since 1985, 108 more patients have been implanted, for a total of 208 from the first implantation in 1979. These include 133 prelinguistically deaf and 75 postlinguistically deaf cases. Further, there have been 79 children (between 4 and 18 years old) implanted, 68 of whom were prelinguistically deaf.

Conservatism in Europe

The earliest concepts for cochlear implants involved multielectrode stimulation. Extracochlear developments appear to have been influenced by a study originating from England (Ballantyne, Evans and Morrison, 1978, 1982). A survey conducted by a group of British investigators summarised the status and findings of teams using permanently placed cochlear implants. One of the more significant conclusions was a recommendation to determine the merit of single-channel cochlear implants over hearing aids and vibrotactile devices. To accomplish this, devices that could stimulate outside the cochlea, potentially causing less damage, might be most appropriate for such experimentation. Before the 1978 survey, only one group – the EPI from London – had been developing an extracochlear device; since that report, 13 additional extracochlear electrodes (single and multi-) have been developed. Even teams which had been convinced of the value of intracochlear stimulation took the option to design extracochlear units, e.g. Clark/Nucleus, Chouard, Hochmair and Marquet/ Peeters. However, progress in sophisticated cochlear implant technology did not cease, it simply diversified. The final recommendation of the report suggested that extracochlear systems were the first step. If these were shown to be effective, then intracochlear implants could be pursued. The authors of this report, have implanted five subjects with an intracochlear, multielectrode device.

The support for a conservative approach to implantation was readily accepted in Europe. This was especially pertinent because most investigators expressed a desire to provide help to deaf children through the application of cochlear implants. Therefore, invasive techniques were to be carefully analysed. The early investigating teams in Bordeaux (1978), Vienna (1977), West Germany (1978) and Toulouse (1980) developed extracochlear implants. Further, deaf-rights groups were beginning to resent the media's representation of deaf individuals as people who could not cope in hearing communities. Thus, it is also not surprising that there was a rush to defend hearing aids and tactile devices.

France: Bordeaux

At the time when the team of Professor M. Portmann developed an interest in cochlear implants, the questions raised by the Ballantyne study and the efficacy of implanting intracochlear devices were unanswered (Portmann, 1990). Although their earliest interest in using direct electrical excitation of the auditory nerve was to investigate tinnitus suppression, they also examined the effects of electrically stimulating totally deaf subjects using temporary electrodes. Observations relating to the aetiology of deafness suggested that there was little relationship between cause of deafness and a patient's ability to respond to auditory sensations, at least at an awareness level, i.e. even long-term deafened subjects could benefit from electrical stimulation (Cazals et al., 1984). As a result of this finding, they developed their own single-channel device, choosing extracochlear to reduce the potential of damaging the structures of the cochlea. The first model became available in 1980. Their results showed that patients could monitor their own voice, could attend to sound, but had very little or no discrimination capabilities for speech (Portmann, Cazals and Negrevergne, 1986). A total of 22 Prelco devices (the Bordeaux implant) were implanted in five different investigating centres; 14 of these were implanted in Bordeaux (Daumon, Bebear and Portmann, 1990). To date, the single-channel implant continues to be placed in subjects whose cochleae are completely ossified; however, in most cases the choice is a multichannel implant (Portmann, 1990).

France: Toulouse

Interest in Toulouse first arose in 1979 when the mood in France was strongly against intracochlear implantation of children. Professor Bernard Fraysse and his colleagues decided to embark on the development of a single-channel, extracochlear system. They observed that the House system might have some problems with stabilisation of the implant itself, and sought a better means of fixation in the cochlea. They also wished to reduce chances of infection and provide more convenience to the patient. Therefore, their implanted electronics were placed in the thoracic area where there would be no potential postauricular problems and the implanted portion would be aesthetically pleasing because it was unseen. Further, there was a large area available for implantation. This made a small-sized implanted receiver-stimulator a less important factor and also technologically easier to implement. They associated themselves with a French pacemaker company, Medtronics, in 1980. The processing approach was straightforward, using bandpass filtering and compression of an analogue signal (Fraysse et al., 1987). The first patient was implanted at the end of 1981 in Toulouse and the last patient in early 1988 after a total of 22 patients, including those from five other investigating centres. Their findings indicated poor speech results and problems with the extracochlear placement, and so the decision was made to discontinue implanting a single-channel device. Further, 25% of the patients had very high thresholds with a resultant small dynamic range (B. Fraysse, 1990, personal communication). The Toulouse centre continues to implant multichannel devices in their patients.

Czechoslovakia: Prague

Tichy and his colleagues began their first development in 1979 with an extracochlear, single-channel neuroprosthesis and used this with four patients (V. Raisova, 1990, personal communication). Later, two patients were implanted with the Implex (Hortmann), eight-channel, extracochlear system. A great deal of time was spent gathering together a complete implant team and developing test materials, as none of the materials being used for comparative studies could be applied to their language. Some technical difficulties were experienced with both devices: inadequate sealing of the implantable electronics resulted in the Czechoslovakian unit having a short life expectancy, and one of their two Implex patient's implanted auricular antenna failed. The team discontinued implantations in 1989, but intend to pursue the development of a multichannel device.

The 1970s came to an end with three extra- and three intracochlear devices having been implanted in a total of about 60 individuals in France, Australia, Austria, West Germany, Switzerland and England. This period of research brought both controversy and confirmation to the field of auditory prostheses.

Clinically Applied Implants

Most of the implant systems developed in the 1970s underwent, and continue to undergo, technological advances. Six systems have assumed clinical status, moving beyond experimental or investigatory applications. For the purposes of classification, this means that at least 50 or more subjects have received a particular device. Further, each has affiliated with a manufacturing company making it possible for the devices to become commercially available. The characteristics of the six are listed in Table 3.2. It can be seen that there is only one newcomer to the early researchers; this is the UCH/RNID device from London.

England: London (UCH/RNID)

This group, spearheaded by Fraser, Graham and Gray, essentially developed their system out of necessity. They had originally begun cooperative work in early 1983 with the Michelson device from San Francisco. When that device ran into production problems they used the Vienna device. One patient was implanted with the SF device and 5 were implanted with the Vienna extracochlear system. Unfortunately, the Vienna system, having been taken over by 3M, ran into some challenges relating to US FDA regulations and delivery problems arose. At this point, the University College Hospital team decided that there was an urgent need for a

Table 3.2 Description of commercially available cochlear implant systems that have been designed in Europe and Australia

In clinical use[a,b]

Principal investigator	Manufacturer	Available configurations[c]	Processing		Coding		Signal		Timing		Transcutaneous link	Programmable memory
			Analogue	Digital	Feature	Filter	Analogue	Pulsatile	Sequential	Single-		
Banfai	EMG	3		X		X		X	X	X	X	X
Chouard	MXM	3		X	X	X		X	X	X(F0)	X	X
Clark	Nucleus	2		X	X			X	X	X	X	X
Fraser	Finetech	2	X			X	X			X	X	
Hochmair	Med-El	3	X			X	X			X	X	
Hortmann	Implex	3		X		X		X	X	X	X	X

[a]Systems which have been developed outside the Americas.
[b]Clinical use defined as more than 50 patients implanted.
[c]Configurations refers to extra-/intra-/single/multi-.

reasonably priced, European-made, cochlear implant (Fraser, 1989b). They developed their own system, in association with the Royal National Institute for the Deaf, based on the principles of the Viennese device, i.e. a broad-band analogue approach to coding and a single ball electrode. The implanted receiver-stimulator utilised a different type of encapsulation process: a high-grade Silastic, rather than epoxy. This method of encapsulation had been demonstrated to be effective in other applications by the Medical Research Council Neurological Prostheses Unit. At the time of publication, 65 adults and one postlinguistically deafened child have received this system. The team intends to continue the manufacturing of their single-channel unit, and also to develop a multichannel European system. They are convinced that an analogue approach is the most effective for profoundly deaf implantees and will use that coding strategy in their speech processor. The goal remains the same: to provide an affordable cochlear implant system which is European-made (Fraser, 1989a).

Experimental Cochlear Implants

Single-channel devices

Although the controversy surrounding single- vs multichannel devices had lessened, single-channel implants continued to be developed and research- ed because of their technical simplicity, relative ease in manufacturing and minimal insertion requirements into the cochlea. The underlying motiva- tion for these developments, with a few exceptions, appears to be mainly financial. Single-channel implant systems have been designed in China (Chen, Lee and Lin, 1985), Czechoslovakia (Valvoda, Betka and Hruby, 1987), East Germany (Gerhardt and Wagner, 1986) and Thailand (Kanchanarak, Siriratwatanakul and Boonyanukal, 1989). This latter group, from Chaing Mai, reports that they have modified a House/3M device with material costs of only US$25.00. They modified the circuit and removed the AM modulated circuit, thus consuming less power and requiring fewer transistors. They also used a new and simple technique for coating the implanted coil. Another team − Gersdorff and Sneppe at the Université Catholique de Louvain − developed their own single-channel device in order to conduct comparative studies. It had a ball electrode for stimulation transcutaneously linked to an analogue processor. The first electrodes were implanted extracochlearly, with the ground electrode located near the round window. Later some of the same subjects were reimplanted intracochlearly with the same electrode because difficulties with the placement, most importantly the securing of the electrode, developed. Eventually, a total of five patients received the MSR-UCL device. Comparative evaluations with these patients, and with others who had

received the Bordeaux (Prelco) device, concluded that significant differences were shown by intracochlear subjects who showed better voice
modulation and a 'more favourable perceptual quality to sound sensations'
(Gersdorff et al., 1987). However, the MSR-UCL device is no longer
produced, mainly because of the manufacturing expenses and the problem
of servicing already implanted patients. Currently the MSR group has
chosen to implant the Nucleus 22-electrode, intracochlear device.

One last single-channel development presents an interesting alternative
to the intracochlear/extracochlear placements. Frachet and his colleagues
(Frachet, Vormes and Despreaux, 1987) have suggested placement of an
electrode on the oval window. Their motivation for development was
concern over the fixation of extracochlear round window electrodes and
the often poor anatomical landmarks for the round window as compared
to the oval window. The electrode is 'cupula-shaped, placed at the end of
an incudovestibular prosthesis'. It is not clear how many devices have been
implanted. However, it has been reported that some subjects demonstrated
results similar to those obtained by patients with round window or
promontory implants (Frachet, Vormes and Despreaux, 1987).

Multichannel devices

Few new systems are under development, but two are worthy of mention.
The first has been implanted in five subjects and was developed with the
support of the Project Ear Foundation in London. The initial outcome of
the project, headed by A. Morrison, A. Shalom and E. Evans, resulted in the
design of a versatile research implant system (E. Evans, 1990, personal
communication). Five electrodes are available: four placed within the
cochlea and one placed at the round window; thus both extra- and
intracochlear stimulation can take place. The receiver-stimulator is
implanted in the thorax and has the capability of stimulating simultaneous
or sequential, analogue or digital, monopolar or bipolar. When stimulating
in an analogue fashion, its function is similar to the Ineraid device. Due to
the teams' aims being both experimental and clinical, they intend to
continue conducting comparative investigations between the different
configurations and coding strategies possible in their system, and also to
broaden the population of implanted subjects.

The second new multichannel system is under development in Spain
(Bosch et al., 1989). The designers reported on a six-bipolar electrode
implant, which appears to be implanted as independent electrodes in the
promontory, where frequency-to-electrode relationship is between 200
and 4000Hz. The transmission is to be transcutaneous. The pulse width,
pulse rate, pulse train and pulse amplitude will be adjustable. Acoustic
frequencies between 100 and 4000Hz will be fast Fourier transform

analysed. They claim that their simulations using cochlear experimental modelling have demonstrated new methods for utilising 'the coding of pulse frequency'. This device – called BARNA – has not been implanted in human subjects at this time.

Summary

The very first worldwide developments were directed towards designing an implant and processor that would successfully provide speech understanding. A turn towards conservatism in the mid-1970s in Europe led to extensive research and development of extracochlear electrodes. More than 40% of implants designed outside North America have been single channel and 17 of the 38 different electrode configurations have been extracochlear (Figure 3.1 and see Table 3.1). In contrast, only one single-channel and four intracochlear systems have been fabricated in North America. In general, this has been because single electrodes were considered safer in the earlier years of cochlear implant research, were easier to manufacture and often could be used with already existing speech processors. By the mid-1980s, however, most independent clinical reports had shown that all cochlear implants had the capacity to provide detection of environmental sounds, recognition and discrimination of voices and comprehension of basic speech elements. More advanced multichannel devices, however, could provide sufficient information to allow some

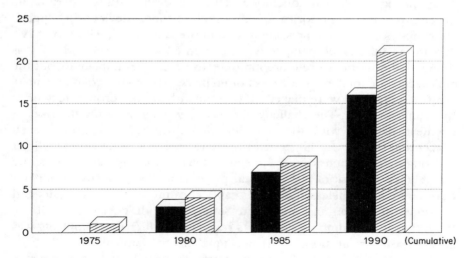

Figure 3.1. Cochlear implant device configurations: total number of implant devices developed outside the Americas; cumulative from 1975 to 1990 (as of February 1990). ■ Single electrode; ▨ multielectrode.

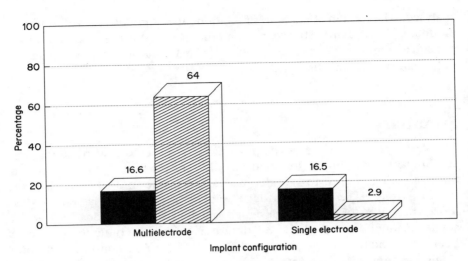

Figure 3.2. Cochlear implants: percentage of implanted population. Comparison of extracochlear-to-intracochlear implant recipients and single-to-multichannel implant recipients. ■ Extracochlear; ▨ intracochlear. (As of February 1990.)

understanding of ongoing speech without lipreading (Shallop and Meck-lenburg, 1988).

In Europe, support for implanting multichannel devices was provided by a comparative study designed to evaluate speech perception abilities of subjects using single- and multichannel French implant systems. The study, sponsored by the French National Commission, was conducted from 1985 through 1988 and concluded: 'The comparative study...permits us to confirm the superiority of the multichannel device for speech discrimination without lipreading' (Roulleau and Matha, 1989, p. 419). Perhaps an interesting perspective is presented in Figure 3.2 where it is shown that not only were more multielectrode devices implanted, but the multielectrode implants were most often placed within the cochlea; single-electrode implants were placed more frequently on the promontory or at the round window. The challenge in Europe was rationalising the risks of cochlear damage with the benefits gained through open-set speech perception. Figure 3.3 illustrates the trend to accept that the benefit of potential comprehension of spoken language through audition alone outweighed the risk of intracochlear placement. The majority of implant developers nevertheless remained sceptical of multichannel benefits and continued to design and investigate single-electrode devices, in spite of the fact that the number of subjects receiving multichannel implants was always greater than those receiving single-channel implants.

Single-channel results, in most cases, indicated that supplemental information to timing and intensity were needed for speech understanding and that added cues to speech were more possible with multielectrode

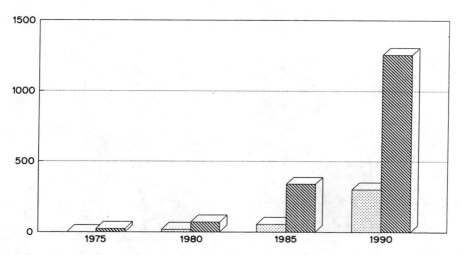

Figure 3.3. Cochlear implant recipients (cumulative): total number of implanted subjects outside the Americas: cumulative form 1975–1990. ▨ Single electrode: ▨ multielectrode. (As of February 1990.)

implants. Still, implantation in adults proceeded slowly until after 1985 when more valid evidence supporting the effectiveness of multichannel devices had been gathered. The earliest implants in children did not take place until the 1980s, when multichannel devices were implanted by Chouard and Banfai; Clark began implanting children in 1984. Although extracochlear implant arrays continue to be used, findings from psychophysical research have shown that better frequency specificity is obtained when multichannel arrays are placed within the cochlea. Thus, the largest number of implant recipients (81%) have multielectrode devices either intracochlear (67%) or extracochlear (33%) (Figure 3.4). It is not surprising, then, that by 1990 three of every four patients implanted received a multichannel device in spite of the large number of single-channel systems available.

The decade of the 1980s saw implantation increase from approximately 60 adults to 1600 adults and children. The progress in the area of implant design has been remarkable. Devices have faster processing, less power consumption requirements, improved access to useful speech information, increased reliability, make greater use of space-age 'chip' technology and have been significantly miniaturised. Better understanding of anatomical considerations has evolved, along with improvements in surgical approach, intraoperative testing, reduction of medical complications and enhanced rehabilitation techniques. The question of whether or not cochlear implants are a safe and effective means of stimulating the auditory nerve of deaf individuals has been answered to a relative degree. Still, some safety

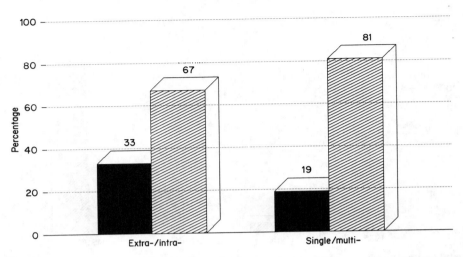

Figure 3.4. Cochlear implants: percentage of implanted population. Comparison of total extra-/intra-implant recipients and single-/multichannel implant recipients. (As of February 1990.)

issues await resolution, such as the long-term effects of electrical stimulation, the longevity of implanted electronics and electrodes, explantation and reimplantation of extra- and intracochlear electrode arrays, interface problems from the electrical stimuli to the auditory nerve and problems of isolating individual electrodes. Future research and development will lead to a more complete understanding of processing acoustic speech information, further miniaturisation resulting in more 'wearer-friendly' external components, more natural-sounding signals, simplified fitting procedures, intraoperative testing and device setting, more cost-effective manufacturing and the identification of predictive factors for successful use of a particular cochlear implant configuration. Thus, whilst today's cochlear implants are an accepted clinical tool, the future holds great promise for improved applications.

Acknowledgements

Special thanks are given to those researchers who responded so quickly to requests for updated information about their devices. These include: Professor S. Peeters (Antwerp), Professor C. Chouard (Paris), G. Hortmann (Germany), Mr E. Douek (London), Mr J.G. Fraser (London), Professor P. Banfai (Düren), Dr N. Dillier (Zürich), H. McDermott (Melbourne), Dr R. Dauman (Bordeaux), A. Faulkner (London) and H. Cooper (London).

References

BALLANTYNE, J.C., EVANS, E.F. and MORRISON, A.W. (1978). Electrical auditory stimulation in the management of profound hearing loss. Report to the Department of Health and

Social Security on visits in October 1977 to centres in the USA involved in cochlear implant prosthesis. *J. Laryngol. Otol.* (suppl. 1), 1–117.

BALLANTYNE, J.C., EVANS, E.F. and MORRISON, A.W. (1982). Electrical auditory stimulation in the management of profound hearing loss. An updated report to the Department of Health and Social Security. *J. Laryngol. Otol.* **96**, 811–816.

BANFAI, P., HORTMANN, G., KARCZAG, A., KUBIK, S. and WURSTROW, F. (1984). Results with eight-channel cochlear implants. *Adv. Audiol.* **2**, 1–18.

BANFAI, P., KARCZAG, A., KUBIK, S., LÜERS, P., SÜRTH, W. and WEISKOPF, P. (1987). In: Banfai, P. (ed.), *Cochlear Implant: Current Situation*, pp. 557–579. Proceedings from the International Cochlear Implant Symposium, Düren, West Germany.

BOSCH, J., COLOMINAS, R., AGUILO, J. and VILLA, R. (1989). The 'BARNA' cochlear implant. Paper presented at the International Symposium on Acquisitions and controversies in cochlear implants held in Toulouse, June 9–10.

BURIAN, K., EISENWORT, B., HOCHMAIR, E.S. and HOCHMAIR-DESOYER, I.J. (1984). Clinical experiences with the 'Vienna cochlear implant'. *Adv. Audiol.* **2**, 19–20.

CAZALS, Y., ARAN, J.M., NEGREVERGNE, M. and PORTMANN, M. (1984). Activation and inhibition of hearing with electrical stimulation of the ear. *Adv. Audiol.* **2**, 30–35.

CHEN, C.W., LEE, P.M. and LIN, M.D. (1985). Preliminary results of four-electrode cochlear implants. Cochlear Implant Symposium and Workshop, Melbourne 1985. *Ann. Otol. Rhinol. Laryngol.* **96**(suppl. 128), 139.

CHOUARD, C.H. (1978). *Entendre Sans Oreille*. Paris: Laffont.

CHOUARD, C.H., MEYER, B., FUGAIN, C., CHABOLLE, F. and WEBER, J.C. (1987). Introduction. In: Banfai, P. (ed.), *Cochlear Implant: Current Situation*, pp. 327–330. Proceedings from the International Cochlear Implant Symposium, Düren, West Germany.

CLARK, G.M. (1987). The University of Melbourne-Nucleus multi-electrode cochlear implant. *Adv. Oto-Rhino-Laryngol.* **38**, 124–126.

DAUMON, R., BEBEAR, J.P. and PORTMANN, M. (1990). Cochlear implant in Bordeaux: past to present strategy. Paper presented at the Politzer Society, Courchevel, France, March 11–16.

DILLIER, N., LEIFER, L. and FISCH, U. (1976). Design of a portable system for chronic stimulation of the auditory nerve, a hearing aid for the sensory deaf. From the proceedings of IIIrd Audio Symposium held in Zürich, pp. 57–69. 6–7 February.

DILLIER, N. and SPILLMANN, P. (1978). Elektrische Stimulation des Gehörs beim Menchen. *HNO* **26**, 77–84.

DILLIER, N. and SPILLMAN, P. (1984). Results and perspectives with extracochlear round window electrodes. *Acta Oto-Laryngol. Suppl.* **411**, 221–229.

DILLIER, N., SPILLMANN, P. and DE MIN, N. (1987). Ten years experience with cochlear implants: Results with single and multielectrode systems. In: Banfai, P. (ed.), *Cochlear Implant: Current Situation*, pp. 197–215. Proceedings from the International Cochlear Implant Symposium, Düren, West Germany.

DJOURNO, A. and EYRIES, C. (1957). Prosthese auditive par excitation electrique a sistance du nerf sensoriel a l'aide d'un bobinage inclus a demeure. *Presse Med.* **35**, 14–17.

DOUEK, E.E. and FAULKNER, A. (1987). Speech pattern stimulation for the totally and profoundly deaf: The work of the External Pattern Input (EPI) group. In: Banfai, P. (ed.), *Cochlear Implant: Current Situation*, pp. 237–239. Proceedings from the International Cochlear Implant Symposium, Düren, West Germany.

EPSTEIN, J. (1989). *The Story of the Bionic Ear*. Melbourne, Australia: Hyland House.

FRACHET, B., VORMES, E. and DESPREAUX, G. (1987). Electrical stimulation of the oval window. In: Banfai, P. (ed.), *Cochlear Implant: Current Situation*, pp. 657–662. Proceedings from the International Cochlear Implant Symposium, Düren, West Germany.

FRASER, J.G. (1989a). The University College Hospital/Royal National Institute for the Deaf Cochlear Implant Programme. *J. Laryngol. Otol.* (suppl. 18), 1–3.

FRASER, J.G. (1989b). The UCH/RNID cochlear implant programme and the need for European single and multi channel systems. In: Fraysse B. (ed.), *Cochlear Implant: Acquisitions and Controversies*, pp. 385–394. Toulouse: Paragraphic.

FRAYSSE, B., SOULIER, M.J., URGELL, H., LEVY, P., FURIA, F. and DEFRENNES, V. (1987). Extracochlear implantation: Technique and results. *Ann. Otol. Rhinol. Laryngol.* 96(suppl. 128), 111–113.

GERHARDT, H.J. and WAGNER, H. (1986). The Berlin cochlea implant: conception and first experiences. Part I: surgical conception. *HNO-Prax* (Lpz) 11, 187–194.

GERSDORFF, M.C.H., SNEPPE, R., WITTEMANS, S., BARBAIX, M.T., DERUE, L., MONTMIRAIL, C. and VANDERBEMDEN, S. (1987). Our experience in rehabilitation of the severely deaf by means of a monocanal cochlear implant. *Am. J. Otol.* 9, 537–544.

HOCHMAIR-DESOYER, I.J., HOCHMAIR, E.S., BURIAN, K. and FISCHER, R.E. (1981). Four years of experience with cochlear prostheses. *Med. Progr. Technol.* 8, 107–119.

HOCHMAIR-DESOYER, I.J., HOCHMAIR, E.S., ZIERHOFER, C. and STIGLBRUNNER, H. (1989). A family of extra- and intracochlear implant systems. In: Fraysse, B. (ed.), *Cochlear Implant: Acquisitions and Controversies*, pp. 361–372. Toulouse: Paragraphic.

HORTMANN, G. (1990). The development of the IMPLEX cochlear implant system. Unpublished paper, Hortman GmbH:Neckartenzlingen.

HOUSE, W.F. and URBAN, J. (1973). Long term results of electrode implantation and electronic stimulation of the cochlea in man. *Ann. Otol. Rhinol. Laryngol.* 82, 504–516.

HOWARD, I.S. and HUCKVALE, M.A. (1988). Speech fundamental period estimation using a trainable pattern classifier. *Proceedings of Speech '88*: 7th FASE Symposium, Institute of Acoustics, Edinburgh, pp. 129–136.

KANCHANARAK, C., SIRIRATWATANAKUL, N. and BOONYANUKUL, A. (1989). Inexpensive cochlear implant device modified from House-3M cochlear implant device. Paper presented at the XIV World Congress of Otorhinolaryngology, Head and Neck Surgery, Madrid, September 10–15.

LEHNHARDT, E., VON WALLENBERG, E.L. and BATTMER, R. (1990). Preliminary clinical results with a modified coding strategy for the NUCLEUS Cochlear Implant. In: *Proceedings from the XIV World Congress of Otorhinolarnygology Head and Neck Surgery*, Madrid, Sept 10–15, 1989, in press.

LUXFORD, W.M. and BRACKMANN, D. (1985). The history of cochlear implants. In: Gray, R.F. (ed.), *Cochlear Implants*, pp. 1–26. London: Croom Helm.

McDERMOTT, H.J. (1987). Cochlear implant for simultaneous multichannel stimulation. *Ann Otol. Rhinol. Laryngol.* 96(suppl. 128), 67–68.

McDERMOTT, H.J. (1989). An advanced multiple channel cochlear implant. *IEEE Trans. Biomed. Eng.* 36, 789–797.

MacLEOD, P., CHOUARD, C.H. and WEBER, J.P. (1985). French device. In: Schindler, R.A. and Merzenich, M.M. (eds), *Cochlear Implants*, pp. 111–120. New York: Raven Press.

MICHELSON, R.P. (1971). Electrical stimulation of the human cochlea, a preliminary report. *Arch. Otolaryngol.* 93, 317–323.

MOORE, B.C.J., DOUEK, E., FOURCIN, A.J., ROSE, S.M., WALLIKER, J.R., HOWARD, D.M., ABBERTON, E. and FRAMPTON, S. (1984). Extracochlear electrical stimulation with speech patterns: experience of the EPI Group (UK). *Adv. Audiol.* 1, 148–162.

PEETERS, S., OFFECIERS, F.E., MARQUET, J. and VAN CAMP, K. (1990). The LAURA cochlear prosthesis: technical aspects. Internal paper, University of Antwerp.

PEETERS, S., MARQUET, J., OFFECIERS, F.E., BOSIERS, W., KINSBERGEN, J., VAN DURME, M., SOMERS, T.,

DePAEP, K., VAN CAMP, K. and MOENECLAEY, L. (1987). The LAURA cochlear prosthesis: development and description. In: Banfai, P. (ed.) *Cochlear Implant: Current Situation*, pp. 547–555. Proceedings from the International Cochlear Implant Symposium, Düren, West Germany.

PORTMANN, M. (1990). Implants Cochleaires. Internal paper, Laboratoire d'Audiologie Expérimentale, Hôpital Pellegrin: Bordeaux.

PORTMANN, M., CAZALS, Y. and NEGREVERGNE, M. (1986). Extracochlear implants. *Otolaryngol. Clin. North Am.* **19**, 307–312.

ROULLEAU, P. and MATHA, N. (1989). Comparative evaluation of performances obtained with multi- and mono-channel implants: A study on forty patients. In: Fraysse, B. and Cochard, N. (eds), *Cochlear Implant: Acquisitions and Controversies*, pp. 417–426. Toulouse: Paragraphic.

SHALLOP, J.K. and MECKLENBURG, D.J. (1988). Technical aspects of cochlear implants. In: Sandlin, R.E. (ed.), *Handbook of Hearing Aid Amplification*, Vol. I, pp. 265–280. San Diego: College-Hill Press.

SIMMONS, F.B. (1966). Electrical stimulation of the auditory nerve in man. *Arch. Otolaryngol.* **79**, 559–567.

SIMMONS, F.B. (1967). Permanent intracochlear electrodes in cats, tissue tolerance and cochlear microphonics. *Laryngoscope* **57**, 171–186.

VALVODA, M., BETKA, J. and HRUBY, J. (1987). The first experience with cochlear implantations in Czechoslovakia. In: Banfai, P. (ed.), *Cochlear Implant: Current Situation*, pp. 289–290. Proceedings from the International Cochlear Implant Symposium, Düren, West Germany.

WALLIKER, J.R. and HOWARD, I.S. (1990). The implementation of a real-time speech fundamental period algorithm using multi-layer perceptions. *Speech Commun.* in press.

WALLIKER, J.R., DOUEK, E.E., FRAMPTON, S., ABBERTON, E., FOURCIN, A.J., HOWARD, D.M., NEVARD, S., ROSEN, S. and MOORE, B.C.J. (1985). Physical and surgical aspects of external single channel electrical stimulation of the totally deaf. In: Schindler, R.A. and Merzenich, M.M. (eds), *Cochlear Implants*, pp. 143–155. New York: Raven Press.

VON WALLENBERG, E.L., HOCHMAIR, E.S. and HOCHMAIR-DESOYER, I.J. (1990). Initial results with simultaneous analog and pulsatile stimulation of the cochlea. *Acta Oto-Laryngol. Suppl.* **469**, 140–149.

Chapter 4
Cochlear Implant Signal-processing Strategies and Patient Perception of Speech and Environmental Sounds

RICHARD S. TYLER and NANCY TYE-MURRAY

Introduction

This chapter provides an overview of different cochlear implant types and describes the perception of speech and environmental sounds that have been obtained with different cochlear implants. First, we discuss cochlear implant terminology. We then discuss different categories of cochlear implant signal processing, focusing on their rationale. Finally, we review audiological results that have been obtained with these different implants.

It is not possible to review all cochlear implants in use, since the details of some have not been described sufficiently, and newer implants are being developed. Nevertheless, we believe that describing implant categories will provide a general overview of processing schemes and a basis for understanding all schemes, both old and new. We also anticipate that the results obtained with devices using similar schemes will be similar. We focus on our own experience and review the reports of others. In some cases the results will not be directly comparable across different implant types, since the results were obtained under different test conditions and in different countries, often with different languages. Nevertheless, we think that this overview provides a general appreciation for the performance levels that can be expected from *postlinguistically deafened adults.*

Terminology

Electrodes and channels

The electrode pairs represent the positive and negative polarity contacts between which electric current passes. A cochlear implant can have one or several electrode pairs. The stimulating waveforms pass through the electrodes to excite the nerve fibres. A device can have several electrodes, usually placed along the length of the cochlear partition, and this facilitates the stimulation of different neurons.

The word 'channels' is used to designate the number of electrode pairs that are conveying *different* stimulus waveforms. Different stimulus waveforms will excite neurons in different ways. Typically, the number of channels equals the number of electrode pairs. Each electrode receives a different waveform during stimulation. In a few cases, the number of channels is less than the number of electrodes. In this latter case, some (or perhaps all) electrodes receive the same waveform. Thus it is important to distinguish between electrodes and channels.

Single and multiple channels

Following the discussion above, it is now possible to distinguish between single- and multi*electrode* systems, and between single- or multi*channel* systems.

Single electrode systems are limited because they can only be single-channel devices. Multielectrode systems can be either single channel or multichannel. Having more electrodes than channels has the advantage that some selection (for example based on speech recognition perform-ance) can be made among available electrodes. For example, Hochmair and Hochmair-Desoyer (1985) used a four-electrode single-channel device, choosing the 'best' available electrode for stimulation. The Ineraid device (Eddington, 1980) has six electrodes, from which four are selected for stimulation.

In the normal ear, the travelling wave functions to separate the frequency components of speech. Different spectral components stimulate different neurons. This attribute of frequency analysis and differential excitation is what the multichannel systems attempt to simulate.

Extracochlear vs intracochlear

Extracochlear implants have electrodes placed outside the cochlea, usually with the active electrode in the round window niche close to the basal end of the cochlea (although other configurations are possible). Intracoch-lear implants have electrodes placed inside the cochlea, usually inserted through the round window. There is some concern that placing an electrode inside the cochlea might cause bone growth and damage nerve fibres. Although the long-term (30–40 years) effects are unknown, many patients have used cochlear implants for over 10 years with no apparent decrement in performance.

There are also advantages to intracochlear stimulation. Intracochlear stimulation places the electrodes closer to the neurons and may simplify the task of stimulating different nerve fibres. Less current is typically required to stimulate the neurons.

One extracochlear implant (Banfai et al., 1988) attempts to stimulate different places along the cochlea. This is accomplished by placing a plate against the medial wall of the middle ear adjacent to the cochlea. Different electrodes are then adjacent to different turns of the cochlea. Coninx (1988) reported that some patients using this device heard different pitches when different electrodes were stimulated, consistent with the notion that different places were being stimulated. Other patients, however, did not hear different pitches, perhaps because of current spread through extracochlear tissue or intracochlear fluids.

Other stimulation sites are possible, for example, in the auditory nerve, cochlear nucleus (Edgerton, House and Hitselberger, 1982; see also Kiang et al., 1985) or brain. Electrode placement central to the cochlea has the disadvantage that the orderly alignment of neural 'best-frequency' to electrode position is not straightforward. The mapping of electrode to pitch would have to be determined for each patient using psychophysical pitch-scaling procedures. This could be difficult in young children.

Complex modifications to the patterns of neural response occur in the ascending auditory system. Many of these transformations are only poorly understood. If electrodes are placed central to the auditory nerve, then more sophisticated signal processing would be required in the implant's speech processor to optimise performance.

Bipolar vs monopolar

When the electrode's active and ground contacts are close together (bipolar), current travels a short distance. When the contacts are far apart (monopolar), current travels a much larger distance. Since all nerves within the flow of current could be stimulated, bipolar stimulation activates neurons from a more restricted place. This is desirable when the task is to stimulate different fibres with different information. However, because fewer fibres are stimulated, more current may be required to hear the stimulus than would be the case with monopolar stimulation.

Analogue and pulsatile

Current presented on the electrodes can be a continuous analogue waveform or a series of pulses. Analogue waveforms can convey all the information about the speech signal. Different nerve fibres are stimulated at different times of the waveform, depending upon the current reaching the fibre and the fibre threshold.

Pulsatile stimulation means a series of pulses which represents a digitised sample of the original waveform. It typically results in a synchronous neural discharge corresponding to the pulse onset. The pulse width, height or interstimulus interval can be varied. Increasing pulse height and width usually results in an increased perceived loudness. Decreasing interpulse interval results in an increase in the pitch perceived at least up to 300–500 pulses per second, and possibly higher (Townshend et al., 1987).

Feature extraction or wideband signal processing

Two broad categories of signal processing are distinguished. In feature extraction certain assumptions are made about the important features of speech, and these particular features are coded explicitly by the implant. Commonly coded features include fundamental frequency (F_0), first formant frequency (F_1), second formant frequency (F_2), and possibly higher formants. Different features can be presented to different channels. In wideband stimulation no assumptions are made about features. Information about the entire speech signal is presented. This can be presented all on one channel, or can be filtered and presented on different channels.

Simultaneous vs sequential stimulation

Stimuli which are presented simultaneously to two adjacent electrode pairs may not necessarily stimulate two different populations of nerve fibres. This is because current can flow throughout the cochlear fluids and surrounding tissue. This has been called *channel interaction* because the waveform on one channel can influence, or interact with, the waveform on another channel. To avoid this problem some implants stimulate different channels at different times. One approach is to interleave pulses, sequentially stimulating different electrodes and then returning to cycle through the sequence of electrodes again.

Transcutaneous vs percutaneous

There are two general ways of passing the stimulus from the speech processor to the electrode. In a transcutaneous system, a transmitter worn outside the skin is coupled to a receiver placed on the mastoid under the skin. Typically, the two are held in alignment with magnets located in both components. A carrier frequency, which is usually demodulated, is used for efficient transmission.

In percutaneous systems, the signal is directly transmitted through the skin via a wire connection between the processor and a 'plug' inserted into the skull. Systems which utilise a percutaneous connection do not require either a transmitter or receiver. The advantage of this system is that less power is required, it is simple to try new speech-processing designs (it is more 'transparent') and the internal electrode impedance can be checked easily. However, the external plug is susceptible to dirt, moisture and mechanical damage, and it provides an external entrance for infection.

Table 4.1 Important design characteristics for some cochlear implants

Implant	Number of channels	Extra- or intracochlear	Bipolar or monopolar	Analogue or pulsatile	Transcutaneous or percutaneous	Simultaneous or sequential	Coding strategy
Feature extraction							
University College London	1	Extra-	Monopolar	Analogue	Percutaneous	Simultaneous	Fundamental frequency
Nucleus	21	Intra-	Bipolar	Pulsatile	Transcutaneous	Sequential	F_0, F_1, and F_2 High frequency peaks
Wideband processing							
Vienna	1	Intra- or extra-	Bipolar	Analogue	Transcutaneous	Simultaneous	Frequency shaping
Ineraid	4	Intra-	Monopolar	Analogue	Percutaneous	Simultaneous	Four bandpass filters

Strategies of Cochlear Implant Speech Processing

In this section some cochlear implant processing strategies are described and referral is made to specific implant designs that have obtained widespread use or that are good examples of the different systems available. Table 4.1 contains some of the important information that distinguishes the different devices. It is important to appreciate that all these devices are currently undergoing revision, and each manufacturer will probably modify the processing strategies from those that are described here. Nevertheless, understanding how these devices work and why they were designed in a certain way should provide the appropriate framework for appreciating all new designs.

Wideband

Single channel

A single-channel device developed in Vienna by Hochmair and Hochmair-Desoyer (1985) operates similarly to a hearing aid and Figure 4.1 shows a schematic representation. The device provides automatic gain control to limit overstimulation, and frequency-dependent amplification (typically giving high-frequency emphasis). The effect of the high-frequency amplification can be seen (Figure 4.1) by comparing the waveform of the input 'sat' (lower left) to the output (lower right). The initial 's' and the final 't', both containing high-frequency energy, show enhancement relative to the

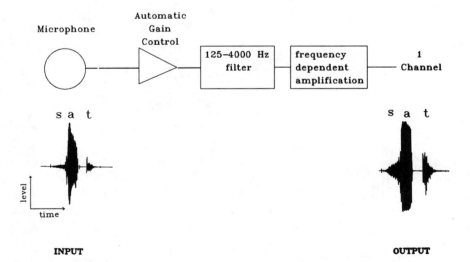

Figure 4.1. Schematic of the Vienna (Hochmair and Hochmair-Desoyer, 1985) single-channel cochlear implant.

vowel. This makes these high-frequency components of speech audible for the implant patients. Both intracochlear and extracochlear versions are available.

The UCH/RNID cochlear implant (Fraser, 1989) was designed to perform in a similar fashion to the Vienna device described above (Conway and Boyle, 1989). It presents a frequency-equalised, compressed analogue signal to an extracochlear electrode.

Multichannel

The Ineraid device (Eddington, 1980) has four channels (Figure 4.2). The incoming signal is separated into four frequency regions by four filters. Each of the four channels stimulates one of the four electrodes. The centre frequencies of the filters are 500 Hz (which stimulates the most apical electrode), 1000 Hz, 2000 Hz and 4000 Hz (which stimulates the most basal electrode). In Figure 4.2, an input signal of three sine waves is shown. These are separated by the filters, and each sine wave stimulates a different electrode. No energy was present in the 2000-Hz filter. With speech as the input, a similar separation of frequency components into different channels would be achieved.

Another wideband device of this type was developed by a team in Düren/Cologne (Banfai et al., 1988). The uniqueness of this device has already been mentioned because it is a multichannel extracochlear device. A plate containing electrode terminals is placed on the medial wall of the

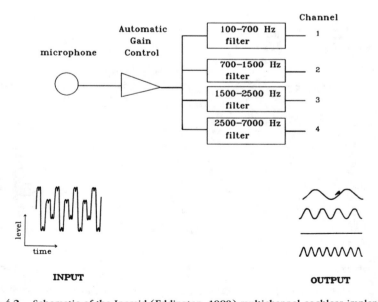

Figure 4.2. Schematic of the Ineraid (Eddington, 1980) multichannel cochlear implant.

middle-ear cavity such that the terminals are adjacent to different turns of the cochlea. This provides two very important potential advantages. First, the electrodes are not inserted into the cochlea, which will limit trauma in situations where a non-functional cochlea is uncertain (for example in a very young child). Secondly, electrodes are positioned adjacent to higher turns in the cochlea (regions that normally respond to the lower frequency components of speech). Sixteen bandpass filters are used to determine spectral peaks. Fixed amplitude and duration pulses are produced sequentially on electrodes that correspond to those filters having spectral peaks. The interpulse interval is determined by the centre frequency of the filter, lower frequency filters corresponding to longer interpulse intervals. The device can also be used as a single-channel device, with only one pair of electrodes in use.

Another example of the wideband multichannel device is the Chorimac implant developed by Chouard et al. (1986). The output of a series of bandpass filters is used to trigger pulsatile stimulation, with the current density proportional to the energy in the filter. The electrodes are stimulated sequentially with the interleaved pulses presented at a very high sampling rate. The exact parameters are set carefully for each patient.

Feature extraction

Single channel

A simple single-channel device, developed by Fourcin et al. (1979) at University College London (UCL), codes the fundamental frequency (F_0) (Figure 4.3). Fundamental frequency is important because it has been shown to enhance lipreading (e.g. Rosen, Fourcin and Moore, 1981; Grant et al., 1985; Breeuwer and Plomp, 1986). Pulses are sent at a rate

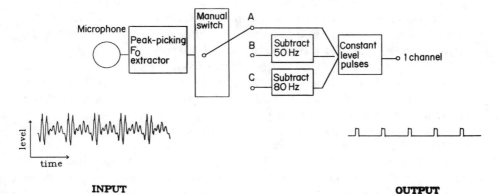

INPUT   **OUTPUT**

Figure 4.3. Schematic of the Fourcin et al. (1979) single-channel F_0-extraction device (UCH).

proportional to the fundamental frequency. With aperiodic stimuli (voiceless sounds), the pulses are aperiodic. The level of the pulses is fixed at a constant loudness, independent of rate. The average F_0 of adult males is 132 Hz, of adult females is 223 Hz and of children is 264 Hz (Peterson and Barney, 1952). The perception of differences in pulse repetition rate for electrical stimulation is poorer at higher frequencies above 150 or 200 Hz, depending on the individual patient. Therefore, this device provides a switch for patients to decrease the repetition rate when females and children are talking.

In Figure 4.3, a vowel is shown as the input. The fundamental frequency (F_0) has been extracted and a pulse train is presented at the F_0 rate. The device has a manual switch to subtract 50 Hz (for female talkers) or 80 Hz (for children). This maintains the stimulating waveform in the low-frequency region where the discrimination of F_0 is good.

Multichannel

The $F_0F_1F_2$ version of the Nucleus 21-channel intracochlear implant codes fundamental frequency (F_0), the amplitudes (A_1, A_2) and frequencies (F_1 and F_2) of the first and second formants (Figure 4.4). F_0 is extracted by a 270-Hz low-pass filter and determines the pulse rate stimulating the electrodes. The current levels correspond to the input amplitudes, and F_1 and F_2 are coded by the place of electrode stimulation. F_1 includes frequencies from 280 to 1000 Hz, and F_2 includes frequencies from 1000 to 4000 Hz. The F_1 and F_2 stimuli are always separated by about a 0.8-ms interval. For unvoiced sounds the pulse rate varies aperiodically around 98 Hz. Figure 4.4 shows the word 'heard' as the input. The output is a series of (biphasic) pulses on a number of different electrodes. The electrode position is designated by F_1 and F_2, with pulse levels at A_1 and A_2. Pulse rate is determined by F_0.

A new processing strategy has recently been introduced by Nucleus in an attempt to provide more high-frequency information. In addition to the F_1 and F_2 electrodes mentioned above, it detects energy in three bands: band 1 (2000–2800 Hz), band 2 (2800–4000 Hz) and band 3 (4000–6000 Hz). For F_1 and F_2, the particular electrodes stimulated can change as a function of time depending on the frequency of F_1 and F_2. However, the electrodes corresponding to the new bands are always the same three electrodes. Although five energy peaks are identified in the spectrum, only four electrodes can be stimulated on any cycle. For voiced sounds, F_1, F_2 and bands 3 and 4 are stimulated at a rate equal to F_0. For unvoiced sounds, F_2, and bands 3, 4 and 5, are stimulated at an aperiodic rate that varies between 200 and 300 Hz. Because it is not always possible for patients to hear any difference between two adjacent electrodes, the electrodes corresponding to the bands are not the three most basal. Instead, the basal,

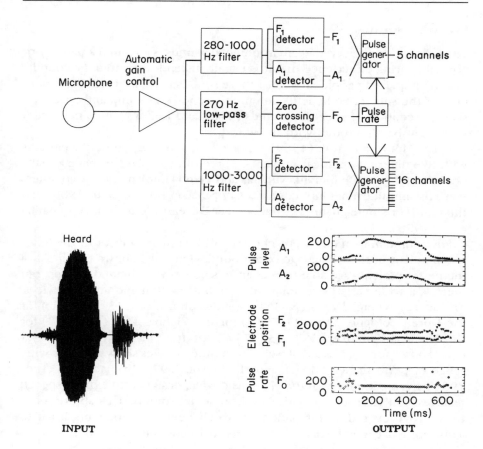

Figure 4.4. Schematic of the Nucleus (Clark et al., 1981) multichannel cochlear implant.

fourth from basal and seventh from basal electrodes are used to represent the bands. Therefore the F_2 electrode may sometimes be assigned a more basal electrode than either band 4 or 5. This could render some speech sounds more difficult to perceive. There is only limited experience with this device presently, and it will be interesting to determine how performance changes with it.

Results

There now follows a discussion of the audiological results in five general categories. These results should give a general appreciation of the performance to be expected with these devices.

Everyday sounds

The perception of everyday environmental sounds is so much a part of our normal hearing experience that it is usually taken for granted. Profoundly hearing-impaired people often miss these sounds in their 'world of silence'. One of the subjective benefits commonly reported by implant patients is their perception of everyday sounds (Tyler and Kelsay, 1990) because it puts them back in touch with the world.

Tyler, Moore and Kuk (1989) reported on some of the better patients with five different cochlear implants. Three of these devices have already been described – the Ineraid, Nucleus and Vienna implants. The two others were the multichannel intracochlear Chorimac (Chouard et al., 1986) and the multi- or single-channel extracochlear Düren/Cologne implant (Banfai et al., 1988).

Environmental sounds were chosen to be appropriate for all patients, independent of their language background. Figure 4.5 shows that most of the better patients are able to recognise some environmental sounds, but there is a wide variation among subjects both within and across devices. The scores averaged 23% (8–36%) for the Chorimac, 21% (8–67%) for the Düren/Cologne, 41% (11–72%) for the Vienna, 44% (25–72%) for the Nucleus/Hannover, 58% (39–75%) for the Nucleus/USA and 83% (56–100%) for the Ineraid. Results from other studies show a similar wide range of performance (Bilger and Hopkinson, 1977; Brimacombe et al., 1984). Even patients with the Nucleus device, designed to extract speech features, can learn to recognise environmental sounds. This ability tends to improve over time for patients with all devices, as patients learn to associate what they hear to the objects that generate the sounds.

Vowel recognition

Tests of vowel recognition indicate how well patients utilise relatively steady-state cues in the speech signal. These cues relate to vowel duration, loudness and spectral composition. A number of subjects have been tested by the authors at the University of Iowa under the continuing cochlear implant evaluation project (Tyler et al., 1986; Gantz et al., 1988). In addition to the cochlear implants already discussed, they included patients using the single-channel House device (House and Urban, 1973; Danley and Fretz, 1982). Twenty-five Ineraid, 32 Nucleus and 9 House patients have completed the authors' vowel test.

The vowel test contains nine /hVd/ utterances spoken by a male talker – the results are shown in Figure 4.6. On average, the Ineraid patients scored 47% (20–94%), the Nucleus patients scored 53% (25–90%), the Vienna patients scored 22% (8–30%) and the House patients scored 16% (8–20%). These findings agree with previous reports. For instance, Dorman et al. (1989a), studying eight of the better Ineraid users (they

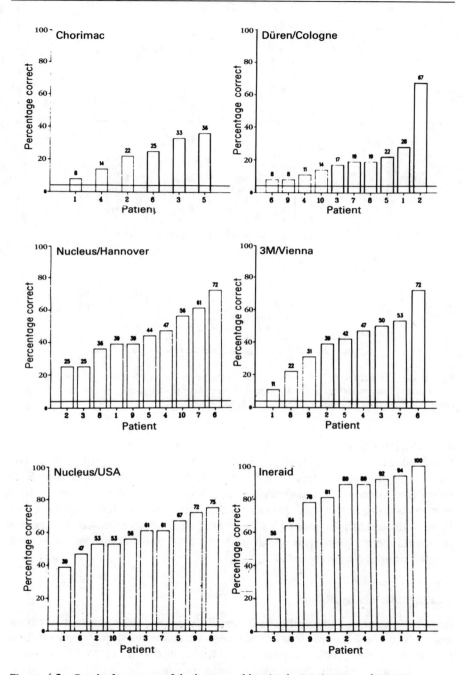

Figure 4.5. Results from some of the better cochlear implant patients on a language-independent environmental sound test. There were 16 sounds, each presented twice. The horizontal bar at 6% correct represents chance performance. (From Tyler, Moore and Kuk, 1989, with permission.)

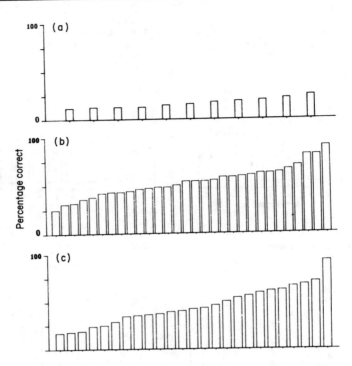

Figure 4.6. Vowel recognition from patients with the House (a), Nucleus (b) and Ineraid (c) cochlear implants measured at the University of Iowa. There were nine different vowels, each presented six times. Chance performance is 11%.

scored better than 70% on a spondee recognition test), reported a mean score of 60% correct (range = 49–79%) for a synthetic vowel test consisting of 12 /bVt/ samples. Blamey et al. (1987) found that five patients using the Nucleus device scored 57% (range = 45–66%) on an 11-item test, consisting of naturally produced /hVd/ utterances. Hochmair-Desoyer, Hochmair and Stiglbrunner (1985) report data on an eight-set vowel test; performance ranged from about 15% to 78% for 12 patients using the single-channel Vienna implant.

Consonant recognition

Another important class of sounds in studying cochlear implant perform-ance is the consonants. Most of the consonants change their frequency and intensity characteristics rapidly over time. Both vowel and consonant recognition are highly correlated to word recognition (Tyler, Tye-Murray and Gantz, 1988a).

Tyler and B.C.J. Moore (1991, unpublished data) also measured consonant recognition in their study of some of the better cochlear implant patients. Eight consonants were selected to be appropriate for talkers of French, German and English. The results, shown in Figure 4.7, again demonstrate the large variations across patients. The average scores were 61% (40–75%) correct for Ineraid, 49% (40–60%) for Nucleus/ USA, 41% (29–52%) for Vienna, 40% (25–58%) for Nucleus/Hannover,

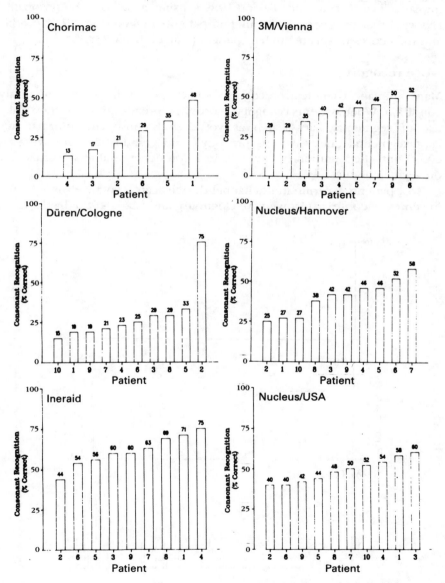

Figure 4.7. Consonant recognition from some of the better patients. There were eight consonants, each presented six times. Chance performance is 13% correct. (Adapted from R.S. Tyler and B.C.J. Moore, 1991, unpublished data.)

29% (15–75%) for Düren/Cologne and 27% (13–48%) for Chorimac. One of the better patients was using the Düren/Cologne device in the single-channel mode. Hochmair-Desoyer, Hochmair and Stiglbrunner (1985) observed scores that ranged from about 18% to 80% on a 16-set consonant test in 12 of their patients with the single-channel Vienna implant. Tye-Murray and Tyler (1989), using a set of 14 consonants, reported that the scores of 10 Ineraid patients ranged from 17% to 58%, and the scores of seven Nucleus patients ranged from 25% to 45%.

Word recognition

Many implant users can recognise some speech in an audition-only condition. When patients recognise words in sentence contexts, they make use of segmental cues (such as vowel and consonant information), suprasegmental cues (such as prosody), and grammatical and syntactic constraints. Recognition of words in isolation depends almost exclusively on segmental cues.

Most patients wearing multichannel devices can recognise some words in sentence contexts (Dowell, Mecklenburg and Clark, 1986; Banfai et al.,

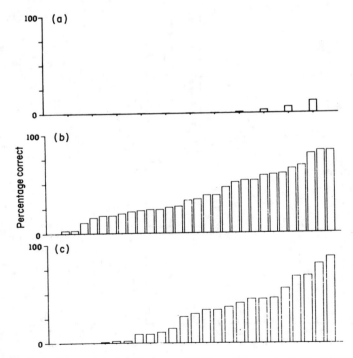

Figure 4.8. Word recognition in sentences on the Iowa Sentence test with (a) House, (b) Nucleus and (c) Ineraid cochlear Implants. Patients were tested at the University of Iowa. There were 100 sentences and 434 words (excluding 'a's and 'the's).

1988; Tyler, Tye-Murray and Gantz, 1988; Dorman et al., 1989b; Tye-Murray and Tyler, 1989) whereas most patients wearing single-channel devices cannot (Owens, Kessler and Raggio, 1983; Tyler et al., 1985; Rosen and Ball, 1986; Rose et al., 1987; Cooper and Carpenter, 1988). Figure 4.8 presents results from our 25 Ineraid, 32 Nucleus and 9 House patients for the Laser Videodisc Sentence Test Without Context (Tyler, Preece and Tye-Murray, 1986). This test presents 100 sentences, with 20 speakers (10 female, 10 male) producing five sentences each. Scores for the Ineraid patients averaged 32% (0–88%), 38% for the Nucleus patients (0–92%), and 1% for the House patients (0–4%).

Recognising words in isolation is a considerably more difficult task than recognising words in sentences (Dowell, Webb and Clark, 1984; Dowell et al., 1985; Mecklenburg, Brimacombe and Dowell, 1987; Dorman et al., 1989b). Scores for tests comprised from the NU-6 list rarely exceed 30% words correct and more typically fall below 20%. Most patients wearing single-channel devices score 0%. However, a few patients wearing the Vienna device have performed relatively well.

Tyler, Moore and Kuk (1989) reported open-set word recognition scores from some of the better cochlear implant patients. Here it is not possible to compare the results directly across patients with different languages. Figure 4.9 shows the performance for all patients. For the French words, the scores averaged 2.5% (0–6%) for the Chorimac patients. For the German words, the scores averaged 17% (0–57%) for the Düren/Cologne patients, 15% (0–34%) for the Vienna patients and 10% (3–26%) for the Nucleus/Hannover patients. For the English words, the scores averaged 11% (3–20%) for the Nucleus/USA patients and 14% (9–20%) for the Ineraid patients. Even for patients using the same device, performance varied enormously. Nevertheless, with all these devices, some open-set word recognition was possible. Open-set word recognition has been reported by others in single-channel patients (Hochmair-Desoyer, Hochmair and Stiglbrunner, 1985; Banfai et al., 1986; Tyler, 1988a,b).

Performance in noise

Listening in a real-world environment is much more difficult than listening in a quiet sound-treated booth, where most audiological testing occurs. In a typical environment, a patient will attend to a talker while voices, footsteps, wind, motor noise and/or music interfere. Almost without exception, implant users are able to understand less speech in these instances than in a quiet condition.

The ability of the Ineraid, Nucleus, Vienna and House patients to understand speech in noise was evaluated with the authors' Minimal Pairs

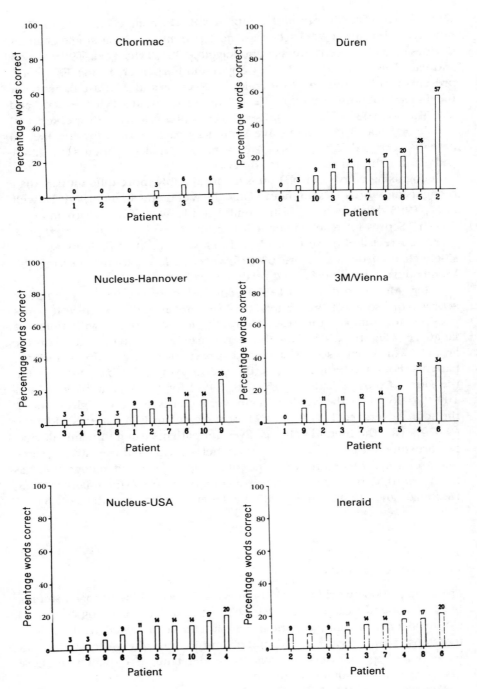

Figure 4.9. Open-set word recognition from some of the better cochlear implant patients. There were 35 words. (From Tyler, Moore and Kuk, 1989, with permission.)

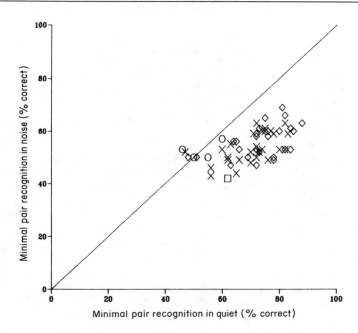

Figure 4.10. Recognition of words in noise when the response set was a 'minimal pair' with (○) House, (□) Vienna, (×) Nucleus and (◇) Ineraid cochlear implants. There were 58 test words, each repeated twice. Chance performance is 50% correct. Patients were tested at the University of Iowa.

Test. The test was administered in quiet and in the presence of competing six-talker babble presented with a signal-to-noise ratio of +10 dB (using the A-weighting scale). The Minimal Pairs Test presents 58 consonant–vowel–consonant word pairs that differ by only one initial consonant feature (e.g. 'pat–bat', 'boat–goat'). The patient's task is to choose which of two words, printed on a computer touch screen, was presented. The test results appear in Figure 4.10. With the exception of two Ineraid, three House and three Nucleus patients, all patients scored above chance in the quiet condition. All of the patients were adversely affected by the addition of noise. On average, all four groups performed at chance level. Others (e.g. Dowell et al., 1988) have also reported that their patients have difficulty hearing speech in noise.

These results suggest that all four groups were severely affected by the presence of background noise, and that none of the cochlear implants utilises adequate noise-reduction circuits.

Speechreading enhancement

The majority of implant users receive speechreading enhancement from their device. Closed-set consonant recognition tests are often used to

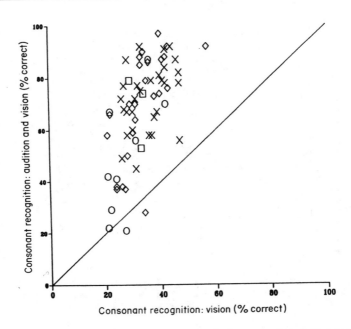

Figure 4.11. Speechreading enhancement on the Iowa Consonant Recognition Laser Videodisc test with (○) House, (□) Vienna, (×) Nucleus and (◇) Ineraid cochlear implants. There were 13 consonants, each repeated 12 times. Chance performance was 8% correct. Patients were tested at the University of Iowa.

evaluate speechreading enhancement because a feature analysis (Miller and Nicely, 1955) can be performed to help elucidate the phonetic perceptions that underlie the confusions. By comparing a vision-only condition to an audition-plus-vision condition, these analyses can indicate which speech cues are conveyed visually and how the transmission of speech cues is enhanced by the addition of the electrical signal.

Figure 4.11 presents the results from the authors' consonant recognition test, where consonants embedded in the /iCi/ context are produced by a male speaker. Each of the 13 consonants is presented 12 times in random order. Ineraid, Nucleus, Vienna and House patients have completed the test in both a vision-only and audition-plus-vision condition. Scores for the vision-only condition are plotted along the abscissa while scores for the audition-plus-vision condition are plotted along the ordinate. Scores falling above the diagonal indicate that the patient received speechreading enhancement from the device. With the exception of two House and one Ineraid patient, all patients received enhancement. Enhancement scores, computed by subtracting the vision-only score from the audition-plus-vision score, averaged 38% for the Ineraid patients, 32% for the Nucleus patients, 37% for the Vienna patients and 21% for the House patients.

Analyses of consonant confusion data indicate that place cues (signalled primarily by spectral information) and frication cues are conveyed by the visual signal relatively well, whereas voicing, nasality and waveform envelope cues are conveyed relatively poorly. Fortunately, the information conveyed by the electrical signal (i.e. envelope, nasality and voicing) complements the visual signal and may serve to resolve visual ambiguities (Blamey et al., 1987; Tyler, Tye-Murray and Lansing, 1988; Tye-Murray and Tyler, 1989).

Ball et al. (1988) showed results from one patient using the UCL single-channel device. Consonant recognition was 30% correct in vision only and 58% in audition plus vision. As expected, information provided by voicing contributed primarily to the enhancement.

Future Directions

There are several new directions that are being pursued in cochlear implant technology. The large benefits in speech perception and lifestyle obtained by some patients have ensured a long-term market. Efforts can now be applied to refining cosmetics, improving performance, exploring new applications and incorporating other technology.

The hardware associated with cochlear implants (internal and external) will be made smaller. Several groups are working towards miniaturising the speech processor and associated components so that all external hardware can fit behind the ear. This will eventually lead to a cochlear prosthesis that is entirely implantable.

Although many patients wearing cochlear implants achieve open-set word recognition, only a few patients achieve high levels of recognition in an audition-only condition. It will be necessary for future devices to focus on providing more spectral information (for example, about the place of articulation), in particular dynamic spectral information.

There is some effort to explore ways of adjusting the implant to optimise its use for individuals. This effort parallels concerns about the inadequacy of the 'one formula fits all' approach used widely for conventional hearing aids (Tyler, 1986). Wilson et al. (1988) have reported that some patients show an immediate improvement in their speech perception when their cochlear implant is adjusted to take into consideration the psychoacoustic limitations of their individual auditory processing abilities. They have explored several different signal-processing approaches and indicated that some patients prefer simultaneous analogue stimulation whereas others achieve higher scores with sequential pulsatile stimulation. This work, together with the efforts of a team in San Francisco (Merzenich, 1985), has led to the development of a new cochlear implant developed by MiniMed, soon to be introduced. It will allow either a pulsatile or analogue strategy to be selected.

Many researchers and manufacturers are attempting to develop new coding strategies. Future devices should be adaptable so that they can accept new coding strategies without changes to implanted hardware. Ideally, external speech processors could be reprogrammed to accommodate new designs. Patients could then benefit from new developments without the inconvenience and expense of another operation or obtaining a new speech processor every time there was a new development in the field.

Many patients desire systems that code better music and environmental sounds. Few groups have focused on these aspects, but they are very important for some patients. It is not unreasonable to expect that music-extraction or music-specific coding strategies will be developed for listening in certain situations.

As mentioned previously, it is necessary to have more effective noise reduction algorithms. This is a common problem among hearing-aid users and appears to be a very difficult problem to solve (Levitt et al., 1986; Tyler, 1988). Nevertheless, the signal processing potential with cochlear implants and the digitisation of conventional hearing aids provide mutual grounds for attacking the problem with a systematic and diverse approach.

It would be desirable to have an inexpensive, reliable cochlear implant. Many patients around the world will not have access to cochlear implant technology unless such devices exist. Considering that high levels of speech perception have been obtained with single-channel devices, it is premature to direct efforts entirely to more sophisticated multichannel devices which are difficult and expensive to maintain.

There is also great interest in providing implants to patients with less severe hearing loss than the profoundly deaf population that was the initial focus. One of the better patients tested by Tyler, Moore and Kuk (1989) also had the most residual hearing. Although not adequately tested yet, it is reasonable to suppose that hearing-impaired patients with more hair cells and more surviving nerve fibres will perform better than those without hair cells and very few nerve fibres. However, these are also the same patients who derive benefit from hearing aids. What needs to be established is the cross-over point of hearing loss severity where the value of the implant no longer exceeds that provided by the hearing aid.

There is some debate about the appropriate strategy for the provision of services for adult and children cochlear implant patients. The evaluation, fitting and follow-up of audiological care requires substantial amounts of time from skilled professionals. Before implantation, members of the team work with parents (and the child) in developing realistic expectations. They usually follow an extensive protocol to establish minimal benefit from a hearing aid, which is a major criterion when considering implanting a young child. This often requires several months. After implantation, a member of the team programs the device and monitors the child's progress over time. Device programming often takes longer with children than adults (several weeks or even months). We use a hospital-centred strategy for fitting the implant and a yearly follow-up. However, we use a school-centred approach for monitoring the implant functioning and audiovisual training. These schools are already responsible for these services for children (including preschool children) with hearing aids. We provide support if needed. The equipment required to set most cochlear implants requires a computer, additional hardware and programming software, which can be expensive. Given the special services required and the high cost of providing these services, it may not be cost-effective for small centres to provide the necessary basic care.

Many unanswered questions remain regarding the appropriateness of cochlear implants in the prelingually deaf. For older children and adults who are part of the deaf culture and who use sign as their primary mode of communication, the ability to provide some limited hearing sensations may not be very helpful. However, for younger prelingually deafened children the ability to provide some level of open-set word recognition has the potential to have a dramatic impact on their entire life. Although preliminary work addressing the amount of hearing to be expected in this population is encouraging (Osberger, 1989; Tyler, 1990), the amount of benefit they receive is not yet well established. We also need to show more understanding of the arguments of the deaf community and to determine if this dramatic impact is in the best interest of the child or not. Is it better to provide limited hearing to deaf children of deaf parents and to subject them to extensive auditory training with perhaps only limited success, or is it better to foster and nurture their growth in the deaf culture?

A greater emphasis needs to be placed on training procedures and their effectiveness. The computer-based device setting of cochlear implants and their specifiable input signal provide an exciting background for the development and verification of efficient training protocols. Training systems which incorporate computers (Sims, 1978; Tye-Murray et al., 1990) and laser video disc technology (Kopra et al., 1985; Tye-Murray et al., 1989) are already being tested. Training should be convenient and relevant to the patient's daily experiences. Some training activities should be implemented in the home or community setting and utilise speech samples produced by the patient's family and friends. Aural rehabilitation usually consists of traditional auditory training and audio-visual speech perception instruction. Newer programmes also emphasise communication therapy (e.g. Erber, 1988). In communication therapy, the patient learns coping strategies and assertive listening behaviours. Ideally, as the patient successfully converses with many individuals and interacts with the environment, the electrical signal becomes increasingly meaningful.

Conclusions

Cochlear implants have been categorised into two primary divisions, either single- or multichannel, and either feature-extraction or wideband signal processing. These are general classifications, and it is necessary to consider the particular signal processing for each system. There are several ways to implement a single-channel, wideband signal-processing cochlear implant, just as there are many ways of implementing a multichannel, feature-extraction scheme.

It appears that there may be an advantage for multichannel over single-channel systems, probably because they attempt to simulate the frequency specificity that is present in the normal auditory system. However, some patients with single-channel systems have been able to obtain excellent open-set word recognition scores.

At present there appears to be no clear advantage of wideband or feature-extraction processing strategies. Excellent results have been obtained with both the multichannel Ineraid and Nucleus devices. It may be that, on average, wideband processing will permit better understanding of everyday sounds and appreciation for music. However, many patients with the feature-extraction Nucleus device perform well on environmental sound tests and report an appreciation of music. These listening skills will probably improve with time.

The cochlear implant has had an enormous impact on the lives of thousands of postlinguistically deafened adults. They recognise many everyday sounds, are better able to speechread, watch the television and, in some cases, carry on a telephone conversation. Relative to normally hearing listeners with similar performance levels in quiet, they are particularly affected by background noise. This is a common problem among the hearing impaired. More work is needed to improve noise-reduction systems. More specifically, computer-based rehabilitation may also help when listening in noise.

Studies of vowel and consonant recognition indicate that patients can utilise cues about the speech envelope, voicing, frication and nasality. Some patients show evidence of processing spectral information.

Acknowledgements

This work was supported by the NIH/NINCDS Program Project Grant N520466, NIH grant RR59 from the General Clinical Research Centers Program, Division of Research Resources, the Burroughs Wellcome Foundation, NATO Grant RF.85/0774, and the Iowa Lions Sight and Hearing Foundation.

References

BALL, V., ROSEN, S.L, WALLIKER, J. and FOURCIN, A. (1988). A speech pattern approach to electrical hearing. In: Banfai, P. (ed.) *Cochlear Implant: Current Situation*, pp. 241–271. Erkelenz, West Germany: Bermann GMBH.

BANFAI, P., KARCZAG, A., KUBIK, S., LÜERS, P. and SÜRTH, W. (1986). Extracochlear sixteen-channel electrode system. *Otol. Clin. North Am.* **19**, 371–408.

BANFAI, P., KARCZAG, A., KUBIK, S., LÜERS, P. SÜRTH, W. and WEISKOPF, P. (1988). Progress in development of cochlear implant from 1978–1987. In: Banfai, P. (ed.) *Cochlear Implant: Current Situation*, pp. 557–582. Erkelenz, W. Germany: Bermann GMBH.

BILGER, R.C. and HOPKINSON, N.T. (1977). Hearing performance with the auditory prosthesis. *Ann. Otol. Rhinol. Laryngol.* **86**(suppl.), 76–91.

BLAMEY, P.J., DOWELL, R.C., BROWN, A.M., CLARK, G.M. and SELIGMAN, P.M. (1987). Vowel and consonant recognition of cochlear implant patients using formant-estimating speech processors. *J. Acoust. Soc. Am.* **82**, 48–57.

BREEUWER, M. and PLOMP, R. (1986). Speechreading supplemented with auditorily presented speech parameters. *J. Acoust. Soc. Am.* **79**, 481–499.

BRIMACOMBE, J.A., EDGERTON, B.J., DOYLE, K.J., ERRATT, J.D. and DANHAUER, J.L. (1984). Auditory capabilities of patients implanted with the House single-channel cochlear implant. *Acta Oto-Laryngol. Suppl.* **411**, 204–216.

CHOUARD, C.H., FOUGAIN, C., MEYER, B. and CHABOLLE, F. (1986). The Chorimac 12: A multichannel intracochlear implant for total deafness. *Otolaryngol. Clin. North Am.* **19**, 355–370.

CLARK, G.M., TONG, Y.C., DOWELL, R.C., MARTIN, L.F., SELIGMAN, P.M., BUSBY, P.A. and PATRICK, J.F. (1981). A multiple-channel cochlear implant: An evaluation using nonsense syllables. *Ann. Otol. Rhinol. Laryngol.* **90**, 227–230.

CONINX, F. (1988). Tonotopically based pitch sensations with multi-electrode extra-cochlear stimulation. In Banfai, P. (ed.) *Cochlear Implant: Current Situation*, pp. 601–603. Erkelenz, West Germany: Bermann GMBH.

CONWAY, M.J. and BOYLE, P. (1989). Design of the UCH/RNID cochlear implant system. *J. Laryngol. Otol.* (suppl. 18), 4–10.

COOPER, H. and CARPENTER, L. (1988). UCH/RNID cochlear implant programme: Post-operative results. In Banfai, P. (ed.) *Cochlear Implant: Current Situation*, pp. 283–296. Erkelenz, West Germany: Bermann GMBH.

DANLEY, M.J. and FRETZ, R.J. (1982). Design and functioning of the single-electrode cochlear implant. *Ann. Otol. Rhinol. Laryngol.* **91**(suppl. 91), 21–26.

DORMAN, M.F., DANKOWSKI, K., McCANDLESS, G. and SMITH, L. (1989a). Identification of synthetic vowels by patients using the Symbion multichannel cochlear implant. *Ear Hear.* **10**, 40–43.

DORMAN, M.F., HANNLEY, M.T., DANKOWSKI, K., SMITH, L. and McCANDLESS, G. (1989b). Word recognition by 50 patients fitted with the Symbion multichannel cochlear implant. *Ear Hear.* **10**, 44–49.

DOWELL, R.C., MECKLENBURG, D.J. and CLARK, G.M. (1986). Speech recognition for 40 patients receiving multichannel cochlear implants. *Arch. Otolaryngol. Head Neck Surg.* **112**, 1054–1059.

DOWELL, R.C., WEBB, R.L. and CLARK, G.M. (1984). Clinical results using a multiple-channel cochlear prosthesis. *Acta Oto-Laryngol.* **28**(suppl. 411), 230–236.

DOWELL, R.C., BROWN, A.M., SELIGMAN, P.M. and CLARK, G.M. (1985). Patient results for a multiple-channel cochlear prosthesis. In Schindler, R.A. and Merzenich, M.M. (eds) *Cochlear Implants*, pp. 421–431. New York: Raven Press.

DOWELL, R.C., PATRICK, J.F., BLAMEY, P.J., SELIGMAN, P.M., MONEY, D.K. and CLARK, G.M. (1988). Signal processing in quiet and noise. In: Banfai, P. (ed.) *Cochlear Implant: Current Situation*, pp. 495–498. Erkelenz, West Germany: Bermann GMBH.

EDDINGTON, D.K. (1980). Speech discrimination in deaf subjects with cochlear implants. *J. Acoust. Soc. Am.* **68**, 885–891.

EDGERTON, B.J., HOUSE, W.F. and HITSELBERGER, W. (1982). Hearing by cochlear Nucleus stimulation in humans. *Ann. Otol. Rhinol. Laryngol.* **91**(suppl. 91), pp. 117–124.

ERBER, N.P. (1988). *Communication Therapy for Hearing-Impaired Adults.* Abbotsford, Victoria, Australia: Clavis Publishing.

FOURCIN, A.J., ROSEN, S.M., MOORE, B.C.J., CLARKE, G.P., DODSON, H. and BANNISTER, L.H. (1979). External electrical stimulation of the cochlea: Clinical, psychophysical, speech perceptual and histological findings. *Br. J. Audiol.* **13**, 85–107.

FRASER, J.G. (1989). The University College Hospital/Royal National Institute for the Deaf cochlear implant programme. *J. Laryngol. Otol.* (suppl. 18), 1–3.

GANTZ, B.J., TYLER, R.S., KNUTSON, J.F., WOODWORTH, G., ABBAS, P., McCABE, B.F., HINRICHS, J., TYE-MURRAY, N., LANSING, C., KUK, F. and BROWN, C. (1988). Evaluation of five different cochlear implant designs: Audiologic assessment and predictors of performance. *Laryngoscope* **98**, 1100–1106.

GRANT, K.W., ARDELL, L.H., KUHL, P.K. and SPARKS, D.W. (1985). The contribution of fundamental frequency, amplitude envelope, and voicing duration cues to speechreading in normal-hearing subjects. *J. Acoust. Soc. Am.* **77**, 671–677.

HOCHMAIR, E.S. and HOCHMAIR-DESOYER, I.J. (1985). Aspects of sound processing using the Vienna intra- and extracochlear implants. In: Schindler, R.A. and Merzenich, M.M. (eds) *Cochlear Implants*, pp. 101–110. New York: Raven Press.

HOCHMAIR-DESOYER, I.J., HOCHMAIR, E.S. and STIGLBRUNNER, H.K. (1985). Psychoacoustic temporal processing and speech understanding in cochlear implant patients. In: Schindler, R.A. and Merzenich, M.M. (eds) *Cochlear Implants*, pp. 291–304. New York: Raven Press.

HOUSE, W.F. and URBAN, J. (1973). Long term results of electrode implantation and electronic stimulation of the cochlea in man. *Ann. Otol. Rhinol. Laryngol.* **82**, 504–517.

KIANG, N.Y.S., FULLERTON, B.C., RICHTER, E.A., LEVINE, R.A. and NORRIS, B.E. (1985). Artificial stimulation of the auditory system. In: Keidel, W.D. and Finkenzeller, P. (eds) *Artificial Auditory Stimulation Theories*, pp. 6–17. New York: S. Karger.

KOPRA, L.L., DUNLOP, R.J., KOPRA, J.A. and ABRAHAMSON, J.E. (1985). Computer-assisted instruction in lipreading with a laser videodisc interactive system. Paper presented at the computer conference of the American Speech-Language-Hearing Foundation, New Orleans, LA.

LEVITT, H., NEUMAN, A., MILLS, R. and SCHWANDER, T. (1986). A digital master hearing aid. *J. Rehabil. Res. Dev.* **23**(1), 79–87.

MECKLENBURG, D.J., BRIMACOMBE, J.A. and DOWELL, R.C. (1987). Performance profile of patients who achieve substantial open-set speech understanding without lipreading. *Ann. Otol. Rhinol. Laryngol.* **96**(suppl. 128), 138.

MERZENICH, M.M. (1985). UCSF cochlear implant device. In: Schindler, R.A. and Merzenich, M.M. (eds) *Cochlear Implants*, pp. 121–129. New York: Raven Press.

MILLER, G.A. and NICELY, P.E. (1955). An analysis of perceptual confusions among some English consonants. *J. Acoust. Soc. Am.* **27**, 338–352.

OSBERGER, M.J. (1989). Speech production in profoundly hearing-impaired children with reference to cochlear implants. In: Owens, E. and Kessler, D.K. (eds) *Cochlear Implants in Young Deaf Children*, pp. 257–282. Boston: Little, Brown & Co.

OWENS, E., KESSLER, D. and RAGGIO, M. (1983). Results for some patients with cochlear implants on the Minimal Auditory Capabilities (MAC) battery. In: Parkins, C.W. and Anderson, S.W. (eds) *Cochlear Prosthesis: An International Symposium*, pp. 443–450. New York: The New York Academy of Sciences.

PETERSON, G.E. and BARNEY, H.L. (1952). Control methods used in a study of the vowels. *J. Acoust. Soc. Am.* **24**, 175–184.

ROSE, D.E., FACER, G.W., KING, A.M. and FABRY, M.A. (1987). Results using 3M/Vienna extracochlear implant in five patients. *Ann. Otol. Rhinol. Laryngol.* **96**(suppl. 128), 114–117.

ROSEN, S. and BALL, V. (1986). Speech perception with the Vienna extra-cochlear single-channel implant: A comparison of two approaches to speech coding. *Br. J. Audiol.* **20**, 61–83.

ROSEN, S.M., FOURCIN, A.J. and MOORE, B.C.J. (1981). Voice pitch as an aid to lipreading. *Nature* **291**, 150–152.

SIMS, D. (1978). Visual and auditory training for adults. In: Katz, J. (ed.) *Handbook of Clinical Audiology*, 2nd edn, pp. 565–580. Baltimore: Williams & Wilkins.

TOWNSHEND, B., COTTER, N., VAN COMPERNOLLE, D. and WHITE, R.L. (1987). Pitch perception by cochlear implant subjects. *J. Acoust. Soc. Am.* **82**, 106–115.

TYE-MURRAY, N. and TYLER, R.S. (1989). Auditory consonant and word recognition skills of cochlear implant users. *Ear Hear.* **10**(5), 292–298.

TYE-MURRAY, N., TYLER, R.S., BONG, B. and NARES, T. (1989). Computerized laser videodisc programs for training speechreading and assertive communication behaviors. *J. Acad. Rehabil. Audiol.* **21**, 143–152.

TYE-MURRAY, N., TYLER, R.S., LANSING, C. and BERTSCHY, M. (1990). Evaluating the effectiveness of auditory training stimuli using a computerized program. *Volta Rev.* **92**, 25–30.

TYLER, R.S. (1986). Adjusting a hearing aid to amplify speech to the MCL. *Hear. J.* **39**(8), 24–27.

TYLER, R.S. (1988a). Open-set word recognition with the Düren/Cologne extracochlear implant. *Laryngoscope* **98**, 999–1002.

TYLER, R.S. (1988b). Open-set word recognition with the 3M/Vienna single-channel cochlear implant. *Arch. Otol. Head Neck Surg.* **114**, 1123–1126.

TYLER, R.S. (1990). Speech perception with the Nucleus cochlear implant in children trained with the auditory/verbal approach. *Am. J. Otol.* **11**(2), 90–107.

TYLER, R.S. and KELSAY, D. (1990). Advantages and disadvantages perceived by some of the better cochlear-implant patients. *Am. J. Otol.* **11**, 282–289.

TYLER, R.S., MOORE, B.C.J. and KUK, F.K. (1989). Performance of some of the better cochlear implant patients. *J. Speech Hear. Res.* **32**, 887–911.

TYLER, R.S., PREECE, J.P. and TYE-MURRAY, N. (1986). The Iowa Phoneme and Sentence Tests (Laser Videodisc). Department of Otolaryngology – Head and Neck Surgery, The University of Iowa, Iowa City.

TYLER, R.S., TYE-MURRAY, N. and GANTZ, B.J. (1988). The relationship between vowel, consonant and word perception in cochlear-implant patients. In: Banfai, P. (ed.) *Cochlear Implant: Current Situation*, pp. 627–632. Erkelenz, West Germany: Bermann GMBH.

TYLER, R.S., TYE-MURRAY, N. and LANSING, C.R. (1988). Electrical stimulation as an aid to speechreading. *Volta Rev. New Reflect. Speechread.* **90**(5), 119–148.

TYLER, R.S., LOWDER, M.W., OTTO, S.R., PREECE, J.P., GANTZ, B.J. and McCABE, B.F. (1984). Initial Iowa results with the multichannel cochlear implant from Melbourne. *J. Speech Hear. Res.* **27**, 596–604.

TYLER, R.S., GANTZ, B.J., McCABE, B.F., LOWDER, M.W., OTTO, S.R. and PREECE, J.P. (1985). Audiological results with two single channel cochlear implants. *Ann. Otol. Rhinol. Laryngol.* **94**, 133–139.

TYLER, R.S., GANTZ, B.J., PREECE, J.P., LANSING. C.R., LOWDER, M.W., OTTO, S.R. and McCABE, B.F. (1986). Cochlear implant program at The University of Iowa. In: Collins, M.J., Glattke, T.J. and Harker, L.A. (eds) *Sensorineural Hearing Loss, Mechanisms, Diagnosis, Treatment*, pp. 369–383. Iowa City: The University of Iowa.

WILSON, B.S., FINLEY, C.C., LAWSON, D.T. and WOLFORD, R.D. (1988). Speech processors for cochlear prostheses. *Proc. IEEE* **76**, 1143–1154.

Chapter 5
The Cochlear Implant Team

GRAHAM FRASER

Introduction

In almost every cochlear implant centre in the world, the initiative for starting a programme of implantation has come from an otologist. It is usually the otologist who sees the patient in the clinic, goes to meetings where cochlear implants are discussed and decides that he or she would like to carry out implants. Usually the otologist is unaware of the amount of work involved in selecting patients and in their rehabilitation. It is not long before he or she discovers that surgery is in fact a rather small part of the whole process and that there is an urgent need for the help of others with different skills. If otologists are working in a department with experience of dealing with the profoundly deaf and deafened, it may be quite possible to do one or two cases with implants with the existing staff. However, as soon as a significant number of implants have been carried out, an overwhelming need for the skills of a dedicated multidisciplinary team becomes apparent. It is the author's firm conviction that only such a team will have the expertise, skills and experience necessary to provide the best possible treatment for deafened patients receiving implants. They will also be in a position to provide the most appropriate form of rehabilitation for those profoundly deafened patients who need help, but who are not suitable for implants.

Setting up the Team

Although cochlear implants have been in use for over 20 years, the early experience is confined to very few centres and it is only in the last 5 years that a significant number of patients have been implanted around the world. In 1988, the British Association of Otolaryngologists recognised cochlear implants as an established therapy, but also insisted that ongoing research and development was necessary. In setting up a team, this must be recognised in selecting and assessing patients and, in planning their rehabilitation, detailed records are necessary to compare different implant strategies. There must therefore be sufficient expertise on the team to take on this time-consuming assessment work as well as the routine work. In ideal circumstances the implant team should be established before any implants are done because, once an implant has been carried out on even one patient, there is a commitment to look after that patient for ever. However, it is often difficult to motivate people until they have some experience of what implants can offer. Once people have met a patient with an implant and have seen the benefit for themselves, they are more likely to fight for the funding necessary to set up a properly staffed unit.

Below a look is taken at the various essential members of the team and their roles.

The otologist

There is no escaping the fact that the otologist has the ultimate responsibility where a surgical procedure is involved. Surgeons are also trained to take decisions about whether to operate or not, which other people may find difficult. In the author's own programme at University College Hospital, two consultant otologists are attached to the team and this has proved to be a most worthwhile arrangement. The interchange of ideas between the two surgeons has allowed development and simplification of the surgical technique and, if one is absent, there is an automatic deputy. It is crucial that there should be an otologist available at all times. We have now reached the point where the registrars (residents) and senior registrars have carried out implants on their own. The junior doctors are also involved at other points in the procedure, such as inserting the electrodes for electrocochleography or promontory stimulation. The insertion of round window electrodes for short-term stimulation is proving one of the most reliable assessment techniques and, once again, this needs the assistance of the otologist or the junior medical staff (Ryan, 1989).

Audiological physician/neuro-otologist

An audiological physician may have considerable experience in the rehabilitation of the profoundly deaf which will be directly relevant, not only to the patients who are implanted, but also to those who are referred and found to be unsuitable for implantation. In the author's own team, the neuro-otologist has a special interest in tinnitus research and tinnitus evaluation has been a standard part of the protocol (Hazell, Meerton and Conway, 1989).

The audiological scientist

An audiological scientist's training makes him or her particularly well suited to integrate all the test procedures. Detailed audiological knowledge is needed for the psychoacoustic tests and many patients with usable residual hearing will not have had an adequate hearing aid trial, which needs to be organised before they are considered for implantation. In the author's own team, the scientific training of the audiological scientist has been essential for the overall management of the research element of the programme so that the test results, which can be overwhelming in number, are collected in a way that is amenable to storage on a computer database. Running the database has been the responsibility of the audiological scientist as well. Setting up such a database and record collection is very time consuming initially, but once properly established, analyses for research purposes are easily achieved (Cooper et al., 1989).

The speech therapist

It is notable how little attention has been given to the speech of the deafened. The effect of being totally deafened is very variable between individuals so that one person may have had no hearing for 40 years and yet have very good speech preservation, whilst another will have very obvious deterioration in his or her speech patterns after a short period without hearing (Read, 1989). A speech therapist is a most crucial member of the team. The speech therapy needed after implantation may be minimal for those with good speech, but for those with very poor speech, they can be trained to use their implant to the maximum advantage and other techniques of feedback such as Visispeech can be combined in training with the information obtained from the implant. The speech therapist also has a crucial role in the supervision of the auditory training programme which is essential after an implant has been provided. This requires very special skills, including in-depth knowledge of speech perception and acoustics.

Teacher of the deaf

The assessment of children and the provision of implants for totally deafened children require very different skills from those needed for adults. If cochlear implants in children are planned, then a teacher of the deaf is an essential member of the team. It is already mentioned that the selection and rehabilitation processes are long ones and much more difficult to organise than surgery. When it comes to children, this is doubly true. It does not take twice as long to assess children; it takes five times as long and needs the sort of patience that comes with training as a teacher of the deaf. A teacher may also participate very usefully in the adult auditory training programme.

Hearing therapist

The training of hearing therapists makes them particularly suitable for active participation in a programme of rehabilitation of the profoundly deaf.

The author's group has found a hearing therapist to be a great asset to the programme. On those occasions when a patient has been through the selection procedure and ultimately been found to be unsuitable for an implant, it has very often proved to be the hearing therapist who has been able to offer some other form of help such as a vibrotactile aid or environmental aids, which have made all the difference to the patient, and the feeling of let down and disappointment is mitigated.

Psychologist and psychiatrist

Many of the standard test batteries for assessment of personality and intelligence designed for hearing people are not suitable for the deaf population. A psychological evaluation is, however, most revealing. The difficulties of communication with totally deaf patients makes it very hard for the clinician to evaluate the psychological status of a patient. Some of the patients about whom we have had our gravest doubts have proved to be the most successful and the opposite is also true. The patients are often isolated and cut off from their friends and family because of their problems of communication. Therefore it is not surprising that they may have some depression. It is important not to reject patients simply because they have had a normal reaction to being deafened. At the same time, it is important not to implant the grossly psychologically disturbed because the implant is likely to be a burden on them and to the implant team. All patients should see a psychologist and have appropriate evaluation to avoid such mistakes. If there is a suspicion of psychopathology, it may be necessary to refer the patient on to a psychiatrist with a special interest in the field and an ability to communicate with the deaf.

Physicist/technician

When only one or two patients are implanted, the back-up needed is very small but once a significant number have been given implants numerous problems arise: the device may be dropped in the bath, eaten by the dog or whatever, and a continuous stream of enquiries may come to the implant team. It is crucial to have a technician who can deal with them as they arise. Once patients have had an implant for a significant length of time, they are devastated by the loss of it and want the repairs done the same day. If a cochlear implant team is concerned with research they will also need a physicist for development with electronics and engineering training.

The Team Approach to Patient Selection

The detailed protocol for patient selection which we have developed is described elsewhere (Fraser et al., 1986). In the early stages of the selection procedure the author's group found themselves performing an unnecessary number of tests over a prolonged period. The reason for this is that such enthusiasm is generated for the work that all the scientists think of just one more test that needs doing. Furthermore, there is a great inclination to generate their own system of records so that many separate records are built up about the same patient. To counter this, a record sheet was designed which travelled round with the patient to each department in turn so that each time the patient had been seen by, say, the speech therapist or audiological scientist, his or her record was completed and the individual records were all stapled together. Furthermore, a time limit was set on the testing so that, if a new test was devised, it could only be used if it fitted in to a total testing time of four working days.

By the end of these four working days the patient has not only been tested thoroughly, but also has a much clearer knowledge of what an implant involves and whether they want an implant or not. It should therefore be regarded as essential that a decision should be made before a patient goes home rather than allowing him or her to leave in doubt. With the author's schedule a panel meeting takes place after the 4-day period. The test results are reviewed and the patient is given a decision there and then. At this panel discussion, one of the otologists and the audiological scientist are always present as well as one of the other scientists who has come to know the patient whilst carrying out their assessments. The author's group also tries to have a representative from the RNID (Royal National Institute for the Deaf) because they are associated with the programme. Thus the decision about who should or should not be offered an implant is a team one, rather than that of the otologist alone. It is most important that members of the rehabilitation team be involved in the selection procedure, otherwise they may feel that the wrong patient has been selected when they are struggling with the difficult rehabilitation later.

The Team Approach to Rehabilitation

If the patient reaches the stage 4 weeks after the operation where there have been no surgical complications, then most of the rest of the work is handed over to the rehabilitation team. The audiological scientist or an assistant makes the necessary adjustments to set up the implant properly at this 4-week stage and it is not until this stage is reached that the need for rehabilitation can be completely assessed. Some patients immediately receive benefit from the implant and go from strength to strength whilst others are disappointed and need much encouragement from all members of the team to persist in its use. Many of these people ultimately do well, but only if they have sufficient support at this early stage.

A team approach is very effective in the training process. Each team member has different skills or a different approach and so they complement each other. The patient is also given variety in experience of different voices. The intensive work involved in training is shared among the team members rather than being all on one person's shoulders.

The rehabilitation team also has the role of treating or advising those patients who have attended with a view to implantation but who have proved unsuitable. Many of these patients are deeply disappointed that they are not to be offered a miraculous 'bionic ear' which will solve all their problems. Much persuasion is needed to get them to try a hearing aid or a vibrotactile device.

Team Cohesion

Regular meetings of the cochlear implant team with a formal agenda and adequate time to discuss knowledge are quite crucial to the cohesion of the team. It is vital in a multidisciplinary team that each member makes some effort to learn something of the language of the other members of the team. A knowledge of phonetics is essential to understand the various tests of lipreading and speech perception that are performed. Similarly, the physicist needs to explain how much information can be transmitted using the device and he or she also needs to explain to the surgeon such concepts as 'critical coupling distance' and 'Q'. The other scientists need to understand the possible surgical complications of the operation and the limitations of surgical technique. They may well be asked by patients about the risks of surgery and they cannot avoid these questions without seeming suspicious. Problems will arise about the management of the patients and simple differences of opinion may give rise to strong feelings unless they are discussed openly.

All these problems can be dealt with by regular team meetings where differences of opinion can be thrashed out. Policy decisions can also be made at such meetings, because it is crucial that every member of the team feels a part of the decision-making process and should not feel that things are decided without his or her knowledge. We have found that, although it is difficult to raise the funds to take people to international meetings, these meetings play a crucial role. Not only does it expose all members of the team to views of other centres and give them new ideas, it also has a more important role of allowing the team to meet informally away from the pressures of everyday life with enough time to talk and think together.

Secretarial back-up

It is impossible to under-estimate the importance of secretarial back-up in the running of an implant programme. With many team members and large numbers of patients coming at different times to see them, the timetabling of visits demands hours of careful work, telephoning and letter writing. Furthermore, when there is a research element the production of papers may falter, not because of the lack of work done by the investigators, but because of lack of secretarial support.

Funding the team

In different countries, the funding for cochlear implants comes from different sources. In some it is part of the normal health service provision, whilst in others it may be funded by insurance companies. In the United Kingdom, we have so far been in the unique position that every cochlear implant has been funded from charitable sources but fortunately this has now changed. The Department of Health has now recognised that implants are an established therapy and have agreed to fund six centres. It may seem that what I have said about the team is extravagant and unrealistic. This is not the case. The deafened are a group that has been woefully ignored in the past. Because they had hearing, they were mostly members of the hearing community and they want to get back into that community. With properly run and funded teams, patients are not only going to escape from their world of isolation and depression, but also will be able to get back to work and be active members of the community once more. The funding situation will be helped when improved and more reasonably priced devices are developed.

It is important to stress that funding for cochlear implants must not take away support for those hard of hearing who need help other than implants. This should not be a danger; indeed, the existence of cochlear implants should help to draw attention to the inadequate resources devoted to all groups of hearing-impaired and make it possible to do more for them. The numbers are not particularly large and, by Health Service standards, the amount of money involved is not huge. Those involved in setting up cochlear implant teams must insist that they are properly staffed and must not be content with a second rate service.

References

COOPER, H.R., CARPENTER, L., ALEKSY, W., BOOTH, C.L., READ, T.E, GRAHAM, J.M. and FRASER, J.G. (1989). UCH/RNID single channel extracochlear implant; results in thirty profoundly deafened adults. *J. Laryngol. Otol.* suppl. 18, 22–38.

FRASER, J.G., COOPER, H.R., HAZELL, J.W.P., PHELPS, P.D. and LLOYD, G.A.S. (1986). The UCH/RNID cochlear implant programme: patient selection. *Br. J. Audiol.* **20**, 9–17.

HAZELL, J.W.P., MEERTON, L.J. and CONWAY, M.J. (1989). Electrical tinnitus suppression (ETS) with a single channel cochlear implant. *J. Laryngol. Otol.* suppl. 18, 39–44.

READ, T. (1989). Improvement in speech production following use of the UCH/RNID cochlear implant. *J. Laryngol. Otol.* suppl. 18, 45–49.

RYAN, R.M. (1989). Pre-operative cochlear implant assessment using a round window ball electrode. *J. Laryngol. Otol.* suppl. 18, 11–13.

Chapter 6
Selection of Candidates for Cochlear Implantation: An Overview

HUW COOPER

Philosophy

Approaches to the selection of candidates for cochlear implantation vary depending on the underlying philosophy of the implant group. Often, there is a tendency to 'hunt' for candidates for implant surgery and to lose interest in those patients who, though profoundly or totally deaf, do not meet predetermined criteria and are therefore 'rejected'. Many professionals working with the hearing-impaired are concerned that this approach will inevitably fail to meet the needs of the rejected patients, and that a disproportionate amount of time and resources will be spent on those suitable for implantation to the neglect of the rest.

A more balanced method is for each patient to undergo careful assessment by a multidisciplinary team, aimed at answering the question 'What is the most appropriate and effective way to help this person?' rather than 'Is this person suitable for a cochlear implant or not?'. Cochlear implants are then seen as just one out of a range of possible prosthetic options (also including hearing aids and vibrotactile aids), from which the most appropriate for each patient is selected based on the results of the assessments. The amount of effort invested in each individual's rehabilitation is then tailored according to his or her needs, regardless of the actual hardware he or she is issued with.

Ultimately, the decision of whether to give each patient a cochlear implant must of course be made by the surgeon, because it involves a surgical procedure. It is clear, however, that a team approach to patient selection is essential: unilateral decisions made by the surgeon without taking the advice of the rest of the multidisciplinary team are most likely to produce a poor outcome for the patient.

Assessment of possible candidates for cochlear implantation has two aims: first, to establish whether each patient meets the criteria for suitability and, secondly, to obtain information which will enable some prediction to be made of the likely degree of success. Each of these aims will be discussed in turn, although they are not entirely separable.

Defining the Population

The crudest definition of a candidate for cochlear implantation is a patient who: (1) is totally or profoundly deaf; and (2) has sufficient functioning auditory nerve for electrical stimulation to produce a sensation of hearing.

As will be seen in the following chapters, only a small proportion of those cases who meet the above criteria would be considered for cochlear implants by most groups. The selection process is complex and far from straightforward. Candidacy for implantation can, however, be boiled down into four main areas which make up the bulk of the assessments that are normally carried out.

Audiological status

The definition of 'total' or profound deafness is not sufficient to characterise the patient group suitable for cochlear implantation on purely audiological grounds. Careful assessment of performance with, and benefit from, amplification is required using a range of perceptual tests, the results of which can then be compared with the average and range of results obtained from cochlear implant users. Angela King details techniques to achieve this in Chapter 7.

Medical fitness

At the end of the day, a cochlear implant is only a viable proposition if: (1) the patient is fit enough to undergo surgery; (2) it is possible to insert an electrode array. Roger Gray describes in depth how these two questions are answered in Chapter 10.

Response to electrical stimulation

Some residual nerve VIII function is required for electrical simulation to produce hearing sensations. How to assess the quantity and quality of surviving neural tissue is one of the most challenging problems in selection. The number of cases where electrical stimulation produces no hearing at all is probably very small and, in view of this, some implant groups now omit any trial electrical stimulation from their selection protocol. However, the results of preoperative electrical stimulation can yield invaluable information about the likely outcome with a 'permanent' implant and so should be included in the selection protocol. Paul Abbas and Carolyn Brown outline the most recent advances in techniques used in the assessment of the status of the auditory nerve in Chapter 8.

Psychological status

As Laurence McKenna describes in Chapter 9, there are many aspects of a patient's psychology that are relevant to their candidacy for cochlear implantation, including motivation, expectations, emotional state, acceptance of their deafness, and so on. Conventional psychometric methods do not necessarily lend themselves to assessment of this population, nor do they provide very useful information in terms of prediction of the benefit a patient might receive from a cochlear implant. Techniques designed specifically for this purpose, and evolved through experience with this patient group, are needed and Laurence describes these.

Results of assessments in the four areas mentioned so far will be sufficient to determine whether a patient is likely to benefit from an implant. In addition to these, there are two other main considerations which effect candidacy, and these are age and age at onset of deafness.

Age

The theoretical lower age limit on purely surgical grounds is around 2 years. There is now a significant amount of evidence to show that children of all ages above 2 years can benefit from cochlear implantation. Of course, although it is no longer considered to be experimental, the application of the cochlear implant in children still raises a number of controversial issues. The most enduring of these, and the one which probably causes the greatest concern among those in the deaf community and elsewhere opposed to the implantation of children, is the issue of consent. Should a child be required to give consent for surgery, or is parental consent sufficient as it is for other surgical procedures? There are strong arguments for both viewpoints. The age of a child is critical in terms of the approach and methods used by the rehabilitation team. Children over the age of around 12–14 years may be treated as young adults, using *broadly* the same methods for assessment and rehabilitation as adults, whilst those younger than this require a very different approach, using a range of skills and techniques which can really only be developed through experience with deaf children. Each implant team, therefore, will formulate its own policy on the lower limits of the age group it wishes to consider for implant surgery, depending on the level of experience and skills in the testing and rehabilitation of hearing-impaired children available to the team. There is no theoretical upper age limit; the main consideration in elderly patients is their fitness to undergo surgery and the postoperative rehabilitation.

Age at the onset of deafness

A period of experience of normal hearing is considered by most groups to be a prerequisite for suitability for cochlear implantation in adults: the outcome of implantation in congenitally deaf people or those deafened at a very young age has generally been found to be poor. In reality, the vast majority of those people coming forward for consideration are deafened adults who have had, at the very least, several years' experience of normal hearing in childhood. In many, this period of experience amounts to nearly their whole lives and can be as long as 50 years.

The term 'postlingual deafness' is often used to describe this entire group, but the use of such terminology is difficult in cases of deafness of very early onset as there is no clear cut-off point between pre- and postlingual deafness: the complete acquisition of language structures may not be complete until around the age of 6 years. A third term, 'perilingual', is used to denote the onset of deafness *during* the process of speech and language acquisition and serves to separate the pre- and postlingual groups. It is probably more appropriate to visualise the development of speech and language as a continuum, rather than trying to categorise it in this way. Most implant groups consider the linguistic ability of candidates for implantation to be worthy of careful assessment and include this in their selection protocol. This is partly to estimate the ability of each patient to understand instructions and participate in training and testing procedures, and partly to give an indication of the probability of a successful outcome (if, as in Vienna, it is considered to be a useful predictor of outcome – Fritze and Eisenwort, 1989). Some patients, deaf from a very young age, may have very poor spoken language but a high level of language competence using manual communication (sign language); those carrying out the assessment need to be aware of this and avoid to making the mistake of thinking that sign cannot achieve the same levels of linguistic complexity as speech.

In children, 'prelingual' or even congenital deafness is not now considered by some groups to be a contraindication to cochlear implantation and it has now been shown that considerable benefit can be provided to very young children with very little or no experience of normal hearing (see Chapters 17 and 18 for more details). It is also clear that, in order to confer the maximum possible benefit to the development of speech and language, the implant needs to be provided as soon as possible after the level of deafness has been confirmed. In this way the greatest advantage is taken of the natural plasticity of the child's neural and cortical structures. The provision of a cochlear implant to congenitally deaf older children and teenagers has generally been found to give a very poor outcome and high incidence of non-use. In these cases, the opportunity to provide a basis for the development of speech and language has been missed and, in many cases, the impetus to go through with implantation has come from the children's parents rather than from the children themselves, even though they are old enough to understand what it is all about and make their own minds up.

Predictability of the Outcome of a Cochlear Implant

Much research effort has been invested in the identification of factors that are predictive of the results of cochlear implantation. The accumulation of these data has two main purposes: first, where resources are limited and an expensive piece of technology is being given to each implanted patient, there is an understandable desire to have a system of priorities whereby those patients most likely to achieve more successful results are implanted before those who are less ideal cases. Secondly, information about the probable outcome for each particular case can be used to counsel the patient about roughly the degree of benefit that they might expect from their implant, although it may be unwise to attempt to make specific predictions based on data from a large and heterogeneous group.

Most effort has concentrated on those variables which require no measurement at all (e.g. age), and those which are amenable to measurement during the selection process. Some work has also been done on the development of new tests designed specifically to be outcome predictors. Essentially, the result of cochlear implantation is dependent on three main variables:

1. The ability of the implant itself to present electrical stimulation to the auditory nerve in such a way as to maximise the transfer of information about the sound input.
2. The quantity and quality of surviving peripheral auditory neural elements, and their ability to respond to the electrical stimulation.
3. The higher level information processing and cognitive abilities of the patient.

The first of these is mainly a function of the design of the implant itself; the second and third are patient variables which can be examined in a number of different ways.

Neuronal survival

On theoretical grounds the degree of survival of peripheral auditory neural elements should be closely related to the outcome of cochlear implantation. It has even been suggested (Otte, Schuknecht and Kerr, 1978) that a minimum ganglion cell population of 10 000 is needed for any speech discrimination to be achieved. Different aetiologies, giving different amounts of neuronal survival, would lead to differing degrees of success following an implant. In general this has not been found to be true: little evidence has been reported of superior results from some aetiologies over others. Studies by Berliner (1985), Fritze and Eisenwort (1989) and Gantz et al. (1988) all found no significant relationship between aetiology and postoperative results. Cooper et al. (1989) and Lehnhardt (1989) produced some data to suggest that meningitic cases were liable to produce a worse result than other aetiologies; this would be consistent with the finding of Otte, Schuknecht and Kerr (1978) that meningitis leads to a poor ganglion cell survival. However, the cochlear ossification produced by meningitis, and the sudden onset of deafness, probably also contribute to the tendency to give a poorer outcome. In fact, it is still not known how important ganglion cell populations are for the success of cochlear implantation; Fayad et al. (1990) showed that fewer ganglion cells than previously thought were necessary to produce hearing sensations from electrical stimulation.

Results of a preoperative trial electrical stimulation have been thought of as a measure of the degree of neuronal survival, but disappointingly few data from such testing have been found to be useful as predictors of postoperative outcome. The exceptions to this are dynamic range, which has been found to be positively correlated with success by some (Soulier et al., 1987; Smoorenburg and van Olphen, 1987), but not by others (Gantz et al., 1988), and the temporal difference limen (Hochmair-Desoyer, Hochmair and Stiglbrunner, 1983; Lindstrom, 1987; Waltzman, 1987). Electrically evoked potentials offer the possibility of a more accurate measure of neuronal survival, and are described in detail in Chapter 8.

Age and duration of deafness

A weak but consistent negative correlation between age and postoperative results has been found by many groups (e.g. Gantz et al., 1988; Fritze and Eisenwort, 1989), but on the whole it should not be thought of as a strong predictor of outcome; suffice it to say that a slight tendency for younger people to achieve a better outcome can be anticipated.

Duration of deafness has been found to be much more significant with, more recently, patients generally achieving greater success (Brimacombe et al., 1987; Gantz et al., 1988, 1990; Cooper et al., 1989). Some have even specified a maximum duration of deafness for a 'successful' outcome (usually meaning the achievement of open-set speech recognition), e.g. Lehnhardt (1989): 10 years; Fritze and Eisenwort (1989): 20 years; Gantz et al. (1990): 6 years. It is doubtful whether such apparently arbitrary cut-off points can really be useful without taking into account all the other variables that are relevant, but nearly all the reports of the best results of implantation (with some notable exceptions) have been from recently deafened cases.

Lipreading ability

On theoretical grounds it might be expected that good lipreaders have developed the cognitive/information processing skills relevant to make use of minimal cues in speech recognition and so obtain an increased benefit from a cochlear implant as compared to poor lipreaders. In fact, the evidence to support this hypothesis is weak. Cooper et al. (1989) found a slight relationship between preoperative lipreading ability and the enhancement of lipreading obtained with a single-channel implant. In contrast, Gantz et al. (1988) found no correlation between lipreading ability and performance with multichannel implants. In this latter case, the measure of performance used was sound-only speech recognition as opposed to enhancement of lipreading, which could explain the discrepancy in the findings.

Residual hearing

It could be assumed that the levels of residual hearing in the implanted ear are directly related to the neuronal survival in that ear. If this is true, then we could expect to find a strong relationship between, for example, the number of recordable hearing thresholds in the implanted ear and the result of implantation. This was found by Gantz et al. (1988). This finding, if it is supported by more data from elsewhere, may have implications for the audiological criteria for selection of implant candidates; the choice between amplification and implant will become a lot more difficult in marginal cases with some residual hearing if indeed it is shown that these cases can obtain more benefit from an implant than those with no residual hearing at all. Unfortunately, there is not yet sufficiently strong evidence to conclude that this is the case. In general, implant groups are becoming less conservative in their audiological criteria and so more data concerning the performance of patients with differing levels of residual hearing will become available in due course.

Statistical Formulae

As seen above, there is no single variable or test result that can be used as a reliable predictor of the outcome of cochlear implantation. The degree of success is clearly dependent on a complex interaction of a range of factors, each with its own weight. There have been a number of attempts to determine which are the relevant factors, and the weight or significance that needs to be attached to each of them, using statistical analysis.

The three most apparently successful statistical analyses are those described by Fritze and Eisenwort (1989), Gantz et al. (1990) and Blamey et al. (1990). The first of these produced a formula incorporating language competence (found to be the strongest single factor), duration of deafness, preoperative speech discrimination scores, and threshold for electrical stimulation. This formula was found to be fairly accurate in predicting the result of implantation. It should be noted, however, that the outcome measure used was based on a largely subjective appraisal made by a linguist and speech pathologist. Patients were allocated into one of six possible categories of performance. Both post- and prelingually deafened patients were included in the study, which might account for the finding that linguistic competence emerged as the most significant variable.

In the second study (Gantz et al., 1990), the only variable in common with the Viennese formula is duration of deafness. A duration of less than 6 years was considered to be a favourable indicator. In addition to this, the other 'indicators' found to be relevant were compliance and motivation, performance on a specially designed cognitive task, lipreading (vision-alone consonant recognition), and the slope of the electrically evoked action potential growth function (thought to be a measure of neuronal survival). The outcome measure used was performance on a sound-only sentence test, which is a rather more concrete indicator of success than the subjective appraisal of a member of the implant team as was used in the Viennese study. It is interesting to note that four of the 'favourable indicators' used in this study were concerned with higher-level cognitive and motivational aspects, rather than with the results of tests aimed at lower levels. It may be that these aspects do in fact account for the variability of the results of cochlear implantation more than factors such as the results of electrical stimulation. In other words, provided a patient has a certain minimum level of neuronal survival, the benefit they obtain from an implant may turn out to be dependent to the greatest extent on the degree of their motivation to succeed and their higher-level cognitive and information-processing abilities.

The third study (Blamey et al, 1990) placed greater emphasis on results of preoperative psychophysical testing (gap detection and frequency discrimination on promontory stimulation) and functioning of the electrode array postoperatively (number of electrodes and dynamic ranges). These factors, along with duration of deafness, were used to devise a regression equation to predict postoperative sentence recognition.

Conclusion

The process of selecting candidates for a cochlear implant is highly complex and should be carried out within the context of determining the most appropriate rehabilitational approach for each individual case. Data are now gathering which should enable reasonably accurate predictions to be made about the degree of benefit each patient is likely to obtain. More data from longer-term studies of implanted patients will help to increase the accuracy of such predictions and inter-transfer of results between different implant groups will be necessary to enable pooling of data for this purpose.

References

BERLINER, K. (1985). Selection of cochlear implant patients. In: Schindler, R.A. and Merzenich, M.M. (eds), *Cochlear Implants*, pp. 395–402. New York: Raven Press.

BLAMEY, P.J., PYMAN, B.C., GORDON, M., CLARK, G.M., BROWN, A.M., DOWELL, R.C. and HOLLOW, R.D. (1990). Factors predicting postoperative sentence scores in postlinguistically deaf adult cochlear implant patients. Preprint from Department of Otolaryngology, University of Melbourne.

BRIMACOMBE, J.A., WEBB, R.L., DOWELL, R.C., MECKLENBURG, D.J., BEITER, A.L., BARKER, M.J. and CLARK, G.M. (1987). Speech recognition abilities in profoundly deafened adults using the Nucleus 22-channel cochlear implant system. *International Cochlear Implant Symposium*, Düren, pp. 487–490.

COOPER, H.R., CARPENTER, L., ALEKSY, W., BOOTH, C.L., READ, T.E., GRAHAM, J.M. and FRASER, J.G. (1989). UCH/RNID single channel extracochlear implant; results in thirty profoundly deafened adults. *J. Laryngol. Otol.* suppl. 18, 22–38.

FAYAD, J., LINTHICUM, F.H., OTTO, S.R., GALEY, F.R. and HOUSE, W.F. (1990). Paper presented at the 2nd International Cochlear Implant Symposium, Iowa.

FRITZE, W. and EISENWORT, B. (1989). Statistical procedure for the preoperative prediction of the result of cochlear implantation. *Br. J. Audiol.* 23, 293–297.

GANTZ, B.J., TYLER, R.S., KNUTSON, J.F., WOODWORTH, G., ABBAS, P., McCABE, B.F., HINRICHS, J., TYE-MURRAY, N., LANSING, C., KUK, F. and BROWN, C. (1988). Evaluation of five different cochlear implant designs: audiologic assessment and predictors of performance. *Laryngoscope* 98, 1100–1106.

GANTZ, B.J., WOODWORTH, G., KNUTSON, J., TYLER, R.S. and ABBAS, P. (1990). Multivariate clinical prediction of success with cochlear implants. Paper presented at the 2nd International Cochlear Implant Symposium, Iowa.

HOCHMAIR-DESOYER, I.J., HOCHMAIR, E.S. and STIGLBRUNNER, H.K. (1983). Psychoacoustic temporal processing and speech understanding in cochlear implant patients. *Proceedings of the 10th Anniversary Conference on Cochlear Implants*, San Francisco.

LEHNHARDT, E. (1989). Can Cochlear Implant results be predicted? Paper presented at Hallpike Symposium, London, June.

LINDSTROM, B. (1987). Electric stimulation, pre- and post-operatively. *International Cochlear Implant Symposium*, Düren, pp. 179–181.

OTTE, J., SCHUKNECHT, H.F. and KERR, A.G. (1978). Ganglion cell population in normal and pathological human cochleae – implications for cochlear implantation. *Laryngoscope* 38, 1231–1246.

SMOORENBURG, G.F. and VAN OLPHEN, A.F. (1987). Pre-operative electro stimulation of the auditory nerve and post-operative results with the House/3M Cochlear Implant. *International Cochlear Implant Symposium*, Düren, pp. 227–229.

SOULIER, M.J.E., FRAYSSE, B., VINCENT, M., SONILHAC, F., URGELL, H. and DEGUINE, O. (1987). Pre- and post-implantation electrophysiological tests. International Cochlear Implant Symposium, Düren, pp. 35–36.

WALTZMAN, S. (1987). Correlation of preoperative round window stimulation and CT scan with cochlear implant performance. *International Cochlear Implant Symposium*, Düren, pp. 509–511.

Chapter 7
Audiological Assessment and Hearing Aid Trials

ANGELA B. KING

Scope of Assessment

One of the apparently inevitable problems of discussing assessment in the context of patient selection for a particular form of treatment is that the question becomes 'Who can we give this treatment to?' rather than 'What form of treatment would best suit this person?'. There is a danger of distorting the proper purpose of assessment, which is to evaluate the individual's condition and requirements and to find the best solution(s) from the range available. If profoundly deaf people are to be invited for assessment within a cochlear implant programme, then alternatives to implants, such as conventional hearing aids, signal processing hearing aids and vibrotactile aids, should also be under consideration and available for trial purposes. There should also be access to information about other technical equipment which may be helpful in everyday life (text telephones, visual or vibratory alarm and alerting systems, Teletext etc).

Audiological Selection Criteria

There is general agreement that cochlear implants are appropriate only for people with profound, bilateral, sensorineural hearing loss who cannot gain significant benefit from electroacoustic hearing aids. This may sound straightforward but it is not. The audiometric entry criteria can be clearly defined but serve only to identify a group of people, some of whom may obtain considerable benefit from hearing aids. As it is not possible to predict aided auditory discrimination from the pure-tone audiogram with any precision, evaluation of performance with an appropriate hearing aid is an essential part of the assessment procedure for those with any residual hearing. Unfortunately, different implant teams have not shared the same working definition of significant benefit from a hearing aid.

Audiological assessment is required not only as part of the selection procedure but also to evaluate performance with the implant. Only in this way can a picture be built up of the level (average and range) of perceptual function which can be expected with a particular type of cochlear implant so that, at the selection stage, any benefit from a hearing aid can be compared with likely benefit from an implant.

Procedures

Pure-tone audiometry

The starting point for audiological assessment is the pure-tone audiogram. It is necessary to use an audiometer which can deliver 130 dB hearing level (HL) without distortion at audiometric frequencies from 0.5 to 4 kHz in order that dynamic range as well as detection thresholds can be determined. Patients who do have auditory (as opposed to vibrotactile) thresholds in excess of 90 dB HL often also have a severely restricted dynamic range and so will show clear uncomfortable loudness levels within the range of the audiometer, which need to be taken into account in fitting an appropriate high-powered hearing aid. A high degree of compression may be required to enable them to obtain adequate amplification without also experiencing discomfort. During audiometry, it should also be established whether the patient has tinnitus at a level that makes thresholds difficult to determine and whether, as occurs in a small proportion of patients, acoustic stimulation exacerbates his or her tinnitus. These people are unlikely to be able to use hearing aids (and in the author's experience may also suffer the same problem with electrical stimulation). Abnormal adaptation (tone decay) should also be investigated using a sustained tone at 5 dB above threshold.

People who have auditory (as opposed to vibrotactile) thresholds at more than one audiometric frequency between 250 Hz and 4 kHz, with the 500-Hz threshold at 110 dB HL or less, should be given a hearing aid trial provided that they do not have severe tinnitus or rapid abnormal adaptation (King and Martin, 1986).

Before considering hearing aids, it should be mentioned that a significant relationship has been found between pure-tone thresholds (average of threshold at 0.5, 1.0 and 2.0 kHz) and results on electrical promontory stimulation (Brokx, Hombergen and Coninx, 1988). Those with higher pure-tone thresholds had a smaller dynamic range on electrical stimulation and poorer discrimination of duration differences (i.e. a larger 'temporal difference limen'). Those with pure-tone average threshold better than 115 dB HL showed a temporal difference limen better (shorter) than 130 ms. It has been suggested that these people are likely to do well with an implant, but they may also gain significant benefit from hearing aids, and so it is particularly important for them that evaluation of aided performance is part of the audiological assessment procedure. In fact, recent evidence has not confirmed earlier indications that people with some residual hearing achieve better results with implants than those with none, and promontory stimulation has been largely discredited as a predictor of performance with an implant.

Evaluation of benefit from hearing aids

A small range of appropriate high-powered aids needs to be available for hearing aid trials. Compression is a useful feature to cater for restricted dynamic range, provided that it does not compromise the amount of gain available for input sounds of moderate intensity. For people with residual hearing at or above 1 kHz, aids which selectively compress only the low frequencies may be an advantage. For those with hearing only in the frequency range below 1 kHz, aids with an extended low frequency response are appropriate, but it may be found that some of these patients can receive more benefit from signal processing hearing aids which extract certain features, in particular voice pitch, and map them onto the frequency range of maximum audibility for the individual concerned. An example of such a device is the SiVo aid (Rosen et al., 1987). The SiVo has application particularly when residual hearing with a reasonable dynamic range occurs only below 500 Hz. Care is required in the selection and fitting of hearing aids in order to take full advantage of residual hearing without causing the patient discomfort in listening, and without assuming that hearing at all frequencies is equally useful when it comes to discrimination of speech. It is also essential to be able to provide very well-fitting, comfortable ear moulds to prevent acoustic feedback at the high gain levels which are required.

The question of how benefit from hearing aids should be evaluated is a crucial one. Although there is general agreement that cochlear implants are appropriate only for those who cannot gain significant benefit from hearing aids, different teams have different working definitions of significant benefit. It is clear that, for most profoundly deaf people, hearing aids are at best a means of enhancing lipreading and providing awareness of environmental sound; significant speech recognition is not often possible through auditory perception alone. But the same is true of single-channel implants in all but a minority of exceptional cases. Hearing aids can provide speech information which, though limited, substantially complements the visual information obtained through lipreading. Booth-royd (1989) provides confirmation of this in an analysis of profoundly deaf children's performance on auditory speech perception tests with amplification. Those with 91–100 dB HL average loss received auditory information on intonation, vowel contrasts and some consonant contrasts (perceiving whether consonants were voiced or not and whether they were stops or continuants), as well as perceiving intensity, duration and rhythm. Those with 101–110 dB HL average loss perceived some intonation and vowel cues as well as intensity, duration and rhythm.

An aided warble-tone audiogram including uncomfortable listening levels, obtained in a calibrated sound field, is the first step in evaluating benefit from hearing aids. A word of caution is required here: with high-powered aids, warble tones can sometimes create distortion products in the aid such that the user, though not perceiving the tone, can hear a 'chuffing' sound corresponding to the modulation frequency. Ideally, this should be checked by listening to the attenuated output from the aid as well as by questioning the patient. Some teams have drawn conclusions about hearing aid benefit from the aided audiogram alone, examining its relationship to the typical intensity levels of speech sounds at different frequencies. This is inadequate, both because discrimination ability cannot be predicted precisely from measures of sensitivity, and because it has been demonstrated that profoundly deaf people can make use of low frequency acoustic cues to enhance their lipreading performance. A more logical view is that the aided audiogram should be used primarily as a check on the hearing aid fitting strategy and that aided speech perception must be separately assessed.

Psychoacoustic measures (with amplification to comfortable listening level), such as gap detection, temporal difference limen and frequency discrimination, provide useful research data which can be compared with similar measures for electrical stimulation and with speech perception ability, but are not essential for evaluation of aided benefit. What is important is to employ a set of tests of aided performance which assess the perception of speech at different levels, from the most basic prosodic features such as syllable number and intonation, through perception of vowel and consonant contrasts (i.e. segmental features), to recognition of words in isolation and in sentences. The tests of consonant identification and word recognition should be presented audiovisually as profoundly deaf people are unlikely to achieve significant scores without the support of lipreading; it is the comparison between aided and unaided performance on these tasks which provides a measure of benefit from hearing aids. This kind of test battery, giving a profile of speech feature perception at different processing levels, has been used systematically in the Swedish cochlear implant project (Agelfors and Risberg, 1989).

A comprehensive test battery for assessment of aided speech perception is given in Table 7.1. It may not be practicable to use all the tests listed, but it is important to select tests that cover a range of perceptual levels including aided/unaided lipreading. For children, it will be necessary to select or devise a small number of tests at an appropriate linguistic level.

Table 7.1 Tests for assessment of aided speech perception

Task	Response-type*	Type of test material	Mode of presentation
1 Identifying number of syllables in a word:		Recorded/synthesised speech:	Auditory
(a) easy	C	(a) using voiceless stop consonants	
(b) difficult	C	(b) using range of consonants	
2 Identifying stressed syllable in a word	C	Recorded/synthesised speech	Auditory
3 Identifying intonation pattern:	C	Recorded/synthesised speech	Auditory
(a) rise/fall or question/statement			
(b) locating important word in a sentence			
4 Identifying man/woman/child's voice	C	Recorded/synthesised speech	Auditory
5 Vowel identification (equal length vowels)	C	Recorded/synthesised vowels equalised for subjective loudness	Auditory
6 Consonant identification	O	e.g. 12 intervocalic consonants test (see Faulkner et al, 1989 and Chapter 16)	Audiovisual: aided/unaided
7 Isolated word recognition			
(a) closed set	C	Recorded spondee word lists	Auditory
(b) open set	O	Videotaped standard word lists	Audiovisual: aided/unaided
8 Recognition of words in sentences	O	(a) Audio version of BKB sentence lists (Bench and Bamford, 1979)	Auditory
		(b) Video version of BKB sentence lists (Rosen and Corcoran, 1982)	Audiovisual: aided/unaided
9 Connected Discourse Tracking	O	(See de Filippo and Scott, 1978)	Audiovisual: aided/unaided

*C = closed set; O = open set.

Criteria for Significant Benefit from Hearing Aids

Faced with the results on tests of aided speech perception, criteria are required for the level of aided benefit which is unlikely to be exceeded by a cochlear implant, and which is therefore taken to exclude the patient from being offered an implant. It has already been mentioned that criteria vary between different implant teams and that some draw conclusions from the aided audiogram alone. The San Francisco team (Owens, Kessler and Schubert, 1982) considered that any degree of open-set auditory speech recognition, or a combination of good vowel recognition with definite aided improvement in lipreading, contraindicates a single-channel device. The trouble with this criterion is that it takes a level of performance with hearing aids which is not very likely to be *matched* by a single-channel implant, let alone exceeded by it. It could therefore be argued that the criterion should be lower, for example, identification of syllable number and syllable stress, some perception of intonation and aided improvement in lipreading: this is significant benefit in that it compares with what can be expected with a single-channel device.

Lipreading improvements are shown in Figure 7.1 for a group of profoundly deaf people with hearing aids compared with that shown by a

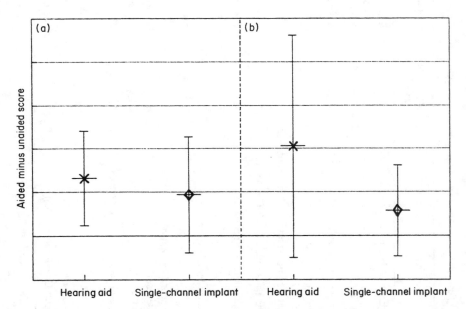

Figure 7.1. Effect on lipreading of using a hearing aid or a single-channel implant (profoundly deaf users). (a) Discourse tracking (difference in words/min); (b) BKB sentences (difference in number of keywords correct out of 50). X = Mean for group with hearing aids; ◇ = mean for group with single-channel implants. One standard deviation each side of the mean is shown.

group with single-channel implants. It can be seen that most of the hearing aid users obtained at least as much benefit as that gained by single-channel implant users.

Criteria in relation to multichannel implants tend to be more stringent, most teams demanding some open-set auditory speech recognition as evidence of 'significant' hearing aid benefit. For example, the Iowa team requires at least 4% correct on word lists or 10% correct words on their sentence test to conclude that the person does too well with a hearing aid to be considered for an implant (Gantz, 1989). The problem here is the variability of performance with multichannel implants, which makes it difficult to predict, with confidence for any individual, that speech perception with an implant will be a substantial improvement on that with hearing aids.

The success or otherwise of a hearing aid trial will finally depend as much on the person's subjective assessment of benefit, including aware-ness and recognition of environmental sounds, as it will on the results of formal tests of perception. But formal tests, as well as providing objective data, can be useful in demonstrating to the individual the amount of help they can get from hearing aids (or from vibrotactile aids – see Aleksy, 1989) in relation to the benefit that can reasonably be expected from a particular type of cochlear implant.

Summary

In summary, the purpose of audiological assessment is given by the following points:

1. Discover whether the patient has any residual hearing.
2. Establish the range of residual hearing in both the frequency and the amplitude dimension, and assess any abnormal adaptation or tinnitus-related effects of acoustic stimulation.
3. Decide whether a hearing aid trial is indicated and which hearing aid features would be most appropriate.
4. Evaluate aided sensitivity and auditory discrimination; in particular assess perception of speech at different processing levels, and the difference between aided and unaided lipreading performance.
5. Compare aided benefit with that which can reasonably be expected from a particular type of cochlear implant.
6. Consider the patient's subjective assessment of benefit (including awareness of environmental sounds) and help him or her to choose the treatment – hearing aid, implant, vibrotactile aid or none – which will best suit his or her particular requirements.

References

AGELFORS, E. and RISBERG, A. (1989). Speech feature perception by patients using a single-channel Vienna 3M extracochlear implant. *Speech Transmission Laboratory – Quarterly Progress and Status Report*. Stockholm, Sweden: Royal Institute of Technology.

ALEKSY, W. (1989). Comparison of benefit from UCH/RNID single-channel extracochlear implant and tactile acoustic monitor. *J. Laryngol Otol.* suppl. 18, 55–57.

BENCH, J. and BAMFORD, J. (eds) (1979). *Speech Hearing Tests and the Spoken Language of Hearing-impaired Children*. London: Academic Press.

BOOTHROYD, A. (1989). Hearing aids, cochlear implants, and profoundly deaf children. In: Owens, E. and Kessler, D.K. (eds), *Cochlear Implants in Young Deaf Children*. Boston: College-Hill Press.

BROKX, J.P.L., HOMBERGEN, G. and CONINX, F. (1988). Relations between audiometrical thresholds of potential cochlear implant patients and their performance in preoperative psycho-physical tests with electrical stimulation. *Scand. Audiol.* 17, 217–222.

DE FILIPPO, C.L. and SCOTT, B.L. (1978). A method for training and evaluating the reception of ongoing speech. *J. Acoust. Soc. Am.* 63, 1186–1192.

FAULKNER, A., POTTER, C., BALL, G. and ROSEN, S. (1989). Audio-visual speech perception of intervocalic consonants with auditory voicing and voiced/voiceless speech pattern presentation. *Speech, Hearing and Language: Work in Progress, UCL* 3, 87–106.

GANTZ, B.J. (1989). Issues of candidate selection for a cochlear implant. *Otolaryngol. Clin. North Am.* 22(1), 239–247.

KING, A.B. and MARTIN, M.C. (1986). Audiological assessment in the selection of cochlear implant candidates. *Br. J. Audiol.* 20, 19–23.

OWENS, E., KESSLER, D.K. and SCHUBERT, E.D. (1982). Interim assessment of cochlear implants. *Arch. Otolaryngol.* 108, 478–483.

ROSEN, S. and CORCORAN, T. (1982). A video-recorded test of lipreading for British English. *Br. J. Audiol.* 16, 245–254.

ROSEN, S., WALLIKER, J., FOURCIN, A. and BALL, V. (1987). A microprocessor-based acoustic hearing aid for the profoundly impaired listener. *J. Rehabil. Res. Dev.* 24, 239–260.

Chapter 8
Assessment of the Status of the Auditory Nerve

PAUL J. ABBAS and CAROLYN J. BROWN

Introduction

The decision as to whether or not a given hearing-impaired person should receive a cochlear implant is an important one. There is a wide range of medical, audiological and psychological tests that can be used to assess cochlear implant candidates. One type of test which is used is to evaluate the response of the subjects to electrical stimulation of the ear before implantation. In this chapter, the methods for performing such measures are discussed, together with the possible usefulness of the results of such tests in making decisions concerning implantation.

The effectiveness of the implant may depend on a number of factors, including the status of the auditory nerve and central auditory pathways in addition to the relationship between the surviving neural elements and the stimulating electrodes. Loss of hair cell function can result in degeneration of the neurons in both the auditory nerve and brain-stem nuclei (West and Harrison, 1973; Spoendlin, 1975; Gulley, Wenthold and Neises, 1978). If degeneration is complete and there are no viable neurons in the auditory nerve, then implantation would certainly not be useful. Histological studies of both animal and human temporal bones reveal that some surviving spiral ganglion cells are present in subjects evidencing some hearing capacity in response to electrical stimulation through an intracochlear device (Pfingst et al., 1981; Johnsson, House and Linthicum, 1982; Pfingst and Sutton, 1983). Thus, preoperative electrical stimulation has been suggested as a test that can be used to indicate the presence of viable auditory neurons (House and Brackmann, 1974; Chouard and MacLeod, 1976).

The purpose of preoperative assessment need not be limited to whether or not there are viable auditory neurons. Clearly, there can be a middle ground, cases where only parts of the auditory nerve survive. A number of studies with animals have shown that performance with a cochlear implant may be related to the number of surviving neurons in the auditory nerve (Pfingst et al., 1979; Clopton, Spelman and Miller, 1980). It is presumed that the number of surviving auditory neurons determines the amount of information that can be carried by the auditory nerve and, therefore, the number of surviving neurons may correlate with performance. A method is needed to estimate neuron survival in pre-implant candidates. Some studies have shown a relationship between the recency of hearing loss and the degree of auditory nerve survival (Bergstrom, 1975; Otte, Schuknecht and Kerr, 1978). Other studies have shown that the relationship between aetiology and the degree of nerve survival is not clear cut (Hinojosa and Marion, 1983). Thus, whilst the medical history of a patient may provide some indication of the state of the auditory system, it is probably not adequate to assess accurately the degree of neuron survival. As a result, there have been a number of attempts to identify experimental measures that correlate with nerve survival. If these measures have the potential to predict nerve survival, then they may also be used to predict an individual's performance with the implant.

Finally, when there is degeneration of the auditory nerve, the functioning of the neurons may be affected even though they are still viable. Varying degrees of degeneration may affect the condition of surviving auditory neurons and also the integrity of the surrounding myelin sheath. Such changes in neuronal condition are significant because they may affect the response of the neuron to stimulation. For example, the refractory properties of the surviving neurons may be altered. Refractory properties refer to the effect of one stimulus on subsequent stimulation. These properties may be particularly important in determining the ability of the neurons to reproduce complex time patterns of stimuli that may be necessary to code speech. The degree to which pre-implant testing can assess the functional properties of surviving neurons may be particularly important in predicting the usefulness of the device.

The basic purpose of many preoperative tests is to develop a relatively non-invasive procedure that can be used to predict post-implant performance. Such information may be important in making decisions concerning whether or not to implant and/or which type of cochlear implant may be the most appropriate to use with an individual. There have been experiments carried out using several different types of psychophysical and physiological measures of response. Psychophysical procedures, such as measures of the threshold and dynamic range of response to electrical stimulation, can be evaluated in a relatively straightforward manner and would be appropriate for adult, postlingual subjects. The use of objective measures, such as the electrically evoked auditory evoked response (EABR), may be more appropriate for non-cooperative subjects such as young children. Measures such as threshold and/or growth of the EABR may be related to the number of neurons surviving in the auditory nerve.

Responses to different temporal sequences of stimuli may also be determined either with psychophysical or physiological measures and may be related to the functional properties of surviving neurons. Measures which correlate either with the number of surviving neurons and/or their refractory properties may be relevant to the abilities of a particular subject to function with an implant.

Experiments have been performed in both adult implant subjects and experimental animals which are aimed at assessing the efficacy of various testing procedures that evaluate these properties. In experiments with animal subjects, the correlation between physiological measures and nerve survival can be evaluated directly. In experiments with human implant recipients, the correlation of psychophysical and/or physiological measures with performance with the implant can be evaluated. In this chapter, the authors will discuss the techniques used for making these measurements, describe the results of both psychophysical and electrophysiological experiments, and discuss the possible usefulness of these measures as part of an overall evaluation of candidates for cochlear implantation.

Technique

The basic procedure for preoperative electrical stimulation testing involves placing an electrode in the middle ear, either on the promontory or in the round window niche. To accomplish this, some groups have used a needle electrode similar to that used for electrocochleography that is placed through the tympanic membrane directly onto the promontory of the middle ear (Banfai et al., 1984; Gibson, Game and Pauka, 1987; Hochmair-Desoyer and Klasek, 1987). Current is then passed relative to a reference electrode that is placed somewhere outside the ear (on the mastoid process, for example). The resulting current distribution can affect inner ear structures and result in the percept of sound. The procedure can be performed without anaesthesia and the wound in the tympanic membrane heals quickly. The authors have used a slightly more extensive preoperative stimulation procedure as part of the evaluation in the Iowa Cochlear Implant Project (Gantz et al., 1988). In this procedure, a flap is opened in the tympanic membrane and a platinum ball electrode is placed in the round window niche under direct visual observation. Stimulation is accomplished relative to a reference external to the ear. Placement of the electrode onto the round window niche using this procedure has the advantage that the placement is more uniform across subjects and that the electrode is positioned closer to the neural elements that are to be stimulated by the current than is achieved using a promontory electrode. The disadvantage is that the procedure is slightly more invasive and cannot be performed without local anaesthesia. Several variations of these procedures have been reported: several groups report using a procedure in which a temporary electrode is positioned transtympanically into the middle ear and is left in place for several days (Douek et al., 1983; Fourcin et al., 1983; Abel and Tse, 1987; Black et al., 1987). This procedure allows time for the subject to adapt to the new form of stimulation and for more extensive testing of different aspects of the subject's response properties. Finally, several groups have reported results obtained using non-invasive extratympanic electrodes which can elicit an auditory sensation through electrical stimulation of the ear canal (Hochmair-Desoyer and Klasek, 1987; Liard et al., 1988).

Psychophysical Tests

The absence of any perception of sound in response to electrical stimulation of the promontory has been used by several implant groups as a criterion for implantation under the theory that, if there are no stimulable neurons in the auditory nerve, then there would be little chance of success with the implant (House and Brackmann, 1974; Mecklenberg and Brimacombe, 1985). Certainly, if the result of pre-implant electrical stimulation testing is positive (i.e. the subject reports an auditory sensation), then a similar result may be expected with an intracochlear electrode. Most subjects who have been tested with extracochlear stimulation do, in fact, receive some sensation of sound (Brightwell et al., 1985; Chouard, Meyer and Gegu, 1985; Gibson, Game and Pauka, 1987). The authors' own experience has been that, in 57 of the 61 ears of prospective cochlear implant recipients in which pre-implant stimulation has been attempted, the subject did perceive sound. One subject was implanted for whom preoperative electrical stimulation was not successful. This subject also did not receive any significant perception of sound from the implant. In all other cases, whilst there was a clear sensation of sound through the implant, the usefulness of the stimulation provided by the implant to each subject was extremely variable. Some subjects receive little more than awareness of sound in their environment. Others receive enough information to recognise words with only acoustic cues.

Perception of sound in response to pre-implant electrical stimulation has been used by a number of investigators as part of a regular evaluation to determine the appropriateness of a cochlear implant candidate (Meyer et al., 1984; Fraser, 1985). However, many groups who typically perform such a test prior to implementation do not use it as part of their regular pre-implant work-up (Thielemeir, Brimacombe and Eisenberg, 1982; Rothera et al., 1986). The main difficulty with such a test is the possibility of false negatives, i.e. even though the subject could not perceive sound with extracochlear stimulation, stimulation with intracochlear electrodes may be successful (Brown et al., 1983). The position of the stimulating electrode within the middle ear may determine the relative threshold of pain or vibrotactile stimulation as well as the threshold of auditory sensation. Thus, variations in placement of the stimulating electrode during pre-implant electrical stimulation testing may confound the results.

In addition to simply testing for the presence of viable neurons, several researchers have evaluated the potential usefulness of these pre-implant tests as predictors of the subject's performance with the implant. Measurements of the threshold of detection and the maximum comfortable level of current provide an estimate of the available dynamic range (Rothera et al., 1986; Hochmair-Desoyer and Klasek, 1987; Gantz et al., 1988). Relatively few studies have examined correlations to performance and/or histology. In animal studies, Pfingst and Sutton (1983) have demonstrated that sensitivity to low-frequency sinusoids is correlated to auditory nerve survival. Brokx, Hambergen and Coninx (1988) demonstrated a relationship between audiometric thresholds in prospective cochlear implant patients and their psychophysical response properties to promontory stimulation. As part of an extensive discriminant analysis to see what factors accounted for differences in performance, Fritz and Eisenwort (1988) identified threshold of promontory stimulation as contributing at least marginally. In contrast, Fourcin et al. (1979) have observed that threshold measures using round window stimulation correlate poorly with performance with an extracochlear implant. The data on this issue are complicated by the relation between thresholds to extracochlear and intracochlear stimulation. Extrapolation of data that are based on post-implant intracochlear electrical stimulation to the pre-implant case may not be reasonable. Psychophysical responses, such as threshold and dynamic range measurements recorded using pre-implant extracochlear stimulation techniques, may not be strongly correlated with the same measures made using stimulation provided by an intracochlear device. There are a number of reasons for these differences, including electrode placement, the location of neuronal structures to be stimulated relative to the position of the electrodes, and the impedance of the different tissue pathways for current flow in and around the ear. Whilst psychophysical measures of response threshold and dynamic range would be expected to be related to the numbers of neurons, a clear correlation between these measures and eventual performance with the implant has not been shown.

Several different experimental tasks have been used to evaluate the temporal processing ability of subjects with pre-implant stimulation. For gap detection, the subject's task is to detect the presence of a silent interval in a tonal or noise stimulus (Hochmair-Desoyer, Hochmair and Stiglbrunner, 1984; Skinner, 1989). In this paradigm, the primary measure is usually the smallest silent interval that the subject can detect. Other investigators have measured temporal difference limens (DLs); temporal DLs measure the ability of the subject to detect changes in the duration of the stimuli (Black et al., 1987; Hochmair-Desoyer and Klasek, 1987). A third type of temporal processing measure is the ability of the subject to detect a change in the frequency of stimulation or rate DL (Black et al., 1987; Knapp et al., 1989). Finally, a measure of tone decay, or the time necessary for the perception of a continuous tone to become inaudible, has also been used in pre-implant evaluations. Each of these measurements may be tapping a slightly different psychophysical ability of the subject, but all should be related to the degree to which the nervous system can follow the temporal pattern of the input stimulus. Several of these measures, when made with pre-implant stimulation, have shown promising correlations to eventual performance with the implant (Hochmair-Desoyer and Klasek, 1987; Skinner, 1989).

Electrophysiological Tests

There has been a great deal of work in both human and animal subjects recording electrically evoked brain potentials, particularly the electrically evoked auditory brain-stem response (EABR). Recording electrodes, their placement and the averaging processes used are similar to those used with acoustic stimulation. When the auditory system is stimulated by electrical current, the response waveform of the EABR is similar to that evoked by an acoustic stimulus, but the peaks are slightly shorter in latency (Starr and Brackmann, 1979). This latency difference is due to the fact that, with electrical stimulation, the neurons of the auditory nerve are stimulated directly, bypassing the cochlear travelling wave and hair cell–neuron synapse. The interpeak latencies, however, are similar to those recorded using acoustic stimulation, because the sequence of subsequent brain-stem activation is the same in both cases (van den Honert and Stypulkowski, 1986). The amplitude of the peaks in the response grows very quickly with changes in stimulus current, in comparison to similar changes obtained using acoustic stimulation, but the latency of each peak of the EABR changes little as the stimulus current is increased. The large changes in response amplitude are consistent with the observed changes in single neuron responses with electric stimulation as compared to acoustic stimulation (van den Honert and Stypulkowski, 1984; Javel et al., 1987). The small latency changes with intensity which are observed in the electrically evoked ABR are also consistent with single unit data and can be attributed to the lack of travelling wave in the cochlea.

In measuring the ABR using electrical stimulation, there are two issues of particular concern. The first is the elimination or reduction of the large stimulation artefact that is inevitably recorded, and the second is the concern that the responses recorded may be from structures outside the auditory nervous system. Since it is important to avoid passing direct current, the stimulus used to elicit the EABR is typically a biphasic current pulse, a positive square pulse followed by an equal and opposite negative square pulse. Since the stimulus is electric current, the electrodes used to record the EABR will also record the electric potential that results from the presentation of the stimulus. Since relatively high amplification is used, the stimulus artefact which is recorded will generally be much larger than any neural potential. Several methods can be used to ensure that this large stimulus artefact does not interfere with measurement of the EABR. The choice of the position of the stimulating and recording electrodes is critical in determining the amplitude of the stimulus artefact (Gardi, 1985). Since EABR is recorded differentially, if the orientation is such that each recording electrode picks up a similar potential from the stimulating electrodes, the artefact should be minimal. For instance, if bipolar stimulating electrodes, oriented in the proper direction, are used, remote recording electrodes will pick up relatively little stimulus artefact in the recorded potential. This configuration is more easily accomplished with intracochlear stimulation. Typically for pre-implant stimulation, the relative position of the stimulating electrodes is further apart and, consequently, the ability to decrease the recorded artefact is limited. Also, if the duration of the biphasic stimulus is kept relatively short (< 0.5 ms), later response potentials can be recorded that are relatively unaffected by the stimulus artefact. This can be accomplished by using filtering that is as broad as possible. When wideband recordings are made, the stimulus artefact will 'ring' for a shorter time and, consequently, the stimulus artefact will be confined to the very beginning of the recording epoch. In subsequent analysis of the averaged waveform, the artefact can be eliminated and the waveforms digitally filtered to eliminate noise. Some investigators (Black et al., 1983) have used a sample and hold circuit essentially to turn off the amplifier during stimulation. Such a device will avoid saturating the amplifier during stimulation and allow better isolation of the response. The authors have used alternating polarity of stimulation (i.e. present a positive first pulse followed by a negative first pulse) to help eliminate the stimulus artefact from the response (Abbas and Brown, 1988). Since the artefact produced by each alternating pulse is opposite in phase, on average the artefact will tend to cancel. There is no single procedure that will eliminate the artefact completely, but, by using a combination of these techniques, it should be possible to reduce the stimulus artefact sufficiently to record brain-stem potentials adequately.

A second important factor to take into consideration in making measures of electrically evoked potentials is the source of the potentials. When electrical stimulation is used, other non-auditory neural and muscular systems may be stimulated as well. The form of the EABR which is recorded with intracochlear electrical stimulation is consistent across subjects and is similar to that evoked with acoustic stimulation. Experiments with such stimulation in monkeys have indicated that the response is primarily from the auditory system rather than from the facial or vestibular systems (Dobie and Kimm, 1980). Van den Honert and Stypulkowski (1986) demonstrate potentials of vestibular origin that are opposite in polarity and quite different in form from the auditory evoked potential. Muscle activity tends to be longer in latency, but can also be differentiated from the auditory potentials by its large amplitude and rapid rate of growth with stimulus current. Additionally, measures of activity in experimental animals have demonstrated an electrophonic response in ears with normal hair cell populations. This response is due to stimulation through the hair cell rather than via direct nerve stimulation and, as a result, electrophonic potentials have a different threshold, latency and form of response. In general, a good criterion for use in the determination of whether or not the recorded potentials are auditory in origin is that the form of the response and its amplitude are similar to that recorded to acoustic stimulation. This is especially important to consider when measures of the EABR are made using middle-ear stimulation. In the authors' experience with over 40 cochlear implant users, intracochlear stimulation produced consistent response waveforms in all subjects. In a similar population of subjects in which pre-implant, round window stimulation was used, a response was recorded from only about half the subjects. Of those subjects for whom it was possible to record a response, the morphology of the potentials which were recorded was quite variable. These observations are illustrated (Figure 8.1) in the examples of EABR responses recorded from several different subjects with pre-implant stimulation (stimulation at the round window niche), monopolar intracochlear stimulation through the Ineraid cochlear implant (with a reference in the temporalis muscle) and bipolar intracochlear stimulation through the Nucleus implant. In each case, the level of the stimulus was chosen in the upper part of the subject's dynamic range and, in each case, the two averaged applications of averaged response are shown.

Several experiments have been reported in which experimental animals have been used to investigate the effects of cochlear nerve survival on the EABR. The EABR has been used to monitor physiological changes in cats with chronically implanted electrodes (Walsh and Leake-Jones, 1982; Miller et al., 1983). Both bony growth and loss of nerve fibres resulted in decreased EABR amplitudes. Smith and Simmons (1983) measured threshold and growth of the EABR in cats with different degrees of experimentally induced neural degeneration. Threshold proved to be a poor predictor of the number of surviving ganglion cells; slope of the amplitude–current function, however, was shown to be a better predictor. Lusted, Shelton and Simmons (1984) compared electrode sites and demonstrated that a scala tympani placement resulted in clearer changes

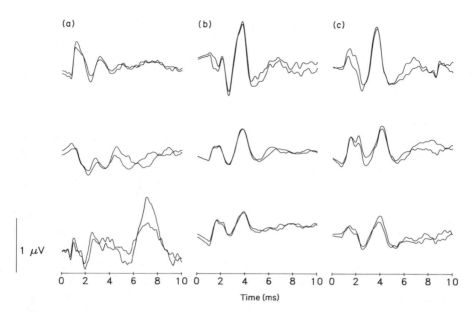

Figure 8.1. EABR waveforms for nine different subjects using direct stimulation of the round window niche (pre-implant) or stimulation through the Ineraid or Nucleus cochlear implant. Stimuli in each case were biphasic pulses and, in each case, the current level was chosen to be in the upper part of the subject's dynamic range. Two averaged traces were measured for each subject and are superimposed in the plot. Pre-implant (a) stimulation was monopolar, with the reference placed on the ipsilateral mastoid process. Stimulation through the Ineraid implant (b) was between the most apical intracochlear electrode and the electrode implanted in the temporalis muscle. Stimulation through the Nucleus implant (c) was bipolar between electrodes 10 and 16. There are 22 electrodes in the array, with 1 being the most basal and 22 the most apical.

in growth of amplitude for different degrees of neuron loss than electrodes placed outside the cochlea. Hall (1989) has recently reported on measures of the early peak in the EABR of rats in which he demonstrated a correlation between growth of response magnitude and nerve fibre survival. In contrast to the above findings, there have been several studies in which a strong relationship between evoked potential measures and nerve survival have not been demonstrated (Shepard, Clark and Black, 1983; Steel and Bock, 1984). Thus, while the data from experimental animals are not conclusive, there are some indications that EABR growth may be related to the number of surviving auditory neurons.

In work with human subjects, several groups have included the recording of EABR to stimulation of the middle ear prior to cochlear implantation, in an effort to evaluate the usefulness of such a measure in predicting success with the implant (Meyer et al., 1984; Simmons et al., 1984; van den Honert and Stypulkowski, 1986; Black et al., 1987; Game, Gibson and Pauka, 1987; Gantz et al., 1988). In general, measures of the

EABR made preoperatively have been quite variable and no clear correlation has been found between EABR pre-implant data and post-implant performance. A number of investigators have used intracochlear stimulation (through the implant) to measure EABR responses (Starr and Brackmann, 1979; Gardi, 1985; Waring, Don and Brimacombe, 1985; van den Honert and Stypulkowski, 1986; Abbas and Brown, 1988, 1989). The responses in these cases are much more consistent, both across studies and across implant types. The differences between pre-implant and post-implant studies are interpreted so that they are related to the proximity of the electrodes to the nerve and the consistency of the electrode placement in the cases of intracochlear stimulation. This trend is illustrated in the traces from the Ineraid, and Nucleus users in Figure 8.1 show the same form of response. There are usually up to three peaks in the response with the last having a latency of approximately 4 ms. The amplitude and latency of that peak, which is probably analogous to wave V of the acoustically evoked brain-stem response, is plotted as a function of current level in Figure 8.2. The amplitude of the response generally increases with increasing stimulus level and the latency of the peak shows a tendency to decrease. Stimulation of different electrodes within the Ineraid implant can result in different sensitivity, but all show similar changes of amplitude and latency with current level. The authors have recently investigated the correlation of these measures with the ability of implant subjects to perform with the implant. Measures of threshold and growth of response showed, at best, only modest correlation to scores on tests of word recognition.

The limited success of the EABR as a predictor of implant performance has led some researchers to investigate other physiological responses. Kileny and Kemink (1987) have used the electrically evoked, middle latency response (EMLR) in their measures of pre-implant stimulation. The advantage of this technique is that the stimulus artefact problems are significantly reduced because the neural response occurs at a much longer latency than the EABR, so there is little chance that the stimulus artefact will overlap with the neural potential and contaminate the measurement of the response. Jyung et al. (1989) have recently reported on EMLR measures made in experimental animals in which a good correlation to nerve survival was found.

An alternate approach taken by Brown, Abbas and Gantz (1989) is the recording of the electrically evoked, whole-nerve action potential (EAP) which is a potential whose source is the summed action potentials in auditory nerve fibres. This method has the disadvantage that artefact problems are compounded by the short latency of the response (< 0.4 ms), but has the advantage that the response is a direct measure of the nerve activity and, consequently, may correlate more directly with the state of the nerve. To date, there have been no measures of the EAP in

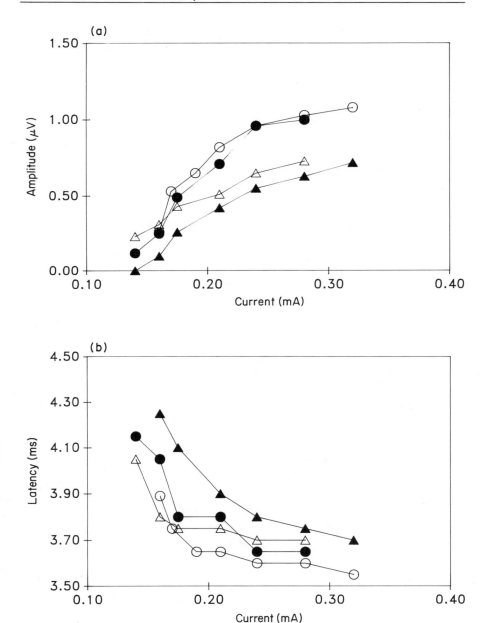

Figure 8.2. Amplitude and latency of the fourth peak (latency about 4 ms) in the EABR are plotted as a function of current level. Stimulation was accomplished through the Ineraid intracochlear electrode array. The subject had been implanted for 18 months before these measurements were made. Parameter on the graphs is the electrode pair used in stimulation. Electrode 1 is the most apical intracochlear electrode and electrode 8 is placed in the temporalis muscle.

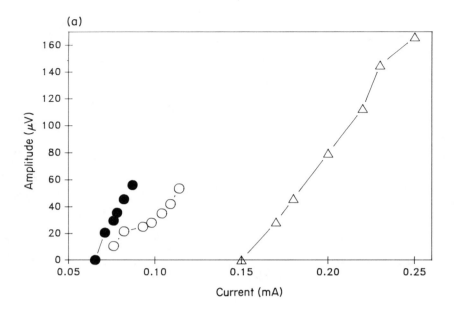

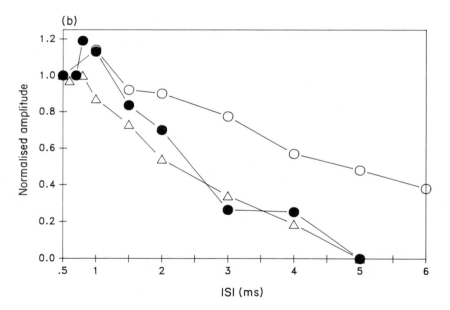

Figure 8.3. (a) This is a plot of amplitude of the EAP as a function of current level. (b) This is a plot of normalised amplitude of the measured response to the second pulse of a two-pulse sequence as function of ISI (the time between the two pulses). Data are shown from three different subjects implanted with Ineraid electrodes. Stimulation is accomplished from electrode 1 to electrode 6. Recordings were made from electrode 4 in the intracochlear array relative to electrode 8 in the temporalis muscle.

human subjects before implantation, but the measures of the EAP made using intracochlear stimulation through the implant have shown some promising results. In that work, the authors measured response growth and also used a two-pulse stimulation paradigm to evaluate recovery from the refractory state. The graphs in Figure 8.3 illustrate growth functions (amplitude vs current level) and recovery from refractory state (normalised amplitude vs interstimulus interval) for three different subjects. In the lower graph, a normalised value of 1 indicates no response to the second pulse in a two-pulse sequence; a value of 0 indicates a normal (unadapted) response. There is variability among subjects in sensitivity, growth of response and rate of recovery. When these variables were compared to the subject's performance with the implant, both the slope of the growth function and the time necessary to recover from the refractory state showed a modest correlation to word recognition scores. These findings are interpreted as meaning that both numbers of neurons and the refractory properties of those surviving neurons may be related to the subject's ability to use the implant.

Summary

There are a number of different pre-implant tests, both psychophysical and physiological, that have been used in the evaluation of cochlear implant candidates. As may be expected from the complexity of the system, none of the tests individually shows a very good correlation with performance. The ability to use the implant successfully is probably dependent on a number of factors, in addition to the condition of the auditory nerve. The type of measures that are discussed in this chapter deal with assessment of auditory nerve stimulability to some degree independent of other factors, such as cognitive abilities and language development. These types of tests will probably find their best use as part of a more extensive assessment procedure which includes medical and audiological history, psychological tests, speech and language assessment, and other relevant information.

References

ABBAS, P.J. and BROWN, C.J. (1988). Electrically evoked brainstem potentials in cochlear implant patients with multi-electrode stimulation. *Hear. Res.* **36**, 153–162.

ABBAS, P.J. and BROWN, C.J. (1989). Electrically evoked brainstem potentials through two different cochlear implant systems. *Abstracts of the Association for Research in Otolaryngology*, Twelfth Midwinter Meeting, Abstr. 330, p. 274.

ABEL, S.M. and TSE, S-M. (1987). Pre-implant evaluation of speech and hearing. *J. Otolaryngol.* **16**, 284–289.

BANFAI, P., HARTMANNE, G., KARCZAG, A. and IVERS, S. (1984). Selection of patients. *Acta Oto-Laryngol. Suppl.* 411, 147–156.

BERGSTROM, L. (1975). Some pathologies of sensory and neural hearing loss. *Can. J. Otolaryngol.* 4(suppl. 2), 1–28.

BLACK, F.O., LILLY, D.J., FOWLER, L.P. and STYPULKOWSKI, P.H. (1987). Surgical evaluation of candidates for cochlear implants. *Ann. Otol. Rhinol. Laryngol.* 96(suppl. 128), 96–99.

BLACK, R., CLARK, G., SHEPHERD, R., O'LEARY, S. and WALTERS, C. (1983). Intracochlear electrical stimulation: Brainstem response audiometric and histopathological studies. *Acta Oto-Laryngol. Suppl.* 399, 1–18.

BRIGHTWELL, A., ROTHERA, M., CONWAY, M. and GRAHAM, J. (1985). Evaluation of the status of the auditory nerve: Psychophysical tests and ABR. In: Schindler, R.A. and Merzenich, M.M. (eds), *Cochlear Implants*, pp. 343–348. New York: Raven Press.

BROKX, J.P.L., HAMBERGEN, G. and CONINX, F. (1988). Relations between audiometrical thresholds of potential cochlear implant patients and their performance in preoperative psychophysical tests with electric stimulation. *Scand. Audiol.* 17, 217–222.

BROWN, C.J., ABBAS, P.J. and GANTZ, B. (1989). Electrically evoked whole-nerve action potentials recorded in cochlear implant users. *Abstracts of the Association for Research in Otolaryngology*. Twelfth Midwinter Meeting, Abstr. 329, 274.

BROWN, A.M., DOWELL, R.C., CLARK, G.M., MARTIN, L.F.A. and PYMAN, B.C. (1983). Selection of patients for multichannel cochlear implantation. In: Schindler, R.A. and Merzenich, M.M. (eds), *Cochlear Implants*, pp. 403–405. New York: Raven Press.

CHOUARD, C.-H. and MACLEOD, P. (1976). Implantation of multiple intracochlear electrodes for rehabilitation of total deafness: Preliminary report. *Laryngoscope* 86, 1753.

CHOUARD, C.-H., MEYER, B. and GEGU, D. (1985). Pre- and per-operative electrical testing procedure. In: Schindler, R.A. and Merzenich M.M. (eds), *Cochlear Implants*, pp. 365–374. New York: Raven Press.

CLOPTON, B.M., SPELMAN, F.A. and MILLER, J.M. (1980). Estimates of essential neural elements for stimulation through a cochlear prosthesis. *Ann. Otol. Rhinol. Laryngol.* 89(suppl. 66), 5–7.

DOBIE, R.A. and KIMM, J. (1980). Braimstem responses to electrical stimulation of the cochlea. *Arch. Otolaryngol.* 106, 673.

DOUEK, E., FOURCIN, A.J., MOORE, B.C.J., ROSEN, S., WALLIKER, J.R., FRAMPTON, S.L., HOWARD, D.M. and ABBERTON, E. (1983). Clinical aspects of extracochlear electrical stimulation. *Ann. N.Y. Acad. Sci.* 405, 332–336.

FOURCIN, A.J., DOUEK, E.E., MOORE, B.C.J., ROSEN, S., WALLIKER, J.R., HOWARD, D.M., ABBERTON, E. and FRAMPTON, S.L. (1983). Speech perception and promontory stimulation. *Ann. N.Y. Acad. Sci.* 405, 280–284.

FOURCIN, A.J., ROSEN, S.M., MOORE, B.C.J., DOUEK, E.E., CLARKE, G.P., DODSON, H. and BANNISTER, L.H. (1979). External electrical stimulation of the cochlea: Clinical, psychophysical, speech–perceptual and histological findings. *Br. J. Audiol.* 13, 85–107.

FRASER, J.G. (1985). Selection of patients for implants. In: Schindler, R.A. and Merzenich, M.M. (eds), *Cochlear Implants*, pp. 343–348. New York: Raven Press.

FRITZE, W. and EISENWORT, B. (1988). Zur Vorhersagbarkert des Ergebnisses nach Cochlearimplantation. *HNO* 36, 332–334.

GAME, C.J.A., GIBSON, W.P.R. and PAUKA, C.K. (1987). Electrically evoked brain stem auditory potentials. *Ann. Otol. Rhinol. Laryngol.* 96 (suppl. 128), 94–95.

GANTZ, B.J., TYLER, R.S., KNUTSON, J.F., WOODWORTH, G., ABBAS, P., McCABE, B.F., HINRICHS, J., TYE-MURRAY, N., LANSING, C., KUK, F. and BROWN, C.J. (1988). Evaluation of five different cochlear implant designs: Audiologic assessment and predictors of performance. *Laryngoscope* 98, 1100–1106.

GARDI, J.N. (1985). Human brainstem and middle latency responses to electrical stimulation: Preliminary observations. In: Schindler, R.A. and Merzenich, M.M. (eds), *Cochlear Implants*, pp. 351–363. New York: Raven Press.

GIBSON, W.P.R., GAME, J.A. and PAUKA, C.K. (1987). Transtympanic electrically evoked auditory sensations. *Ann. Otol. Rhinol. Laryngol.* 96(suppl. 128), 94–94.

GULLEY, R.L., WENTHOLD, R.J. and NEISES, G.R. (1978). Changes in the synapses of spiral ganglion cells in the rostral anteroventral cochlear nucleus of the waltzing guinea pig following hair cell loss. *Brain Res.* 158, 279–294.

HALL, R.D. (1989). Electrically evoked auditory brainstem response in the rat: Its use in estimating spiral ganglion cell populations and the effects of facial nerve activation. *Abstracts of the Association for Research in Otolaryngology*, Twelfth Midwinter Meeting, Abst. 24, p. 24.

HINOJOSA, R. and MARION, M. (1983). Histopathology of profound sensorineural deafness. *Ann. N.Y. Acad. Sci.* 405, 459–484.

HOCHMAIR-DESOYER, I.J. and KLASEK, O. (1987). Comparison of stimulation via transtympanic promontory electrodes, implanted electrodes, and salt electrodes in the ear canal. *Proceedings of the International Cochlear Implant Symposium*, Düren, West Germany.

HOCHMAIR-DESOYER, I.J., HOCHMAIR, E.S. and STIGLBRUNNER, H.K. (1984). Psychoacoustic temporal processing and speech understanding in cochlear implant patients. In: Schindler, R.A. and Merzenich, M.M. (eds), *Cochlear Implants*, pp. 291–304. New York: Raven Press.

HOUSE, W.F. and BRACKMANN, D.E. (1974). Electrical promontory testing in differential diagnosis of sensory-neural hearing impairment. *Laryngoscope* 84, 2163–2171.

JAVEL, E., TONG, Y.C., SHEPHERD, R.K. and CLARK, G.M. (1987). Responses of cat auditory nerve fibers to biphasic electrical current pulses. *Ann. Otol. Rhinol. Laryngol.* 96(suppl. 128), 26–80.

JOHNSSON, L.-G., HOUSE, W.F. and LINTHICUM, F.H., JR (1982). Otopathological findings in a patient with bilateral cochlear implants. *Ann. Otol. Rhinol. Laryngol.* 91(suppl. 91), 74–89.

JYUNG, R.W., CROWTHER, J.A., MARSAL, S. and MILLER, J.M. (1989). Prediction of eighth nerve survival using the electrically-evoked middle latency response. *Abstracts of the Association for Research in Otolaryngology*, Twelfth Midwinter Meeting, Abstr. 30, p. 29.

KILENY, P.R. and KEMINK, J.L. (1987). Electrically evoked middle latency auditory evoked potentials in cochlear implant candidates. *Arch. Otolaryngol. Head Neck Surg.* 113, 1072–1077.

KNAPP, R.B., SHANNON, R.V., GERONA, B., TOWNSHEND, B., DENT, L.J. and COTTER, N.E. (1989). Relating speech perception and psychoacoustic test results in cochlear implant patients. *Abstracts of the Association for Research in Otolaryngology*, Twelfth Midwinter Meeting, Abstr. 326, p. 272.

LIARD, P., PELIZZONE, M., ROHR, A. and MONTANDON, P. (1988). Noninvasive extratympanic electrical stimulation of the auditory nerve. *J. Otorhinolaryngol. Related Specialties* 50(3), 156–161.

LUSTED, H.S., SHELTON, C. and SIMMONS, F.B. (1984). Comparison of electrode sites in electrical stimulation of the cochlea. *Laryngoscope* 94, 878–882.

MECKLENBURG, D.J. and BRIMACOMBE, J.A. (1985). An overview of the Nucleus cochlear implant program. *Semin. Hear.* 6, 41–51.

MEYER, B., DRIRA, M., GEGU, D. and CHOUARD, C.H. (1984). Results of the round window electrical stimulation in 400 cases of total deafness. *Acta Oto-Laryngol. Suppl.* 411, 168–176.

MILLER, J., DUCKERT, L., MALONE, M. and PFINGST, B. (1983). Cochlear prostheses: Stimulation-induced damage. *Ann. Otol. Rhinol. Laryngol.* **92**, 599–609.

OTTE, J., SCHUKNECHT, H.F. and KERR, A.G. (1978). Ganglion cell populations in normal and pathological human cochleae. Implications for cochlear implantation. *Laryngoscope* **88**, 1231–1246.

PFINGST, B.E., DONALDSON, J.A., MILLER, J.M. and SPELMAN, F.A. (1979). Psychophysical evaluation of cochlear prostheses in a monkey model. *Ann. Otol. Rhinol. Laryngol.* **88**, 613–624.

PFINGST, B.E. and SUTTON, D. (1983). Relation of cochlear implant function to histopathology in monkeys. *Ann. N.Y. Acad. Sci.* **405**, 224–239.

PFINGST, B.E., SUTTON, D., MILLER, J.M. and BOHNE, B.A. (1981). Relation of psychophysical data to histopathology in monkeys with cochlear implants. *Acta Oto-Laryngol.* **92**, 1–13.

ROTHERA, M., CONWAY, M., BRIGHTWELL, A. and GRAHAM, J. (1986). Evaluation of patients for cochlear implant by promontory stimulation. *Br. J. Audiol.* **20**, 25–28.

SHEPARD, R.K., CLARK, G.M. and BLACK, R.C. (1983). Chronic electrical stimulation of the auditory nerve in cats. *Acta Oto-Laryngol. Suppl.* 399, 19–31.

SIMMONS, F.B., LUSTED, H., MEYERS, T. and SHELTON, C. (1984). Electrically induced auditory brainstem response as a clinical tool in estimating nerve survival. *Ann. Otol. Rhinol. Laryngol.* **93**(suppl. 112), 97–100.

SKINNER, M.A. (1989). Relation between pre-operative electrical stimulation and post-operative speech recognition performance with a cochlear implant. Paper presented at the Annual Conference of the New Zealand Audiological Society, Hamilton, New Zealand.

SMITH, L. and SIMMONS, F.B. (1983). Estimating eighth nerve survival by electrical stimulation. *Ann. Otol. Rhinol. Laryngol.* **92**, 19–25.

SPOENDLIN, H. (1975). Retrograde degeneration of the cochlear nerve. *Acta Oto-Laryngol.* **79**, 266–275.

STARR, A. and BRACKMANN, D.E. (1979). Brainstem potentials evoked by electrical stimulation of the cochlea in human subjects. *Ann. Otol.* **88**, 550–560.

STEEL, K.P. and BOCK, G.R. (1984). Electrically-evoked responses in animals with progressive spiral ganglion degeneration. *Hear. Res.* **15**, 59–67.

THIELEMEIR, M.A., BRIMACOMBE, J.A. and EISENBERG, L.A. (1982). Audiological results with the cochlear implant. *Ann. Otol. Rhinol. Laryngol.* **31**(suppl. 91), 27–34.

VAN DEN HONERT, C. and STYPULKOWSKI, P.H. (1984). Physiological properties of the electrically stimulated auditory nerve. II. Single fiber recordings. *Hear. Res.* **14**, 225–243.

VAN DEN HONERT, C. and STYPULKOWSKI, P.H. (1986). Characterization of the electrically evoked auditory brainstem response (ABR) in cats and humans. *Hear. Res.* **21**, 109–126.

WALSH, S.M. and LEAKE-JONES, P.A. (1982). Chronic electrical stimulation of auditory nerve in cat: Physiological and histological results. *Hear. Res.* **7**, 281–304.

WARING, M., DON, M. and BRIMACOMBE, J. (1985). ABR assessment of stimulation in induction coil implant patients. In: Schindler, R.A. and Merzenich, M.M. (eds), *Cochlear Implants*, pp. 375–378. New York: Raven Press.

WEST, C.D. and HARRISON, J.M. (1973). Transneural cell atrophy in the congenitally deaf white cat. *J. Comp. Neurol.* **151**, 373–391.

Chapter 9
The Assessment of Psychological Variables in Cochlear Implant Patients

LAURENCE McKENNA

Introduction

The use of a cochlear implant can be expected to place great demands upon an individual's psychological abilities. In addition, the use of an implant may lead to changes in psychological functioning; indeed if it does not, the value of the procedure can be questioned. The importance of psychological variables in this context has long been recognised (Clark et al., 1977; Miller et al., 1978; Crary et al., 1982; Wexler et al., 1982) and continues to be advocated by many groups (Chouard et al., 1987; Risberg et al., 1987; Knutson, 1988). Gantz (1989) points out that candidate rejection from a cochlear implant programme is less often due to medical and surgical considerations than to other factors such as the patient's psychological profile. Berlin et al. (1987) state that the majority of the dropouts from their programme withdrew for reasons other than audiological and medical ones, and they suggest that the emotional and psychological impact of implantation must be given equal weight with the audiological and medical results. Lehnhardt (1989) reported that patients with better psychosocial status require less postoperative rehabilitation.

Psychological assessment may therefore be regarded as an integral part of the assessment procedure within a cochlear implant programme. This chapter discusses procedures for psychological assessment of candidates for, and of patients who have received, cochlear implants. Procedures used in the UCH/RNID programme, together with some of those from other programmes, which have been outlined in the literature, will be discussed. Historically, much of the effort invested in the psychological assessment of candidates for cochlear implantation and of implant users has been in the application of standardised measurement devices such as intelligence and personality tests. The use of these devices will be discussed first. Following this, techniques which allow a more individualistic and possibly more informative assessment will be discussed.

Personality Characteristics

It has been suggested by a number of workers that candidates should be assessed using standard personality inventories and be excluded if they have personality characteristics which (1) were 'unsatisfactory' (Clark et al., 1977); (2) would 'make programme completion unlikely' (Miller et al., 1978); or (3) showed 'significant signs of psychopathology' (Crary et al., 1982). Crary et al. (1982) consider scores of two standard deviations above the mean on the Minnesota Multiphasic Personality Inventory (MMPI) as evidence of pathology, although there is no guidance about whether such a score on a single MMPI scale is sufficient to classify a candidate as pathological or whether high scores on two or more scales are required. As only candidates with normal personality profiles have been included in implant programmes, the question of whether people with deviant personality profiles are, in fact, poor cochlear implant users remains unanswered. However, Crary et al. (1982) reported that the MMPI scores of 'normal' patients did not predict the number of hours that patients used their implants.

It would certainly seem imprudent to include in a cochlear implant programme someone who shows evidence of personality deviance, however that is defined, particularly where such a programme includes a very high evaluative component. To do so may be to introduce additional variables which would serve to complicate the evaluation. The use of standardised personality inventories in the assessment of cochlear implant candidates was discussed by McKenna (1986) who suggested that the use of such devices was problematic because of their questionable suitability and utility in this setting. The nature of such inventories is that they are dependent upon normative data. Extremely few such data are available for a deafened population. Knutson (1988) states that the MMPI profiles of cochlear implant candidates seen by his group (Iowa) are on average one standard deviation above the mean in areas of depression, suspiciousness and social introversion. There is a need to establish norms before meaningful decisions can be made using such measurement devices. Some caution will be needed in this process. Taylor (1970) states that the content of certain MMPI items is biased against physically disabled people and suggests that, where this is the case, the items should be removed and the scoring of the scales altered accordingly. Thomas (1984) also points out that the content of many of the questions in some inventories, including the MMPI, is loaded against the hearing impaired. Such considerations make interpretation, particularly of marginally deviant scores, difficult.

A number of studies have examined changes in personality profiles following cochlear implantation. Miller et al. (1978) examined changes between pre- and post-implant MMPI scores. They found that 1 year postoperative scores were unchanged from preoperative levels, although most of the patients reported feeling better and made use of the implant. However, decreases were noted in depression and suspiciousness as measured by the MMPI in a subsample of patients at 3–5 years' follow-up. A later paper from this group (Crary et al., 1982) reported no changes from preoperative levels in MMPI scores at postoperative assessments. Chute, Parisier and Kramer (1984) reported similar findings.

There are a number of considerations that make the use of standardised personality inventories unlikely to be informative as outcome measures in this setting. These tests seek to assess stable personality traits that are unlikely to be sensitive enough to act as short-term measures. Personality changes may be apparent only over a number of years, during which time the person may have been exposed to many diverse influences. Hallam (1976) points out that changes in personality test scores are known to be responsive to changes in emotional state. Knutson (1988) points out that any changes in such measures should be lagged against changes in audiological competence. He reported on changes in MMPI scores (and other psychometric measures – see below) as a function of changes in audiological ability; the latter was assessed in terms of percentage correct in a noise/voice discrimination test and the percentage correct on a sentence test administered in both a sound-only and a sound-plus-vision format. Change on only one scale of the MMPI – suspiciousness – correlated significantly with changes on the sound-only sentence test and the noise/voice discrimination test. Knutson (1988) noted that change on the depression scale did not correlate with changes on the tests of audiological competence, although changes on another measure of depression (which would be expected to be more sensitive – see below) did correlate with changes in audiological competence.

Crary et al. (1982) point out that to expect scores which are already within the normal ranges to improve significantly may be unrealistic. It must be remembered that such tests are more suited to the assessment of large groups rather than the individual. Whilst there may be value in the detection of group changes or indeed in noting the absence of such changes following implantation, the value of averaged group data, particularly in the selection of the individual candidate, may be very limited (Hersen and Barlow, 1976).

When the UCH/RNID programme was first instigated, the Eysenck Personality Questionnaire (EPQ) (Eysenck and Eysenck, 1975) was used in the assessment of patients. However, the use of the EPQ was discontinued as the scores did not seem to facilitate decision making in the selection of candidates and also there was insufficient variation in scores for it to be a useful outcome measure. Information about the individual's personality and behaviour is obtained from interviewing the person and, whenever possible, other significant people. Formal tests are resorted to when such information is inconsistent or unobtainable.

During a symposium on cochlear implantation, Luxford (1984) pointed out that the use of personality measures is no longer part of the routine assessment procedures of the House (San Francisco) group. Chute, Parisier and Kramer (1984) have also discontinued routine use of the MMPI in the selection of candidates. Knutson (1988) suggests that the abandonment, in this field, of standardised psychological measures such as the MMPI is premature. He points out that successful prediction requires sufficient variance in both predictor and outcome measures. However, he states that it is apparent from the variance in his own data, and those reported by others, that in order to identify predictors and document change using such measures more data will be necessary than have been available to date. A larger data set would certainly help to reveal effects which, because of their size, are not apparent from consideration of small groups of subjects. However, an appeal to variables which are discernible only through use of large data sets may be of limited assistance when making decisions about individuals. The generalisability of findings, presumably a primary reason for using standardised tests, may well be lacking, particularly in the matter of the selection of the next candidate.

Emotional State

Consideration of the candidate's emotional state is likely to yield information which may contribute to the decision-making process. Intuitively, it would seem unwise to select for implantation candidates suffering from psychoses. As Ramsden (1989) pointed out during a recent symposium, 'the last thing that one would wish to do is to put an electrode into the ear of a paranoid schizophrenic'. These ideas suppose that the psychological risk/benefit ratio involved in having an implant is unfavourably altered for psychotic patients. Whether or not this is the case is not known. However, consideration of psychotic subjects at this stage in the history of cochlear implants would complicate the evaluation. Psychotic patients are likely to present for cochlear implantation less frequently than candidates suffering from lesser psychological disorders.

Lezak (1976) points out that a poor emotional state can affect task performance resulting in 'such mental efficiency problems as slowing, scrambled or blocked thoughts and words, and memory failure' (p. 111). Mathews and Eysenck (1987) also review evidence pointing to the influence of emotional state on cognitive processing. It is therefore conceivable that a state of emotional distress may affect the person's ability to carry out the tasks involved in learning to use an implant. Emotionally distressing states are often assessed using standard questionnaire measures such as the Beck Depression Inventory (BDI) (Beck et al., 1961) or the General Health Questionnaire (GHQ) (Goldberg, 1978). The GHQ is one of the most frequently used devices for detecting emotional disorders in patients seen in non-psychiatric medical settings. Some information is available on its use in audiological settings (Singerman, Reidner and Folstein, 1980; O'Connor et al., 1987; Berrios et al., 1988; McKenna, L., Hallam, R. and Hinchcliffe, R., 1991, unpublished data). However, the question raised above – of the applicability of standardised measures in this context – is again relevant and, as a minimum, a careful analysis of individual items within such devices is advisable.

Many people coming forward as candidates for cochlear implantation are likely to be suffering from at least some degree of emotional upset. McKenna, Hallam and Hinchcliffe (1991, unpublished data) reported that 27% of neuro-otology outpatients who complained of a hearing loss showed evidence of significant psychological disturbance. The prevalence among the population of people seeking a cochlear implant might be higher. There may be some concern that to exclude people on the basis of emotional disorder would be to exclude so many candidates as to make the programme unworkable. However, the high prevalence of emotional disorders should not be considered a reason for excluding it from the selection criteria. It should be noted that emotional states may change; how quickly this happens depends on the reasons for that state. It may be that a candidate whose emotional state excludes him or her from the programme at one time could be considered suitable at a later date. Counselling may contribute to such a change. It may be assumed that a poor emotional state reflects a set of circumstances which are unhappy or worrying for the person. These circumstances merit careful consideration as they may form part of the context within which the cochlear implant is being sought and is to be used (see below).

Measures of emotional distress are likely to be reasonably sensitive and changes are likely to occur more rapidly than changes in personality traits. Emotional state may therefore provide a more appropriate outcome measure than would measures of personality characteristics. Knutson (1988) reported that changes on the BDI following cochlear implantation were found to correlate with changes in measures of audiological ability. Miller et al. (1978) reported that many of their patients stated that they felt emotionally better following cochlear implantation. Similar reports have been obtained from many of the patients implanted by the UCH/RNID team and at least one patient has reported a reduction in the frequency of episodes of depression following cochlear implantation. Further systematic evaluations in this area may well be fruitful. However, a note of caution may be struck; some candidates may regard an implant as an alternative to, or preferable to, more conventional psychotherapeutic methods. This is clearly unwise, as much so as considering cochlear implantation without due recourse to more established audiological rehabilitation methods.

Intellectual Status

Given that cochlear implant programmes involve educational schemes, a considerable amount of testing requiring the subject's cooperation, postoperative training and rehabilitation etc. (all of which will place at least some intellectual demands upon the person), it seems reasonable to suppose that the person's intellectual ability should be taken into account. Miller et al. (1978) suggested that on a priori grounds candidates should show no evidence of brain damage or of mental handicap. A number of authors (Miller et al., 1978; Crary et al., 1982) have considered formal psychometric assessment of candidates' intellectual status to be relevant to the assessment procedure and reported that all of their patients who had received implants were within normal ranges of intellectual functioning. Gantz et al. (1988) reported that cognitive assessment measures were not predictive of auditory performance using a multichannel device. Gantz (1989) questions the use of IQ measures as selection devices, particularly for those who are within normal ranges, and he points to the audiological success of several people with 'modest intellectual ability' and to the limited gains of some with 'excellent intellectual ability'. He suggests that some people with mild learning disability may benefit from 'the additional opportunities afforded by some access to an acoustic environment'.

The usefulness of tests of general intellectual function does seem questionable for the same reasons mentioned in the discussion of personality variables. In addition, the fact that the most popular intelligence tests, such as the Wechsler Adult Intelligence Scale, are heavily dependent upon verbal administration may disadvantage deafened subjects. At the very least, the testing is likely to be more time consuming than for those with adequate hearing and accordingly more fatiguing. The results are therefore likely to be less valid and reliable. Such considerations will again make interpretation, particularly of marginal scores, difficult. Tests which are not dependent upon verbal administration, such as the Raven Progressive Matrices, may avoid some of these difficulties. Knutson (1988) reported that the Raven Progressive Matrices correlated significantly with changes in acoustic competence as measured by a noise/voice discrimination (N/V) test. However, in a later paper Gantz et al. (1988) reported that the Raven Progressive Matrices were not predictive of ability to use an implant to process sound.

Miller et al. (1978), Crary et al. (1982) and Chute, Parisier and Kramer (1984) report no significant changes in intellectual status at post-implant assessments. This is perhaps not surprising because, like personality tests, most tests of general intellectual function are robust instruments sensitive only to larger changes. Again any expectation of an improvement in scores already within normal ranges may be unrealistic. Crary et al. (1982) point out that there is no evidence of cognitive deterioration resulting from prolonged use of an implant. Luxford (1984) stated that the House Group no longer routinely use IQ tests; Chute, Parisier and Kramer (1984) report that they have also discontinued the use of such tests.

Within the UCH/RNID programme, some attention is given to the matter of intelligence. However, less reliance is placed on psychometric testing than on indicators such as educational and occupational achievement and the person's general level of functioning within his or her environment. When an appeal to psychometric testing is necessary because of incomplete or inconsistent information from other sources, then non-verbal tests such as the Raven Progressive Matrices are used. Those who have received cochlear implants within the UCH/RNID programme have all been of at least average intellectual ability. To date, no candidate has been rejected on the basis of low intellectual ability. There is no evidence to suggest that any changes in intellectual ability have taken place postoperatively.

Knutson (1988) reported that laboratory tests of information processing including a vigilance task requiring subjects to identify changes in patterns and a symbol cancellation task correlated with ability on the N/V test. The application of such tests of more specific cognitive function would seem more likely to be fruitful in identifying predictor variables than would the use of more general tests of intellectual ability.

The Functional Context/The Patient's Expectations

The use of a cochlear implant may be regarded as a behaviour subject to the same laws as any other behaviour. In order for behaviour to occur and to be maintained, it is necessary for that behaviour to be reinforced. Reinforcement is any event which makes the recurrence of the behaviour more likely. In essence, behaviour will be reinforced, and therefore will be likely to continue, if it serves some useful function for the individual. Behaviour which is not reinforced or which is punished will stop. The reinforcement may be an overt gratification or it may be more subtle. What constitutes reinforcement of a useful function will vary with each individual. Owens and Ashcroft (1982) give an account of functional analysis in applied psychology. When considering whether or not a candidate is suitable for cochlear implantation, information should be gathered about whether the candidate's use of the implant is likely to be reinforcing for him or her. The consequences which the candidate expects from his or her use of the device need to be considered and judged against the collected wisdom about what changes are possible and likely.

The issue is not simply confined to what the candidate expects the quality and level of the new acoustic input to be. In addition, an assessment is needed of what the candidate expects to be different about his or her life after cochlear implantation. Most candidates hope for improvements in their lives. Whether the candidate's use of the implant and the new acoustic input which this will bring will lead to the expected improvements is the point at issue. The changes in lifestyle hoped for by some candidates seem less likely to be fulfilled than those of others. A candidate seen within the UCH/RNID programme hoped for an improvement in her poor relationship with her husband. However, careful interviewing of the couple revealed that the discord between them lay primarily in matters unconnected with her hearing loss and that the discord had in fact predated the hearing loss. To expect a cochlear implant to resolve problems unconnected with the person's hearing loss would seem overambitious and unlikely to be fulfilled. This candidate was considered unsuitable for this and other reasons. She went on to apply to other implant programmes. Another candidate applied for a cochlear implant in the expectation of a reduction in her sense of isolation and her level of stress. She had little contact with the world outside her family and also described herself as cut off from her family and unable to respond to their demands. It transpired that the family did not have good communication skills, e.g. they did not face her when speaking to her. Without a change in the family's behaviour, it would seem unlikely that her use of an implant would be fruitful. The provision of basic communication skills training was a more appropriate direction to follow. Further, part of her motivation in seeking an implant was to please her family. To undergo such a procedure primarily for the benefit of others distances the possible sources of reinforcement, making them less accessible and less predictable, and may raise difficult ethical issues. This is a consideration that has been raised with a number of candidates. Such a situation would be clearly untenable when the aspirations of others are in conflict with those of the candidate. The latter circumstance has been encountered locally only once. However, a candidate's answer to the question 'Who suggested that you ask for a cochlear implant and why?' may produce useful information.

One candidate (C1) was in the process of divorce when he asked to be considered for an implant. His legal advisers had told him that his hearing impairment made it unlikely that he would win custody of his children and therefore of the family home. He believed that if he were to obtain an implant this would influence the divorce court in his favour. This constituted his primary motivation for undergoing the procedure. It seemed very questionable whether an implant would decisively influence a court. This man was suffering from a mild depressive episode as a result of the marital dispute. Therefore the functional context within which this man was seeking an implant was at best unstable, but more probably unlikely to be such as to sustain his use of the device. However, he was considered suitable in all other respects and did receive an implant. Postoperative assessment at 1 year revealed that he had not achieved his ambitions in the divorce court; the implant was frequently broken and he described it as of little value to him when it was working and he did not often use it. A separate assessment, using a Repertory Grid technique, confirmed that he perceived the implant as having made no difference to his life (see below).

Another candidate (C2) who was considered suitable from all points of view for cochlear implantation, and who received an implant, went on to find little use for the device and rarely wore it. The main reason for this was a change in his circumstances. Some months after the operation he lost his job. The job loss meant that he had little opportunity to communicate with others; improved communication had been his main focus when seeking the implant. His use of the device therefore was not reinforced. The change in circumstances was not foreseen. A Repertory Grid assessment was also carried out with this patient (see below).

The case examples of C1 and C2 highlight the importance of the functional context within which the implant is to be used. If the use of a cochlear implant by a person does not serve the function that was expected of it, not only is its use likely to stop but it may also have a negative emotional impact on the person. Unfulfilled expectations can constitute a loss that may, in turn, render the person vulnerable to emotional problems, such as depression. Candidates who are already emotionally distressed may be particularly susceptible to this.

Within the UCH/RNID selection procedure, considerable emphasis is placed upon the assessment of the likely functional value of an implant for each candidate. Information is gathered from interviews about the handicaps that the candidate is experiencing, both as a result of his or her hearing loss and for any other reason, and about the changes that the candidate envisages. A structured interview is used in which these factors are reviewed for each major area of the patient's life, e.g. home, work, social life etc. Candidates are considered suitable when it is thought likely that there is an opportunity for an implant to serve a useful function, i.e. when there appears to be a high probability that the act of using the device will be reinforced.

Postoperative Interview Data

On the basis of interview data, Miller et al. (1978) reported that postoperatively most patients felt better and made routine use of their cochlear implant. They suggested that after an initial 'high' during which new sounds were tested, a period of disillusionment follows which may last for up to a year, after which patients become more realistic about the device and go on to develop skills in its use. Patients reported feeling less cut off from their environment and more able to take part in social events because of improved speechreading, better voice monitoring and more awareness of when others are speaking.

In addition to the psychometric assessments mentioned above, Crary et al. (1982) gathered information from clinical interviews with patients. Consistent with the findings of Miller et al. (1978), they found that patients reported an initial sense of disappointment (each hoping to have become a star patient) followed by an acceptance of the limitations of the device and a regaining of enthusiasm. On the basis of the clinical interviews, they went on to suggest that cochlear implants help to reduce patients' sense of isolation, restore their confidence about interpersonal functioning, improve their speechreading and make them aware of valuable warning sounds.

Patients within the UCH/RNID programme are interviewed postoperatively at regular intervals. The rationale and structure behind such interviews are those outlined above in the discussion of the functional context within which the implant is to be used. An assessment is made of the value which the implant has given and of the associated behavioural and other resulting changes. As in the assessment of candidates, each major area of the patient's life — family, social life, employment situation etc. — is reviewed and an assessment is made of any behavioural and other changes. Reference is made to the expectations that the patient expressed during initial candidacy interviews and a review is conducted of the extent to which these have been fulfilled. A number of changes are widely reported. Most patients report a greater awareness of environmental sounds and this appears to be intrinsically pleasurable for many patients, although a very small number are disappointed at the quality of the sound. This greater awareness leads to certain changes in behaviour, e.g. the patient answers the door rather than someone else or the patient is free to carry on with other activities while waiting for the kettle to boil or for the washing machine to finish. Many patients report a reduction in the sense of isolation, and some also report a heightened sense of safety when out of their homes; in some patients this is matched by a greater preparedness to go out alone. Improvements in communication are reported by many, although not by all patients using the UCH/RNID device. Many patients report an increase in the quantity of communication, with fewer reporting an improvement in quality; indeed it has been noted that a small number of patients complain of an initial reduction in their ability to understand what is being said to them because the new auditory input from the cochlear implant distracts them from their speechreading; this difficulty eases with time and practice.

The interview data suggest that improvements in communication are most consistently noticed in the home. It is likely that this is due to the greater familiarity with the people involved and to the opportunity to communicate. Patients report spending more time in conversation with their families and taking a more active part in conversations. This seems to be facilitated by gains in temporal perception of sounds, which allows a greater awareness of gaps in the conversation, and by improvements in voice level control. Some patients report a change in the mode of communication used, with a reduction in writing and a corresponding increase in spoken communication. Whilst such changes are generally unequivocally welcomed, in at least one patient it was likely that they contributed towards marital breakdown; improved communication permitted discussion of painful marital disputes previously left dormant because of perceived communication difficulties. It is helpful if the cochlear implant team is aware of such difficulties so that they can proceed with appropriate sensitivity and provide support.

Improvements have also been reported in the sphere of patients' social lives. However, there is a greater range in the extent of such improvements. Whilst some patients have reported very small changes in their social lives, e.g. exchanging greetings with a neighbour, others have told of increases in the number of parties given and attended and a resumption of attendance at church services and theatre performances. Again such patients have reported a greater preparedness to take a more active role, e.g. speaking directly to strangers rather than allowing their partners to interpret during social events or when simply out shopping.

A smaller number of patients have reported benefits from using their cochlear implants while at work, e.g. more fluent one-to-one communication with colleagues, a slight improvement in ability to follow proceedings during business meetings. To date, no more specific employment advantages have been reported. However, at least one patient expects promotion; this expectation appears to stem as much from the employer's review of policy regarding the employment of hearing-impaired people, as from a greater ability to perform the job because of increased auditory input. A number of patients have reported being unable to use their implants at work because of ambient noise levels. These patients have tended to be in 'blue collar' jobs.

In addition to the reduced sense of isolation and increased sense of safety mentioned above, patients commonly report improvements in their sense of confidence. This sense of improved confidence is reported in varying degrees by most patients and across many areas of life. Such improvements may be considered natural consequences of increased activity and are likely to help sustain such increases.

Some of the changes noted may be due to factors other than the additional acoustic input provided by the cochlear implant. Many patients report changes in the behaviour of others towards them; in particular patients state that there is an increase in others' expectations of them. From interview accounts, it is clear that the novelty of the operation leads to others expressing a greater interest in patients and having more interaction with them. One patient reported that he became a local celebrity following the operation, with people in his community involving him, for the first time, in social activities and even stopping him in the street, talking to him and wishing him well. Such changes inevitably broaden patients' experience and lead to an increase in their sphere of activity which can be maintained by naturally occurring positive consequences. One patient has had a clear broadening and increase in his activity levels in spite of having repeated and long lasting malfunction of his device. Clearly some account needs to be taken of such non-specific effects; these may be difficult to discover and measure other than through interview. Unfortunately, it is not uncommon for others to believe initially that cochlear implant patients have had their hearing totally restored; realisation that this is not the case can lead to some loss of interest on the part of others.

Questionnaire Measures of Change

Wexler et al. (1982) point out that the ultimate arbiter of the value of any medical advance is the consumer. They suggest that, in striving for objective measures of the efficacy of procedures, phenomenological evidence is often ignored. They take the position that, since recipients of treatment are concerned with the improvement that the treatment brings about in their lives, their perceptions about such changes should be included in the data used to evaluate the procedure. Accordingly, Wexler et al. (1982) used pre- and post-implant questionnaire measures to assess the impact of cochlear implants on both patients and their relatives. The questionnaires were compiled from data obtained from extensive interviews with patients and focused on eight main themes: sense of safety, emotional reactions, nature of interpersonal relationships, social activities, sense of isolation, communication problems, employment, and involvement with hobbies and recreational activities. They reported that, postoperatively, the greatest improvement was seen in answer to questions concerned with feelings of isolation, issues of safety, comfort at social events, difficulty in communication and participation in solitary activities such as going to shops or restaurants alone. They reported less benefit in the areas of employment and involvement with hobbies and recreational activities. No change was reported in the number and quality of patients' friendships. Relatives perceived improvements in the patients' emotional reactions, level of frustration in communication, the quality of the patients' voice and their concern about the patients' safety. Relatives also noted that there was an increase in the number of social events they attended with the patients. Wexler et al. (1982) point out that their patients did have implants at the time of the assessment which was therefore necessarily retrospective.

East and Cooper (1986) devised a questionnaire to assess the subjective benefits and problems encountered at 1 year post-implantation by patients in the UCH/RNID programme. They reported that an awareness of environmental sounds and improved speech modulation were the most significant subjective benefits. Improvements in speechreading ability were less noted.

Dinner et al. (1989) reported on the employment implications of having a cochlear implant. Using a self-report questionnaire they surveyed people in the USA who had received any one of the four major designs of cochlear implant. The questions used are contained in the paper. They noted improvements in quantity and quality of spoken communication at work and significant changes in the major communication modes used at work; lipreading remained the most commonly used mode of communication, but hearing through the implant replaced writing as the second most frequently cited mode. Job satisfaction was improved in the majority of their target population. Few of their subjects reported a change in income or job promotion as a result of their use of their implant; however, over half of their subjects reported an increase in overall job performance. However, it should be noted that the conclusions of Dinner et al. (1989) refer only to that subgroup of their originally larger sample who used their implant while at work. Many of their subjects were in employment but did not use their implants while at work. It is possible that those subjects did not use the device at work because they did not find it beneficial in that setting, in which case their conclusions may be slightly over-optimistic. The majority of their subjects who were employed were in 'white collar' jobs, were college educated, had stable job histories and had lost their hearing postvocationally.

Repertory Grid Analysis

A more recent development in the UCH/RNID programme has been the introduction of the Repertory Grid technique into the assessment of cochlear implant patients. The Repertory Grid technique provides a means for a more systematic description of changes in the individual's conceptual-isation of him- or herself and others. The technique provides a means of determining what dimensions the individual holds as important when considering the world and where he or she stands with respect to these dimensions. From this, a more careful evaluation of the person's expecta-tions and motivation, and of the impact of cochlear implantation on the patient's psychological domain, can be obtained. To date in this pro-gramme, a greater emphasis has been given to the use of this technique as part of the postoperative assessment.

The technique stems from the Personal Construct Theory – a framework developed by Kelly (1955) as a means of understanding and assessing personality. Within Kelly's (1955) theoretical framework humans are seen as scientists. In the same way that a scientist develops concepts to interpret and predict events so 'man as scientist' develops constructs through which he or she understands the world. It is suggested that people perceive similarities and differences among others and among events, and that they use constructs to impose order on these phenomena. Each individual develops a unique set of constructs which he or she uses to understand and structure his or her own environment. Kelly's emphasis is on the individual as a whole and this distinguishes his position from other approaches to the understanding of personality which highlight the importance of parts of the individual or of the group. It is not necessary to wholeheartedly accept Kelly's position in order to make use of the Repertory Grid technique that has been based on it. Even without a strong commitment to Kellian theory, the technique can be fruitful. It was found to be informative in the postoperative assessment of another patient population (Fisher, 1985). There is a variety of forms that the Repertory Grid can take – these are described by Fransella and Bannister (1977).

The Repertory Grid technique allows the patient to state what factors are important and therefore need to be assessed. For the sake of clarity, it may be helpful to outline one form of Repertory Grid technique that seems appropriate to the present context. In essence, the procedure involves the following: the individual is asked to consider a list of people that he or she knows; these people are referred to as 'elements'. In this context, the list includes him- or herself at different points in time: past, present and future, and an ideal self. A list of typical core elements is given in Table 9.1.

Table 9.1 Typical core elements used in a Repertory Grid assessment of a cochlear implant candidate and postoperatively of an implant user

Candidate	Implant user
Me prior to hearing loss	Me prior to hearing loss
My spouse/best friend	My spouse/best friend
Me now	Me prior to implant
A person I admire	Me now
A person I dislike	A person I admire
Me with a cochlear implant	A person I dislike
My ideal self	My ideal self

Other elements may be included in order to broaden and balance the assessment. The person is then presented with three of these elements at a time, e.g. 'Me prior to my hearing loss', 'My spouse' and 'Me now'. The person is asked to say how any two of the three are alike and different from the third. The answer, e.g. the first and second are confident with people while the third is not confident, is considered to be one dimension in the person's construction of the world, i.e. it is one of that individual's 'constructs'.

The procedure is repeated until a list of such constructs has been elicited. Such constructs are bipolar in nature, e.g. confident/not confident, happy/sad, part of the family/isolated from the family. The elements and bipolar constructs are arranged into a grid and the person is then asked to complete the matrix by rating each element against each construct using a numerical scale. The result is an expression of the person's perception of him- or herself at the present time vis-à-vis other people and him- or herself at different points in time (Figure 9.1). This technique allows the assessment of factors that are pertinent to each individual and avoids the use of more generalised and possibly irrelevant and insensitive items. To some extent, this technique allows the investigator a view of the world from where the patient stands and, as such, it may represent a very important measure.

A comparison can then be made of the relative ratings, e.g. 'Me now' compared with 'Me with a cochlear implant' in the case of preoperative assessment, or 'Me now' and 'Me prior to implant surgery' if it is a postoperative assessment. Such a comparison would provide information about the candidate's expectations of change or about the patient's perception of change as measured along factors that he or she has described as important. The resulting data may be considered in a number of ways with varying levels of complexity. A straightforward visual inspection of the data can be very informative. Alternatively, a principal component analysis can be carried out and the two main orthogonal factors used as axes describing factor space within which the relative positions of the elements and/or constructs can be plotted (Figure 9.2).

The use of the Repertory Grid technique in the preoperative assessment of patients is not yet validated. To date, no systematic study has been possible. It seems reasonable to suppose that the use of Repertory Grids adds information about the areas in which candidates expect change to take place and about the level of that change. However, it is still necessary to compare and contrast this information against the collected wisdom about what to expect from a cochlear implant. It may be that as the body of data grows, the process will become more precise. However, the technique offers itself more immediately to the postoperative assessment of patients.

Lynch (1987) used a Repertory Grid technique in the postoperative assessment of five patients within the UCH/RNID programme. However, as the process of eliciting constructs in the way described above is undoubtedly time consuming, she employed a frequently used method of shortening the technique by imposing a set of constructs which the investigator considers to be relevant. She used a set of imposed constructs

IF THIS SIDE IS MORE TRUE OF AN ELEMENT USE NUMBERS 1 VERY MUCH APPLIES 2 MODERATELY APPLIES 3 APPLIES A LITTLE	(E L E M E N T S)							IF THIS SIDE IS MORE TRUE OF AN ELEMENT USE NUMBERS 7 VERY MUCH APPLIES 6 MODERATELY APPLIES 5 APPLIES A LITTLE
	ME PRIOR TO HEARING LOSS	SPOUSE	ME PRIOR TO IMPLANT	ME NOW	SOMEONE I ADMIRE	SOMEONE I DISLIKE	MY IDEAL SELF	
CONFIDENT WITH PEOPLE	1	2	5	3	1	2	1	NOT CONFIDENT WITH PEOPLE
PART OF A FAMILY	2	1	5	3	1	1	1	CUT OFF FROM FAMILY
AWARE OF SURROUNDINGS	3	2	7	5	2	3	2	MISSES OUT ON SURROUNDINGS
CALM	1	3	6	2	1	3	1	WORRIED
SECURE JOB	1	2	2	2	3	5	1	INSECURE JOB
ABLE TO COMMUNICATE	1	1	6	3	2	2	1	POOR COMMUNICATION SKILLS
ACHIEVES MANY THINGS	3	2	6	5	2	5	2	ACHIEVES LITTLE
A NORMAL PERSON	1	2	6	5	1	3	1	DIFFERENT FROM OTHERS
INDEPENDENT	1	1	5	3	2	3	1	RELIANT ON OTHERS

Figure 9.1. Repertory Grid of implant user: each element is rated along each bipolar construct continuum.

which she had gathered from interviews with a population of profoundly deafened adults. These patients had been using their implants for at least 1 year. She did include an opportunity for eliciting some additional constructs from these patients. This led to the provision of no more than one or two extra constructs in any one case. She found that three of the five patients perceived themselves to have undergone positive change following the implant and rehabilitation procedures. For these patients, the

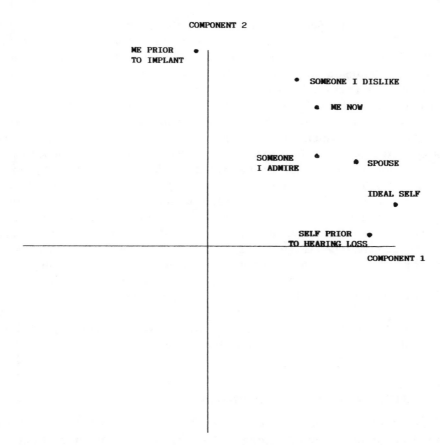

Figure 9.2. Plot of elements within each factor space following principal component analysis of Repertory Grid assessment of a cochlear implant user.

distance in factor space between the elements 'Me now' and 'My ideal self' was smaller than that between 'Me before implantation' and 'Ideal self'. This was also true when 'Me before hearing loss' was substituted for 'My ideal self'. In these patients, the greatest change was seen in a positive direction along constructs concerned with 'awareness of the environment', 'self-confidence' and 'being calm'. The Repertory Grids from the other two patients indicated little change. One of the two patients who showed little change was C1, discussed above. A functional analysis approach to assessing his motivation and expectations had suggested that his use of the implant was unlikely to be reinforced. Lynch's (1987) results provide some validation for that assessment system. The other of these two patients (C2) had been considered suitable at preoperative assessment. However, his circumstances changed so that there was little opportunity for his implant to be of value to him, and these changes could not have been predicted.

Whilst the use of imposed constructs has the advantages of simpler and quicker administration and is to be commended for this, it lacks the relevance and sensitivity associated with the use of elicited constructs. Lynch (1987) herself points out that the use of imposed constructs necessarily constricts the individual's comments and that this is opposed to the freedom which the technique purports to offer and which it is suggested represents the superiority of Personal Construct Theory over other schools of personality assessment. L. McKenna and C. Denman (unpublished data) are employing a Repertory Grid analysis, using elicited constructs obtained by the method described above, in the postoperative assessment of a consecutive series of patients using the UCH/RNID device. It is not possible, as yet, to comment in full on this study. However, preliminary results indicate that most patients perceive improvements in their psychological well being. Further work needs to be carried out before more definite conclusions can be drawn from this study. However, in so far as the use of the Repertory Grid technique provides a measure of consumer evaluation of the overall product, the findings to date are favourable. In the end, the efficacy of any intervention will be judged by the subjective benefit that it brings the recipient.

Summary and Conclusions

To date, much of the effort in the psychological assessment of cochlear implant candidates and patients has focused on the evaluation of people on standard measures of personality and intellectual function. Such evaluations have been valuable in establishing that prolonged stimulation through the use of a cochlear implant does not lead to deleterious changes in intellectual function or personality (Crary et al., 1982). As predictors of implant use, they are largely untested but would seem to be able to add little to the decision making in selection of a candidate and are unlikely to be sensitive as outcome measures. More specific tests of cognitive function, such as the vigilance tests mentioned by Knutson (1988), are more likely to be informative in this setting. Measures of emotional state are also likely to be more relevant to the assessment than measures of personality.

One of the single most important factors in the assessment of a candidate is a determination of the likely value of an implant in terms of the reinforcements that its use will bring to the patient. If the use of an implant cannot or does not effect changes in lifestyle which the candidate seeks or comes to regard as valuable, then the use of the implant will stop. This is a crucial issue because many candidates seek changes that are unlikely to be fulfilled. This matter is most usefully assessed through face-to-face discussion with the candidate and, if possible, with relatives. Postoperatively, the discussion can review the circumstances in which the implant is used and the changes in behaviour that accompany this. Interview data collected by the UCH/RNID group and others (Miller et al., 1978; Crary et al., 1982) point to improvements in the lot of most implant recipients. Interview data are clearly important, permitting relevant assessments of each individual and allowing documentation of events that more quantitative measures might overlook. However, it has the disadvantage of being anecdotal and is clearly not the most systematic method of data collection. Questionnaire measures developed by individual groups (Wexler et al., 1982; East and Cooper, 1986; Dinner et al., 1989) have confirmed the interview findings concerning outcome in a more systematic way.

One method of collecting data which offers the possibility of being both sensitive and relevant to each individual is the Repertory Grid technique. By permitting the patient to determine which variables are important and having him or her make numerical statements about these variables, the technique can offer a 'patient's eye-view' of his or her situation which is available for mathematical expression. The application of the technique in the assessment of cochlear implant candidates and patients is still very much in the developmental stage. Systematic studies concerning the predictive validity of the technique, in this context, still need to be carried out. From the work which has been carried out to date using the technique as an outcome measure (Lynch, 1987; L. McKenna and C. Denman, unpublished), it would seem likely that it will prove to be an appropriate tool. The data from these studies suggest that the majority of implant recipients perceive important and beneficial changes in their psychological domain. However, there is scope for more controlled studies.

Whilst the importance of psychological factors has been recognised for some time, the development of a precise understanding of the nature and operation of psychological factors in this field, and of tools for their assessment, has occurred at a slower pace than that of other variables. Given the proliferation of published material about cochlear implants in recent years, the number of papers concerned either entirely or even in part with psychological variables is extraordinarily small. In spite of statements to the effect that psychological variables are among the principal determinants of attrition from cochlear implant programmes and of the amount of rehabilitation that a patient will need following surgery, some authors (Berlin et al., 1987; Lehnhardt, 1989) give no details about what protocol they employ when evaluating these variables. There is clearly a critical need for further research into the determination of psychological predictors of successful implant use. Similarly, the elucidation of measures of psychological outcome, arguably the ultimate determinant of the value of cochlear implants, deserves further investment.

References

BECK, A., WARD, C., MENDELSON, M., MUCK, J. and ERBAUGH, J. (1961). An inventory for measuring depression. *Arch. Gen. Psychiatr.* **4**, 561–571.

BERLIN, C., JENISON, V., HOOD, L. and LYONS, G. (1987). Patient selection for multichannel electronic prostheses. *Ann. Otol. Rhinol. Laryngol.* (Suppl.) **128**, 104–106.

BERRIOS, G., RYLEY, J., GARVEY, T. and MOFFAT, D. (1988). Psychiatric morbidity in subjects with inner ear disease. *Clin. Otolaryngol.* **13**, 259–266.

CHOUARD, C.H., MEYER, B., CHABOLLE, F. and FUGAIN, C. (1987). Preoperative assessment of multichannel cochlear implant patients. *Ann. Otol. Rhinol. Laryngol.* (Suppl.) **128**, 95–96.

CHUTE, P., PARISIER, S. and KRAMER, S. (1984). The cochlear implant. Part 2. Assessing candidacy for cochlear implants. *Hear. Rehabil. Q.* **9**, 13–16.

CLARK, G., O'LOUGHLIN, B., RICKARDS, F., TONG, Y. and WILLIAMS, A. (1977). The clinical assessment of cochlear implant patients. *J. Laryngol. Otol.* **91**, 697–708.

CRARY, W., BERLINER, K., WEXLER, M. and MILLER, L. (1982). Psychometric studies and clinical interviews with cochlear implant patients. *Ann. Otol. Rhinol. Laryngol.* (Suppl.) **91**, 55–81.

DINNER, M., ACKLEY, R., LUBINSKI, D., BALKANY, T., REEDER, P. and GENERT, L. (1989). Vocational implications of cochlear implants. *J. Am. Deaf. Rehabil. Assoc.* **22**(3), 41–47.

EAST, C. and COOPER, H. (1986). Extra-cochlear implants: The patient's viewpoint. *Br. J. Audiol.* **20**(1), 55–60.

EYSENCK, H. and EYSENCK, S. (1975). *Manual of The Eysenck Personality Questionnaire*. London: Hodder & Stoughton Educational.

FISHER, K. (1985). Repertory Grids with amputees. In: Beail, N. (ed.) *Repertory Grid Techniques and Personal Constructs: Applications in Clinical and Educational Settings*. New York: Croom Helm.

FRANSELLA, F. and BANNISTER, D. (1977). *A Manual for Repertory Grid Technique*. London: Academic Press.

GANTZ, B. (1989). Issues of candidate selection for a cochlear implant. *Otolaryngol. Clin. North Am.* **22**(1), 239–247.

GANTZ, B., TYLER, R., KNUTSON, J., WOODWORTH, G., ABBAS, P., McCABE, B., HINRICHS, J., TYE-MURRAY, N., LANSING, C., KUK, F. and BROWN, C. (1988). Evaluation of five different cochlear implant designs: Audiologic assessment and predictors of performance. *Laryngoscope* **98**, 1100–1106.

GOLDBERG, D. (1978). *Manual of the General Health Questionnaire*. Slough: National Foundation for Education Research.

HALLAM, R.S. (1976). The Eysenck Personality Scales: Stability and change after Therapy. *Behav. Res. Ther.* **14**, 369–372.

HERSEN, M. and BARLOW, D. (1976). *Single Case Experimental Designs: Strategies for Studying Behaviour Change*. New York: Pergamon Press.

KELLY, G. (1955). *The Psychology of Personal Constructs*, Vols 1 and 2. New York: Norton.

KNUTSON, J.F. (1988). Psychological variables in the use of cochlear implants: Predicting success and measuring change. Presented at NIH Consensus Development Conference, May 2–4, Washington DC.

LEHNHARDT, E. (1989). Can cochlear implant results be predicted? Paper presented at XVth Hallpike Symposium, Cochlear Implants and Rehabilitation. Institute of Neurology, London, June.

LEZAK, M. (1976). *Neuropsychological Assessment*. Oxford: Oxford University Press.

LUXFORD, W. (1984). The House Ear Institute programme on intracochlear implantation. Paper presented at the Symposium on Cochlear Implantation at Middlesex Hospital Medical School, London.

LYNCH, C. (1987). *Postoperative psychological change in cochlear implant recipients.* Unpublished research thesis, Institute of Sound and Vibration Research, University of Southampton.

McKENNA, L. (1986). The psychological assessment of cochlear implant patients. *Br. J. Audiol.* **20**, 29–34.

MATHEWS, A. and EYSENCK, M. (1987). Clinical anxiety and cognition. In: Eysenck, H. and Martin I. (eds) *Theoretical Foundations of Behaviour Therapy.* New York: Plenum.

MILLER, L., DUVALL, S., BERLINER, K., CRARY, W. and WEXLER, M. (1978). Cochlear implants: A psychological perspective. *J. Oto-Laryngol. Soc. Austr.* **4**, 201–203.

O'CONNOR, S., HAWTHORN, M., BRITTEN, S. and WEBBER, P. (1987). Identification of psychiatric morbidity in a population of tinnitus sufferers. *J. Laryngol. Otol.* **101**, 791–794.

OWENS, G. and ASHCROFT, J. (1982). Functional analysis in applied psychology. *Br. J. Clin. Psychol.* **21**, 181–189.

RAMSDEN, R. (1989). Results with a multichannel device. Paper presented at XVth Hallpike Symposium, Cochlear Implants and Rehabilitation, Institute of Neurology, London, June.

RISBERG, A., AGELFORS, E., BREDBERG, G., LINDSTROM, B. and OSSIAN-COOK, B. (1987). Preoperative testing of cochlear implant patients. *Ann. Otol. Rhinol. Laryngol.* (Suppl.) **128**, 109–110.

SINGERMAN, B., RIEDNER, E. and FOLSTEIN, M. (1980). Emotional disturbance in hearing clinic patients. *Br. J. Psychol.* **137**, 58–62.

TAYLOR, G., (1970). Moderator variable effects on personality item endorsements of physically disabled patients. *J. Consult. Clin. Psychol.* **35**, 183–188.

THOMAS, A. (1984). *Acquired Hearing Loss: Psychological and Psychosocial Implications.* New York: Academic Press.

WEXLER, M., BERLINER, K., MILLER, L. and CRARY, W. (1982). Psychological effects of cochlear implants: patients and index relatives perceptions. *Ann. Otol. Rhinol. Laryngol.* (Suppl.) **91**, 59–61.

Chapter 10
Cochlear Implants: The Medical Criteria for Patient Selection

ROGER F. GRAY

Introduction

The aim of the medical evaluation in selection of candidates for cochlear implantation is essentially to answer two questions:

1. Is the patient in a suitable physical condition to undergo implant surgery?
2. Will it be possible to insert the electrode array?

Age

Any age may be considered, but most surgeons are unwilling to operate on children under 2 years because of the thinness of the skull (Simms and Neeley, 1989) or elderly patients due to the risk of complications. The hazards of thrombosis, pneumonia and disorientation are greatly increased over 70 years of age, especially with an operation lasting 2–3 hours. However, the possibility of significant improvement to the quality of life in such patients may advance a good case for running some risks in an attempt to relieve the isolation of total deafness.

General health

Failure of any main organ so that continuous support or medication is required is a contraindication to implantation. Disorders of immunity (AIDS or immunosuppressive drugs, e.g. due to a previous transplant) or active sepsis pose a significant risk of wound infection. Diabetes is a relative contraindication, as is obesity and excessive smoking. If a patient can be cured, beyond reasonable doubt, of a major disease such as cancer, then implantation may be considered. In short, the potential implant user must have a reasonable life expectancy and be fit enough to concentrate on the task of rehabilitation without undue distraction. A great deal of travel is often required.

Cerebral damage

Head injury may cause cortical damage as well as deafness. Cerebral abscesses may be associated with meningitis and episodes of hypoxia are likely to cause damage to the brain and cochlea alike. Although a relationship between IQ and success of cochlear implantation has not been documented, mental handicap may pose significant problems for the rehabilitation team. Preoperative evaluation of the patient's ability to participate in testing and training procedures is clearly an essential part of the selection process.

Diseases of the nose or throat

Long-standing nasal or sinus infection is a cause of otitis media and eustachian tube obstruction, and should be investigated and cleared up if possible. The risk of otitis media is always present in young children and prior removal of enlarged or infected adenoids is recommended. This may be planned for the same day as the implant itself to spare the child two anaesthetics. The same applies to decaying teeth.

Clinical Examination of the Ears

The pinna or auricle

A deformity of the outer ear is no contraindication to implantation but sufficient protruding ear remnant must be present for those devices, such as the Nucleus or Ineraid multichannel implants, which use an ear hook. This resembles a behind-the-ear hearing aid and is the physical support for the ear level part of the device.

Outer ear

Otoscopic examination of the external meatus should reveal otitis externa, if present. This should be extinguished in both ears with appropriate treatment before implant surgery is contemplated.

Middle ear

Chronic otitis media with an open middle ear is a contraindication to implantation. In a series of 48 patients referred to Cambridge for cochlear implants, 6 were rejected because of middle-ear sepsis which had caused the deafness. All infection must be eradicated and cholesteatoma removed, if present. If the tympanic membrane is perforated, this must be treated by myringoplasty in order to close off the middle ear. In the case of very large or subtotal perforations, there will be a somewhat smaller probability of a successful closure and the other ear would be selected for implant surgery.

Vestibular function

Many patients with profound deafness have lost all balance function originating in the labyrinth and rely on visual references and proprioceptive input from the joints and muscles that maintain upright posture. Labyrinthine failure is easily verified by the Dix–Hallpike bithermal caloric test or simply by irrigating the ears with 10 ml of water at room temperature. There is none of the usual vertigo or nystagmus in response to the test if the labyrinth is dead. The test may be repeated with water at 20°C. If there is a response to caloric testing in either ear (indicating normal or reduced vestibular function), then there is a risk of temporary loss of balance following implant surgery due to perilymph leakage. In view of this, the only functioning labyrinth should not be selected for implant surgery, where possible. If it is not possible to operate on the ear without vestibular function for other reasons, or if there is function on both sides, the patient should be counselled preoperatively about the probability of temporary postoperative loss of balance.

Visual function

Assessment of visual acuity should be included in preoperative testing, as uncorrected poor vision could hamper lipreading.

The deaf blind are a small but important group who, it has now been shown, can benefit greatly from cochlear implantation (Boyd et al., 1990), although their rehabilitation does present some additional challenges. Only multichannel implants would be considered suitable for this group as they offer the possibility of speech recognition without visual cues.

Previous Ear Surgery

Mastoidectomy

Many patients with profound deafness caused by chronic infection will have had bilateral mastoidectomies. The eardrum may be absent or rudimentary and a large cavity present where the middle-ear space and mastoid space have been united by surgery. It is rare for such cavities to be completely uninfected and clean. They are a serious obstacle to cochlear implantation because of infection and exposure of the path of the electrode.

However, some surgeons have successfully attempted to insert a cochlear implant in such cases. A vascularised temporoparietal flap was used by East and Brough at University College Hospital, London, to close off a mastoid cavity prior to cochlear implantation (Cooper, personal communication). A retroauricular flap has been used successfully to cover a radical cavity prior to implantation by Hermes (1989).

Complete obliteration of the middle ear with a free fat graft and closure of the ear canal as a blind pit has been practised by Fisch, Fagan and Valvanis (1984) as a technique for closure after excision of lesions at the base of the skull.

This technique can be used to close off a chronically infected mastoid or fenestration cavity after eliminating the infection. Some months later the ear should be prepared for implantation in the usual way: an electrode pathway tunnelled under the belly fat previously used to obliterate the cavity. Both the surgeon and patient must be prepared for a disappointment if there is still a pocket of pus in the middle ear and implantation has to be postponed.

Fenestration cavities

In the 1950s and 1960s, the technique of fenestration of the most superficial of the semicircular canals was popular for the treatment of deafness caused by otosclerosis. In most cases the operation was a short-term success and a long-term failure. The cavity invariably became infected and hearing and balance function were lost when pus entered the labyrinth through the fenestra. Such patients are now coming forward for implantation. The same problems apply to these open cavities as they do to mastoidectomies.

Failed stapedectomies

From the 1960s, otosclerosis was treated by stapedectomy and some surgeons performed thousands of operations. Over the succeeding years, a significant proportion of these have failed and bilateral profound deafness with a fenestration on one side and a stapedectomy on the other is sometimes encountered in the implant clinic. The silver-coloured piston can occasionally be seen through the eardrum with an auriscope. There is no contraindication to implantation of an ear with a failed stapedectomy; the piston can usually be left undisturbed.

Inner Ear

Radiological examination

The cochlea cannot be examined directly and must be assessed radiologically before surgery (Phelps, Annis and Robinson, 1990). High resolution CT scans through the cochleae are arguably the single most important investigation after the audiogram.

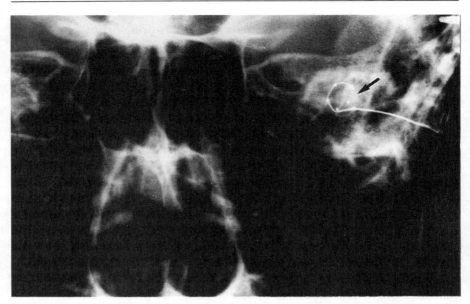

Figure 10.1. Plain X-ray of temporal bone viewed through orbit. Six 0.5-mm platinum ball electrodes are spaced out within the scala tympani (Ineraid electrode, arrowed).

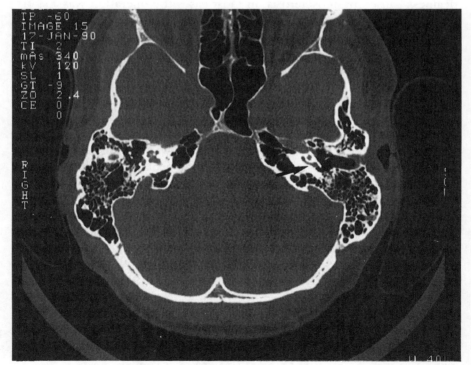

Figure 10.2. Ultra high definition CT scan showing widely patent cochlear ducts. The basal turn and round window areas of interest to the surgeon are arrowed on the right.

The surgeon would hope to see a clear cochlear duct especially in the first or basal turn of the cochlea (Figure 10.2). Balkany, Gantz and Nadol (1988) and Harnsberger et al. (1987) found that, of patients otherwise suitable for a cochlear implant, about one-fifth had radiological evidence of new bone formation partly or completely obliterating the cochlea. This precludes easy insertion of a long multichannel electrode array, but good results may still be obtained with experience. Figure 10.1 shows the successful placement of intracochlear electrodes.

Partial obliteration of the cochlea

Balkany, Gantz and Nadol (1988) also describe successful implantation of 15 patients with partly obliterated cochleae. Eleven of these had been predicted by CT scan (Figure 10.3). Their technique is to drill out the basal turn of the cochlea from the round window forward until a clear passage is encountered. Electrodes were completely inserted in 14 patients and results differed little from those of patients with no partial obliteration.

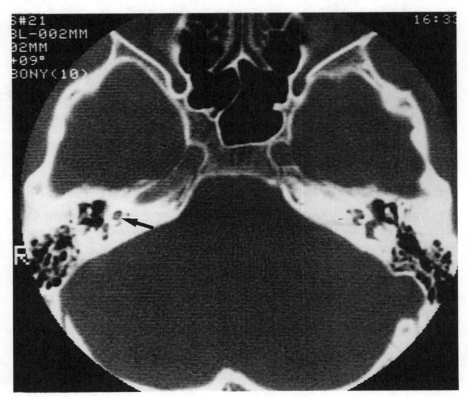

Figure 10.3. High definition axial CT scan showing partly obliterated cochlea duct (arrowed on left) as compared with normal right side.

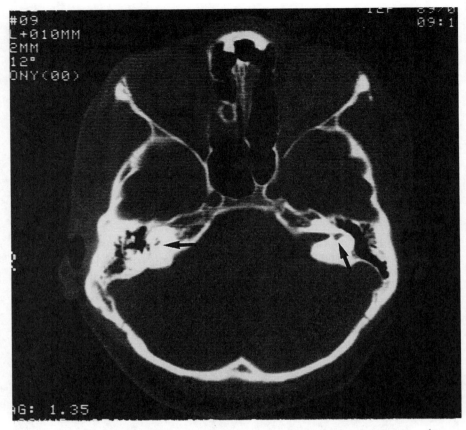

Figure 10.4. High definition CT scan showing almost complete obliteration of cochleae 20 years after bacterial meningitis.

Total obliteration of the cochlea

When the cochlea appears completely white on CT scan (Figure 10.4), it is possible to skeletonise the central spiral of the modiolus by drilling (blue lining the modiolus). Within the modiolus lie the residual cell bodies of the first-order fibres of the auditory nerve. The electrode is curled around the modiolus like a snake around a stick. Zimmerman-Phillips et al. (1990) report four children implanted in this way with complete bony obliteration of both cochleae. Most surgeons beginning an implant service would wish to avoid such a situation until more experienced. Good radiology is therefore a priority.

Arrested development of the cochlea

Some profoundly deaf children have severe deformities of the cochlea. Until interest in implants arose, few profoundly deaf children underwent radiographic examination of the cochlea but now we are becoming aware of a variety of severe cochlear deformities. At a gestational age of 4 weeks, the cochlea is a single common cavity (the otocyst), the contents of which are in free communication with cerebrospinal fluid. At 5 weeks, the semicircular canals of the balance organ are visible and at 6–7 weeks' gestation one and one half turns of the cochlea are visible. Novak et al. (1990) report the implantation of two deaf children in whom cochlear development had been arrested at the 4-week stage. There was auditory perception and some speech production as a result.

Fractures through the temporal bone

These may cause profound deafness by traversing the cochlea or by traversing the internal auditory meatus. In the first case the fracture heals by a fibrous tissue union which can be seen on appropriate X-rays many years later. This is no contraindication to an intracochlear implant but careful postoperative X-rays are needed to make sure that the electrode has not passed out through the fracture line. In the second case, the auditory nerve is usually severed (also, but not always, the facial nerve) and there will be no response to an electrical stimulation. Promontory or round window trial stimulation would give a negative result.

Conclusion

It is understandable and entirely praiseworthy that surgeons at the start of new programmes of cochlear implantation will adopt a cautious attitude. Those with more experience will gain the confidence to carry out implant surgery in more technically difficult cases (e.g. the ossified cochlea). The frontiers of implant surgery are being continuously pushed back and, as a result, the incidence of cases where implantation is ruled out due to medical considerations is decreasing.

References

BALKANY, T., GANTZ, B. and NADOL, J. (1988). Multichannel cochlear implants in partially ossified cochleae. *Ann. Otol. Rhinol. Laryngol.* 97, 3–7.

BOYD, P.J., VIDLER, M., HICKSON, F.S., ALPIN, D.Y., HESKETH, A., RAMSDEN, R. and DAS, V.K. (1990). Rehabilitation of deaf blind patients using a multichannel cochlear implant. Paper presented at the Second International Cochlear Implant Symposium, Iowa.

FISCH, U., FAGAN, P. and VALVANIS, A. (1984). The intratemporal fossa approach for the lateral skull base. *Otolaryngol. Clin. North Am.* 17, 513–552.

HARNSBERGER, H.R., DART, D.J., PARKIN, J.L., SMOKER, W.R. and OSBORNE, A.G. (1987). Cochlear implant candidates: assessment with CT and MR imaging. *Radiology* 164, 53–57.

HERMES, H. (1989). Cochlear implants in patients with radical cavities. In: Fraysse, B. and Cochard, N. (eds), *Cochlear Implant Acquisitions and Controversies*, pp. 119–121. Toulouse: Paragraphic.

NOVAK, M., FIRSZT, J., BROWN, C. and REEDER, R. (1990). Cochlear implantation in severe cochlear deformities. Paper presented the Second International Cochlear Implant Symposium, Iowa.

PHELPS, P.D., ANNIS, J.A.D. and ROBINSON, P.J. (1990). Imaging for cochlear implants. *Br. J. Radiol.* **63**, 512–516.

SIMMS, D.L. and NEELEY, J.G. (1989). Thickness of the lateral surface of the temporal bone in children. *Ann. Otol. Rhinol. Laryngol.* **98**, 726–731.

ZIMMERMAN-PHILLIPS, S.R., KEMINK, J.L., KILENY, P.R., FIRSZT, J.B. and NOVAK, M. (1990). Cochlear implantation of children with complete cochlear ossification. Paper presented at the Second International Cochlear Implant Symposium, Iowa.

Chapter 11
Surgery for Single-channel Cochlear Implantation

JOHN M. GRAHAM

Introduction

Since the early 1970s, there has been both choice and competition between multi- and single-channel cochlear implants. Among the systems now available, multichannel implants offer the greatest potential benefit for a deafened adult with a patent bony cochlear duct for whom the money to pay for a multichannel device is available. However, at the time of writing, both economic and clinical considerations may make multichannel implants inaccessible on grounds of cost or inadvisable because of the risk to residual hearing, obliteration of the scala tympani or caution on the part of those caring for a congenitally deaf child. In the UCH/RNID Cochlear Implant Programme, an additional reason for choosing an extracochlear single-channel device is its suitability for research on the electrical suppression of tinnitus (Hazell, Meerton and Conway, 1989).

Of single-channel implants, the one designed by House and Urban has been the most widely used, with about 750 implanted in adults and 294 in children since it was first introduced in 1972. A robust electrode design, simple speech-processing strategy, transcutaneous transmission of the signal and straightforward, safe surgical technique enabled this implant to be developed early and manufactured relatively easily. By the early 1980s, once it had been proved by extensive use in adults, it was considered safe to apply the device to children.

Most other single-channel devices have been similar in design to the House implant: speech-processing strategies have been similar, using analogue signals; transmission has been transcutaneous using a wireless signal; a single receiver coil has decoded the signal using passive circuitry; the compound used to encapsulate the circuitry has been silicone rubber or epoxy resin. The buried electronics are placed on the squamous temporal bone and platinum wire connects them with a ball electrode placed in the scala tympani or just outside it. An indifferent electrode is placed deep to the temporalis muscle or in the orifice of the eustachian tube where it enters the middle ear.

Apart from differences in design of the various single-channel implants, the surgical technique used by each team varies a little. Since the author's main experience is with the technique employed for the UCH/RNID implant, this chapter will mainly describe this technique and the problems and complications encountered with it. Parallels will, however, be drawn, from the publications of House, and Burian, using the Vienna single-channel device, and other units. Some of the material in this chapter is drawn from a previous account of the surgical technique (Graham, East and Fraser, 1989). The author's own approach has been to simplify the technique as far as possible so that the operation takes no longer than a standard mastoidectomy, can be performed by surgeons in training and causes as little disruption as possible to the routine work of a busy ENT unit. The current surgical technique consists of a standard postaural incision, a simple cortical mastoidectomy and a generous posterior tympanotomy. The main body of the implant is slipped under the temporalis muscle and held in place with Histoacryl glue and a single stitch; the active electrode is secured in the mastoid bowl with another suture and its tip kept in place by the natural spring of the electrode cable. The procedure generally takes between 1.5 and 2 hours and allows time for other routine cases to be booked for the same operating list.

Preoperative Assessment

The main difficulties which may be encountered during implant surgery are related to previous chronic suppurative otitis media, obliteration of the round window niche and obliteration of the bony cochlea. The aetiology of the patient's deafness, if known, may indicate potential problems of surgical access. For example, in advanced otosclerosis the surgeon may expect to find obliteration of the round window niche. At first, the author's group used hypocycloidal polytomography as the standard radiological investigation, but high resolution CT scanning with 1.5-mm cuts has been

Table 11.1   Problems encountered during surgery in 30 patients

Problem	No.
Absent round window niche	2
Narrow round window niche	3
Posteriorly placed round window niche	2
Scar tissue in middle ear and round window area	1
Total	8 patients

found to provide the best definition of the basal turn of the cochlea, round window area and the course of the facial nerve (P.J. Robinson, J. Anniss and P.D. Phelps, personal communication). The majority of patients, however, have normal temporal bones, and difficulties were encountered during surgery in only 8 of the first 30 patients to be implanted (Table 11.1).

Surgical Technique: Systems using Postaural Receiver Coil linked to Round Window Electrode – Extra- or Intracochlear

Preparation and incision

For the UCH/RNID Implant the patient is prepared for postaural mastoidectomy. There is minimal shaving of the scalp, 3 cm behind and above the pinna. Before an incision is made, the intended position of the receiver coil is marked on the scalp using a template (Figure 11.1). The coil must be well clear of the pinna itself to allow easy placement of the transmitter coil later, when the implant is in use; this is particularly important in patients who wear spectacles.

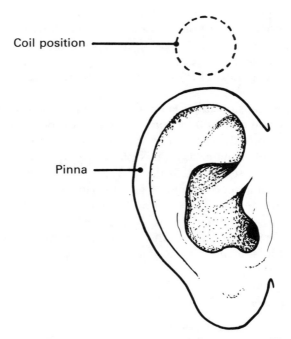

Figure 11.1. Position for receiver coil marked on scalp using template. (Figures 11.1–11.7 reproduced with permission from *Journal of Laryngology and Otology,* suplement 18, 1979.)

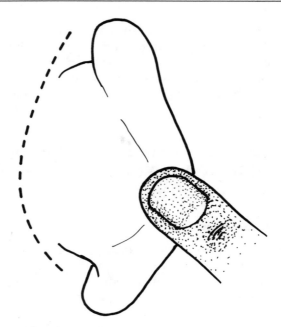

Figure 11.2.   Postaural sulcus incision.

The incision is in or just behind the postaural sulcus (Figure 11.2). A generous amount of temporalis fascia is harvested, which will later be used to cover the electrode cables. Using an elevator, the temporalis muscle and underlying periosteum are lifted from the squamous part of the temporal bone to create a pocket for the receiver coil, between the periosteum and bone.

The sulcus incision heals very reliably and lies anterior and inferior to the receiver coil and well in front of the part of the active electrode cable that passes from the coil over the rim of the mastoid bowl. All the superficial foreign material is thus placed safely *behind* the incision and under the well-vascularized scalp.

The technique recommended for the House implant and the Vienna single-channel device places the incision 1 cm behind and above the coil with a large postaural flap and scalp shave. Once the flap has been raised, for the House device, part of the temporalis muscle is excised and a flat seating on the squamous temporal bone is prepared for the coil, using a 'butterfly' reaming drill.

Mastoidectomy

A cortical mastoidectomy is performed, and a generous posterior tympan-otomy is cut, to expose the whole of the round window niche (Figure 11.3). It is sometimes possible to preserve the chorda tympani in the

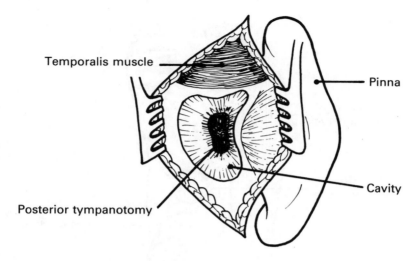

Temporalis muscle

Pinna

Cavity

Posterior tympanotomy

Figure 11.3.   Cortical mastoidectomy and posterior tympanotomy.

dissection, but this should not compromise adequate surgical access. When the round window niche is posteriorly placed, it is safer to identify and skeletonise the vertical part of the facial nerve on the rim of the posterior tympanotomy; identifying the nerve in this way allows the surgeon to drill away the deeper margin of the tympanotomy, beyond the nerve, with greater confidence, to expose a posteriorly placed round window niche.

Removal of the mastoid tip cells is not desirable. If the cortical mastoid cavity is kept fairly small, the cable for the active electrode spirals down its walls before passing through the posterior tympanotomy and approaching the round window membrane from below (Figures 11.4 and 11:5).

Round window: electrode placement

The House implant was originally designed to pass 24 mm into the scala tympani; however, this distance was eventually reduced to 6 mm, mainly to reduce the risk of damage to the basilar membrane. The electrode of the Vienna single-channel implant can be placed outside the cochlea, on the round window membrane, or just inside the scala tympani. Recently, intracochlear placement has proven preferable on the grounds that this gives a superior postoperative result (K. Burian, personal communication). Similarly the UCH/RNID Implant was designed to lie outside the cochlea, on the round window membrane, except in cases of bony obliteration of the round window. Since 1989, it has also been found preferable to place the electrode tip a few millimetres inside the scala tympani in ears with no detectable residual hearing, but not in children and not in patients implanted for tinnitus suppression.

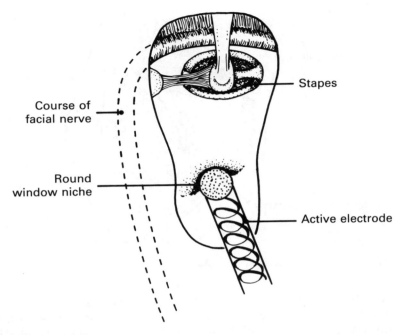

Figure 11.4. Enlarged view of posterior tympanotomy.

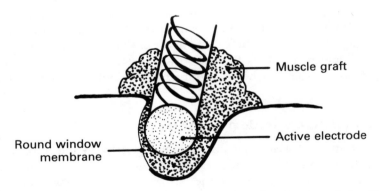

Figure 11.5. Cross-section view of round window niche with active electrode in position and free graft of muscle.

For extracochlear placement, where the round window niche is of normal size, no drilling of the niche is needed. As described above, the electrode cable passes through the inferior part of the posterior tympanotomy and approaches the round window membrane from below, so that the natural spring of the electrode cable holds the tip of the electrode securely in the round window niche. Obliteration or narrowing of the round window niche will involve drilling with a diamond burr.

There should only be enough drilling to allow access for the electrode. If there is no identifiable round window niche, the surgeon must drill in an anterior direction until either the endosteum of the scala tympani is encountered or the scala itself entered. Any leakage of perilymph is sealed with a free graft of temporalis muscle. In view of the nature of the diseases causing profound acquired hearing loss, obliteration or narrowing of the round window niche is relatively common and may occur in up to 50% of cases.

For intracochlear placement, the round window membrane is exposed by drilling away the bony lip of the round window niche to which the lateral and superior rim of the membrane is attached. A small diamond drill is used and care taken not to allow the rotating shank of the burr to touch an exposed vertical portion of the seventh nerve. For the same reason, the drill should not rotate when being passed through the posterior tympan-otomy (House, 1982). The anterior rim of the round window is displaced to allow the electrode to be passed into the cochlea. House (1982) observed that, where the basal turn is obliterated by new bone formation, this new bone is very white in colour and can be distinguished from the surrounding otic capsule. It may then be possible to drill along the core of white bone which may eventually lead to a patent part of the scala tympani. A free graft of temporalis muscle is packed around the electrode cable where it enters the cochlea, to reduce the risk of perilymph leak and of infection entering the cochlea from the middle ear.

Fitting the implant (Figures 11.4–11.6)

The receiver coil of the UCH/RNID Implant is mounted on a square of thin, reinforced Silastic sheeting. This sheeting is trimmed, leaving a flange 0.5–1 cm inferiorly, to take an anchoring suture. The coil is then slipped up under the temporalis muscle and periosteum. Irregularities on the surface of the squamous temporal bone are identified, the coil removed and the bone drilled smooth to allow the coil to lie flat without rocking. The tip of the active electrode is then carefully placed in the round window niche, with the electrode cable spiralling down the walls of the mastoid cavity. The coil of the implant can be shifted in its pocket under the temporalis muscle to allow the cable to lie in a stable position. After the cable to the active electrode leaves the receiver coil, a shallow trough is cut into the bone where the cable crosses the superior rim of the mastoid cavity. This draws the cable medially, as soon as it leaves the coil, and protects it from being moved by external pressure or by contraction of the temporalis muscle. This trough can be undercut in the direction of the natural spring of the cable to hold the cable more securely. A shallow groove is also drilled to accommodate the cable to the indifferent electrode; this cable ends in a flat plate which is tucked under the temporalis muscle towards the root of the zygoma.

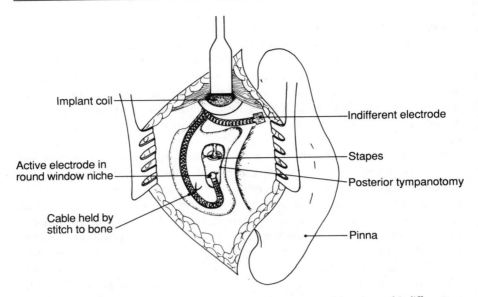

Figure 11.6. Placement of receiver coil, deep to temporalis muscle, active and indifferent electrodes. Active electrode secured in mastoid bowl with suture. The receiver coil is on a base of reinforced Silastic sheeting not shown in the illustration.

The active electrode cable and the Silastic sheeting attached to the receiver coil are each anchored with a silk stitch to 'rat-bite' holes drilled in the mastoid bowl and squamous temporal bone respectively. Before finally anchoring the implant it is important to check: (1) the position of the coil in relation to the pinna and the site previously marked on the scalp (see Figure 11.1); (2) the position of the active electrode tip in the round window niche; and (3) that the active electrode cable sits comfortably in the mastoid bowl. After tying the two silk stitches, the coil is further secured to the squamous temporal bone with Histoacryl glue. The electrode cables are covered by temporalis fascia. Free grafts of temporalis muscle can be used to support the active electrode cable in the mastoid cavity and a tiny piece of temporalis muscle is finally placed around the ball electrode in the round window niche, taking care that this does not form a bridge of soft tissue between the electrode and the horizontal part of the seventh cranial nerve.

The wound is closed in layers without a drain and a pressure dressing is applied for 48 hours. If the ear canal skin was partly elevated, a BIPP pack is left in the canal for 7 days. The line of the postaural scar lies *anterior* to the superficial parts of the implant and reduces the risk of exposure should healing of the wound be delayed.

For the House implant, a circular shallow bed is drilled on the squamous temporal bone, as described above, and part of the temporalis muscle is excised to reduce the tissue between the buried receiver and the external coil. The receiver is prevented from slipping by the ring of its bed cut in the bone and by a single suture across its diameter secured to a pair of 'rat-bite' tunnels in the bone on either side of its bed.

Frachet technique

There have been preliminary reports of a technique described by Frachet in Paris, using a gold 'cupula' electrode placed like a thimble on the tip of a stapedectomy piston, with wires passing from this gold electrode through the mastoid cavity and emerging through the skin of the ear lobe (Frachet et al., 1989). This percutaneous connection uses relatively little power, provided by miniature batteries which can therefore be contained in an ear-level speech processor. It remains to be seen whether this ingenious technique will be free from complications associated with the percutaneous wiring.

Results

The author's own experience reflects the problems that seem common to most devices and most teams.

Peroperative difficulties (see Table 11.1)

In the author's experience, no operation has had to be abandoned because of surgical difficulty. The only purely surgical reason for not selecting a patient for an implant was the presence of bilateral, open mastoid cavities. The only major difficulty encountered during surgery has been complete obliteration of the round window niche. This is now always predicted by radiology. It is helpful to prepare for this situation in advance by practising with a temporal bone, drilling anterior to the round window to find the scala tympani. Even those experienced in performing combined approach tympanoplasty may also find it helpful to practise cutting a posterior tympanotomy on several temporal bones before doing an implant, to establish more confidently the position of the vertical segment of the facial nerve.

Complications (Table 11.2)

None of the first 30 patients implanted with the UCH/RNID device suffered a life-threatening complication and there were no deaths. Major complications were those which prevented use of the implant. In five patients there was a problem that needed surgical correction; in four patients the device itself failed and in one patient the device failed, was replaced, became infected and had to be removed a second time. Apart from this patient, all eight who had their implants replaced now have a functioning device. Most of the surgical failures occurred early in the series before the surgical

Table 11.2 Major complications (requiring removal of implant) and minor ones

Major complications	
Infection	1
Device failure	5
Misplacement or migration of receiver coil	1
Displacement of active electrode	1
Seventh nerve synkinesis	1
Late change in electrode impedance	1
Total	9*
Minor complications	
Minor seventh nerve synkinesis	1
Alteration in taste	3
Seroma in wound	1
Transient seventh nerve weakness with full recovery	2
Disturbance of balance	2
Minor damage to tympanic membrane	2
Total	11

*The total is only nine patients, because one patient had both device failure and infection.

technique was standardised. The device failures also occurred early in the series, and were caused by failure of a single component, now replaced. Minor complications were either transient or had a minor effect on the patients' use of their implants.

Infection rate

This was low with only one patient needing to have the implant removed. In this case, the original device was replaced because it had failed. After this operation, the wound healed but there were signs of persisting middle-ear effusion after 6 weeks. Over the next 2 months the patient experienced intermittent discomfort in the ear and noticed blood in her pharynx. Nasopharyngoscopy showed blood coming from the orifice of the eustachian tube. Finally, a year after the operation, a boggy swelling appeared over the mastoid and a small sinus opened in the wound and discharged pus. The implant was clearly infected and was removed. Tissue cultures grew *Staphylococcus aureus*. The patient has decided not to have another implant.

Coil position

In one patient the implant receiver coil was found to lie too close to the pinna. It was not clear whether the coil had moved or whether it had been put in the wrong place. Since this episode, a simple template has been used to mark on the scalp the correct position of the receiver coil.

Each new implant has also been attached to a sheet of Silastic containing a mesh. This increases the area of contact with the skull and allows an anchoring stitch to the underlying bone. Any change in the position of the coil can be checked with a simple lateral skull X-ray.

Displacement of the active electrode

This occurred in one patient. When the implant was switched on he received very little sound sensation with limited frequency range, even with maximum power from the speech processor. Tympanotomy revealed that the tip of the active electrode had come out of the round window niche and was lying just in contact with the bony promontory. It was not possible to reposition the electrode through the tympanotomy and the operation had to be revised with insertion of a new implant. This episode led to the use of a stitch to secure the electrode cable in the mastoid bowl.

Stimulation of facial nerve

The implant electrically stimulated the facial nerve in two patients, producing synkinetic facial movements. In one patient this was a temporary phenomenon, which slowly disappeared over a period of 3 months. In the second case, the complication was more serious; the thresholds for eighth and seventh nerve stimulation were so close that the patient could not use the device (Figure 11.7a). Since these thresholds did not change over a period of 4 months, the patient's ear was re-explored. The electrode was found in its correct position and the facial nerve was not visibly exposed. The active electrode was then removed from the round window niche and placed first in the attic region, then on the promontory and back in the round window niche. In all these positions stimulation of the implant still produced facial twitching. At this point the scala tympani was opened, through the round window, and the electrode introduced into the cochlea to a depth of 4 mm. The cochleotomy was sealed with muscle packed around the cable. Postoperatively (Figure 11.7b) the thresholds for facial nerve stimulation were unchanged but the hearing thresholds had improved. Although the patient still has facial movement with loud sounds she is able to use her implant.

Imbalance

Both patients who had imbalance after the operation had received drilling into the cochlea. However, all vestibular symptoms settled spontaneously with no need for surgical exploration to exclude a perilymph fistula.

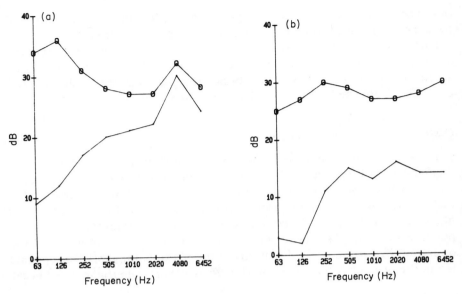

Figure 11.7. Patient with synkinetic movements of the facial nerve. Thresholds for hearing (nerve VIII) (—) and facial nerve stimulation (nerve VII) (–O–). Pulsed stimuli generated by BBC computer and transmitted to the implant. (a) Before revision of surgery; (b) after revision operation, electrode placed 4 mm in scala tympani. Facial nerve stimulation still occurs in response to loud sounds, but the implant is now usable with a moderate dynamic range for sound sensation.

Patients with bilateral open mastoid cavities were excluded from the author's initial series of patients. House (1982) describes a technique of burying the electrode wires with bone paté deep to the skin lining the mastoid cavity, but advocates caution in assessing the short-term results of any mastoid obliteration technique. An operation devised by the plastic surgery unit at University College Hospital has recently enabled one such patient to be implanted using a vascularised temporoparietal flap. This technique, developed to treat persistently infected mastoid cavities, is currently being evaluated (M. Brough, personal communication). Hermes (1989) described a staged operation, turning a postaural skin flap to line the radical cavity and then 6 months later implanting a Nucleus device with the cable buried beneath the skin flap.

Discussion

Patients who receive cochlear implants spend many hours of testing and rehabilitation. The surgery itself, although a major event for the patient, should represent a relatively minor part of their overall treatment. The author's aim has been to simplify surgery and develop a routine operation with a standard technique. Any new project is likely to run into unexpected problems. Some of these are avoidable. Damage to the facial nerve while performing posterior tympanotomy should be avoidable by careful attention to technique. The receiver coil and active electrode are now carefully positioned and anchored in place.

The use of a standard postaural sulcus incision has several advantages. For some implants, it is recommended that a wide anteriorly or inferiorly pedicled skin flap is raised so that the incision lies well behind the site of the receiver coil and electrode cables. The use of such a large skin flap adds to the length of the operation and has been reported to cause necrosis and infection, making removal of the implant necessary (House, 1982; Harris and Cueva, 1987; Cohen, Hoffman and Strosthein, 1988; Robinson and Chopra, 1989). In contrast, a simple sulcus incision is a standard approach to the mastoid with robust healing properties. A skin incision should not directly overlie any buried parts of an implant for fear of sinus formation and infection. A sulcus incision lies well anterior to the implant and so achieves this goal. In the author's single case of infection, the clinical picture strongly suggested that this was secondary to subsequent otitis media.

Prophylactic antibiotics are not used by the author (Robinson and Chopra, 1989). A previous history of chronic suppurative otitis media may cause difficulties. A patient must not be given an implant when there is any suspicion of active middle-ear infection. A perforated tympanic membrane should be dealt with in advance by myringoplasty.

It is not clear why, in two patients, stimulation of the seventh nerve occurred with synkinetic facial movement. In the patient whose ear was re-explored there was no question of direct contact between the electrode and the seventh nerve. Both these patients are postmenopausal women and there was speculation about whether osteoporotic changes might increase electrical conductivity in the temporal bone.

Facial nerve stimulation was mentioned by Cohen, Hoffman and Strosthein (1988) as a major complication leading to removal of the device in one patient of a series of 459 Nucleus Cochlear Implants. In a further three patients in their report, it was possible to prevent facial nerve stimulation by 'programming out' the offending intracochlear electrodes, and Cohen, Hoffman and Strosthein did not speculate on possible mechanisms. In the author's patient in whom the problem resolved spontaneously, the electrical impedance between electrode and seventh nerve increased spontaneously whilst the impedance of current to the eighth nerve did not alter. Conversely, in the second case, burial of the active electrode in the cochlea improved the impedance between electrode and eighth nerve and has allowed the patient to use her implant, although with some narrowing of the dynamic range.

Conclusions

Although in terms of numbers multichannel cochlear implants are now more widely in use world wide than single-channel implants, a place is likely to remain for the latter. A round window electrode can easily be placed outside or just inside the scala tympani without altering the design or length of the electrode and its cable. Simplification of the technique, employing a standard mastoidectomy incision, reduces the risk of skin necrosis and infection that may occur with a more substantial postaural skin flap.

Acknowledgements

Jeanette Sanders kindly typed the manuscript. Angela Scott, of the Department of Medical Illustration, Middlesex Hospital, drew the pictures. The UCH/RNID Cochlear Implant Programme has been supported by grants from the Sir Jules Thorn Trustees and the Clothworkers Foundation.

References

COHEN, N.L., HOFFMAN, R.A. and STROSTHEIN, M. (1988). Medical complications related to the nucleus multichannel cochlear implant. *Ann. Otol. Rhinol. Laryngol.* 97 (Suppl. 135), 8–13.

FRACHET, B., VERSCHUUR, H.P., VORMES, E. and TISON, P. (1989). Extra-cochlear single-channel implant with oval window cupula-electrode and percutaneous earring-connector. In: Fraysse, B. and Cochard, N. (eds), *Cochlear Implant – Acquisitions and Controversies*, pp. 123–131. Proceedings of International Symposium, Toulouse, June 1989.

GRAHAM, J.M., EAST, C.A. and FRASER, J.G. (1979). UCH/RNID single channel cochlear implant: Surgical technique. *J. Laryngol. Otol.* Suppl. 18, 14–19.

HARRIS, J.P. and CUEVA, R.A. (1987). Flap design for cochlear implantation: avoidance of a potential complication. *Laryngoscope* 97, 755–757.

HAZELL, J.W.P., MEERTON, L.J. and CONWAY, M.J. (1989). Electrical tinnitus suppression (E.T.S.) with a single-channel cochlear implant. *J. Laryngol. Otol.* Suppl. 18, 39–44.

HERMES, H. (1989). Cochlear implants in patients with radical cavities. In: Fraysse, B. and Cochard, N. (eds), *Cochlear Implant – Acquisitions and Controversies*, pp. 119–121. Proceedings of International Symposium, Toulouse, June 1989.

HOUSE, W.F. (1982). Surgical considerations in cochlear implantation. In: House, W.F. and Berliner, K.I. (eds), *Cochlear Implants: Progress and Perspectives. Ann. Otol. Rhinol. Laryngol.* Suppl. 91, 15–20.

ROBINSON, P.J. and CHOPRA, S. (1989). Antibiotic prophylaxis in cochlear implantation: current practice. *J. Otol. Laryngol.* Suppl. 18, 20–21.

Chapter 12
Surgery for Multichannel Cochlear Implantation

GRAEME C. CLARK, B.K-H.G. FRANZ, B.C. PYMAN and R.L. WEBB

Introduction

The aim of a multichannel cochlear implant is to take advantage of the spatial representation of frequency in the cochlea so that spectral information in speech can be used to assist patients who are profoundly or totally deaf to communicate. To do this it is preferable to place an electrode array within the scala tympani of the basal turn of the cochlea. There is some biological evidence to indicate that it is better that this electrode array is free fitting (Sutton, Miller and Pfingst, 1980); it is also desirable that it is flexible, smooth and tapered so that it may be withdrawn and another reimplanted if necessary at a later stage (Clark et al., 1987b; Jackler, Leake and McKerrow, 1989). The electrode array is connected to a receiver–stimulator package in the case of the Melbourne/Cochlear (Clark et al., 1977a,b, 1987b) and San Francisco/MiniMed devices (Merzenich, 1985), and the package receives information transmitted through the intact skin by a radio frequency link. On the other hand, the Utah/Ineraid device is connected to a pedestal that is fixed to the mastoid bone, and information is transmitted percutaneously with a plug and socket arrangement (Parkin, McCandless and Youngblood, 1987). Percutaneous plugs were used initially by Pialoux et al. (1979), and Banfai et al. (1985), but have been subsequently replaced by systems using radio frequency links (MacLeod, Chouard and Weber, 1985; Banfai et al., 1987).

In this chapter the principles of cochlear implantation for multichannel devices will be discussed, but specific reference will be made to the techniques for implanting the Melbourne/Cochlear receiver–stimulator (Figure 12.1), as this is the device that is most familiar to the authors. The surgery is covered in more detail by Webb et al. (1990). Surgical procedures discussed will be based on the accumulated experience from our own clinic at the University of Melbourne/Royal Victoria Eye and Ear Hospital (Clark et al., 1979b, 1984) and from discussions with surgeons

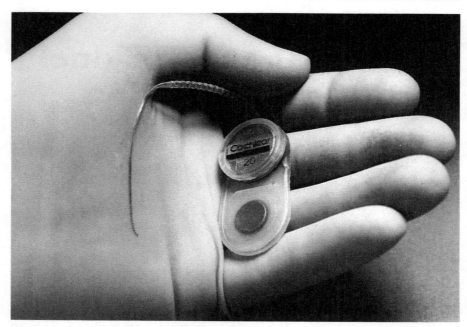

Figure 12.1. A photograph of the Melbourne/Cochlear multichannel receiver–stimulator and electrode array.

implanting the device in other countries and clinics (Cochlear Corporation, *Surgical Procedure Manual*). The Melbourne/Cochlear device has now been implanted in over 3000 patients world wide so there is considerable experience. Furthermore, the incidence of complications is now well documented, in particular from a study of Cohen, Hoffmann and Strosthein (1988) on the experience in the USA with 459 operations, in Hannover for 110 operations and in Melbourne for 100 operations (Webb et al., 1991).

Surgical Anatomy

An understanding of the relevant anatomy is very important for implant surgery, and should also be gained in the temporal bone laboratory. In particular, it is necessary to be completely familiar with the anatomy of the round window and basal turn of the cochlea. In the first instance, the round window membrane may be obscured in its niche by a bony overhang anteriorly and inferiorly. This bony overhang may need to be drilled away to provide adequate exposure of the round window membrane. Occasionally, a fold of mucous membrane may extend across superficial to the round window membrane and be mistaken for it (Nomura, 1984). Failure to recognise this false membrane may lead to the electrode being impacted by the true membrane, and possibly a traumatic insertion. It is also important to understand that the round window membrane is conical and attached superiorly to the osseous spiral lamina. Drilling posterosuperiorly can lead to damage of the spiral lamina and should be avoided if possible (Franz, Clark and Bloom, 1987b). In a proportion of bones there is a hypotympanic cell which opens immediately inferior to the round window niche. This can be mistaken for the round window and the electrode inserted outside the cochlea (Webb et al., 1990). A knowledge of the orientation and direction of the basal turn of the cochlea is critical in establishing the line required for an atraumatic electrode insertion. The scala tympani is narrowed inside the round window membrane by an anteroinferior ridge – the crista fenestrae. This can restrict the electrode insertion and misdirect the electrode to the centre wall and then back to the modiolus and basilar membrane (Figure 12.2). If prominent, the crista fenestrae should be drilled away prior to an electrode being inserted through the round window (Clifford and Gibson, 1987; Franz and Clark, 1987; Webb et al., 1988).

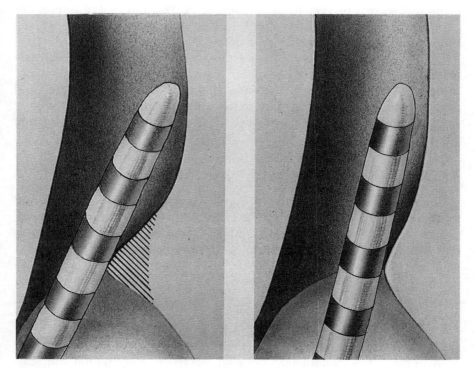

Figure 12.2. Diagrams showing: left – misdirection of the electrode array along the scala tympani of the basal turn of the cochlea due to the crista fenestrae; right – correct insertion of the electrode array after removal of crista fenestrae. (Reproduced with the permission of the Cochlear Corporation, from the *Surgical Procedure Manual*.)

If multichannel implantation is to be undertaken on young children (especially those under 2 years of age), it is important to consider the effects of skull growth as this can lead to an increase in the distance between the round window and package bed of approximately 2 cm. This growth could lead to the electrode array being dislodged. Studies (Shepherd et al., 1987c; Rebscher et al., 1988) are being undertaken on lead wire designs that will accommodate these growth changes. For example, it has been shown that, if redundant lead wire is placed in a Silastic bag, it will not be surrounded by fibrous tissue and progressive lengthening can occur (Shepherd et al., 1987b). It has also been shown that, if a tie is placed around the electrode in the region of the floor of the mastoid antrum, this will help prevent the electrode being withdrawn from the cochlea as the skull grows, as there is relatively little increase in the distance between the round window and the floor of the antrum from year 1 onwards (Shepherd et al., 1987a).

Extracochlear multichannel stimulation may be possible if the bone overlying the cochlea is drilled down to the endosteum (Shepherd et al., 1987b). The thickness of the bone overlying the apical, middle and basal turns was shown to vary from an average of 0.66 mm (s.d. 0.23 mm) to 1.28 mm (s.d. 0.41 mm) (Shepherd et al., 1987b). Another study (Franz and Clark, 1988) has shown that only 1.5–2.0 mm of the apical, 2.8–4.0 mm of the middle, and 4.5–5.0 mm of the basal turns lie directly beneath the medial wall of the middle ear. If electrodes with a diameter of 1 mm were used with adequate spacing for channel separation, it would only be practicable to place five extracochlear electrodes: one over the apical, two over the middle, one over the basal turn and one in the round window.

Applied Biophysics and Physiology

Multichannel cochlear prostheses require electric current to be localised to discrete groups of residual auditory nerve dendrites (peripheral processes) or spiral ganglion cells. Studies have shown (Clark et al., 1987a) that as far as extracochlear multichannel stimulation is concerned, it is necessary to drill down to the endosteal lining before current localisation can be achieved. If bone is left over the cochlea, its impedance is too great for an adequate current output to achieve current localisation. However, in drilling down to the endosteal lining there is a real risk of trauma to the cochlea.

Most experimental studies on current localisation have been concerned with intracochlear stimulation with an electrode array within the scala tympani of the basal turn. These studies have shown that current localisation is best with bipolar stimulation and the current falls away at approximately 3–8 dB/mm (Merzenich, 1974; Black and Clark, 1980).

Satisfactory current localisation can also be achieved with pseudobipolar or common ground stimulation (current flowing between one active intracochlear electrode and the other intracochlear electrodes connected together electronically as a common ground) but is poor with monopolar stimulation (Black and Clark, 1980; Black, Clark and Patrick, 1981).

With bipolar stimulation, studies have shown that the orientation and placement of the electrodes is important for maximal current localisation. If peripheral processes remain intact, current localisation is greatest when a moulded electrode array is used to keep the electrodes just beneath the basilar membrane and spiral lamina. A moulded array was also considered important to reduce the fluid between the array and the wall of the cochlea, and so limit the flow of current away from the peripheral processes. As part of this design, electrodes were placed radially (lying across the scala tympani) as current localisation was better than with a longitudinal placement (lying along the length of the scala tympani) (Merzenich et al., 1979).

It is important to realise, however, that most profoundly–totally deaf people do not have residual peripheral processes (Hinojosa and Marion, 1983; Hinojosa, Blough and Mhoon, 1987) and so an electrode array should not be designed primarily to localise current to the peripheral processes. Experimental studies (Shepherd et al., 1989) have shown that to provide maximal localisation of current to the spiral ganglion cells, the array needs to be placed close to the modiolus.

There are a number of other considerations in the design of electrode arrays. The surface area should be as large as possible. Even with biphasic pulses where the charge is balanced between phases, there is a possibility of platinum corrosion when the charge density is high (Black and Hannaker, 1979). For this reason, a banded electrode was developed to minimise the charge density (Clark, Patrick and Bailey, 1979). Its area is maximised because it is circumferential. This banded electrode array, which is manufactured by Cochlear, is also free fitting, smooth and tapered so that it may be inserted with minimal trauma. Free-fitting, smooth, tapered arrays are equally important requirements if the array is to be explanted and another reinserted. Studies (Clark et al., 1987a) have shown that the banded electrode array is an optimal solution that allows adequate current localisation, but at the same time minimises corrosion and mechanical trauma.

Biocompatibility and Pathology

It is important to ensure that the materials used for the electrode array, lead wire and receiver–stimulator used by each cochlear implant manufacturer are biocompatible. To do this for the Cochlear device, candidate materials were implanted in the subcutaneous tissue and muscle of the experimental animal and, in the case of the materials for the electrode array, in the cochlea. It is also essential that the particular materials used in fabricating devices are tested because their composition may differ or be affected by the manufacturing process. These studies have been carried out at different stages in the development of the Cochlear multichannel implant. They were also required by the US Food and Drug Administration (FDA) prior to granting approval of the device as safe and effective (FDA, 1985; Clark et al., 1987a). The biocompatibility of the materials used in the Cochlear banded array has subsequently been confirmed in a patient who had an implant and died from unrelated causes (Clark et al., 1988).

The electrode array should be atraumatic and, in particular, there should be no damage which could lead to a significant loss of neural elements. In addition, there should be minimal tissue reaction, e.g. new bone growth, because this may result in reduced performance over time. Experimental studies on animals have shown that electrode arrays can be safely inserted into the cochlea providing there is no damage to the spiral lamina or basilar membrane, in which case there will be a loss of peripheral processes and, in turn, of spiral ganglion cells (Simmons, 1967; Clark, 1973, 1977; Clark, Kranz and Nathar, 1975; Schindler et al., 1977; Sutton, Millar and Pfingst, 1980). These studies also indicate that fractures of the spiral lamina are one of the causes of new bone formation. In another experimental study, it was shown that a free-fitting electrode caused less histopathological reaction than a moulded array (Sutton, Millar and Pfingst, 1980). Furthermore, a moulded array cannot readily allow for variations in anatomy and pathology.

The Cochlear multielectrode array has been inserted in human temporal bones to determine the presence of any trauma. The first study (Shepherd et al., 1985a) examined the bones histologically and found that a tear of the spiral ligament occurred quite commonly at a point approximately 10 mm from the round window. This was probably due to a shearing force produced as the electrode passed around the outside of the basal turn. Histopathological studies have shown that this would not lead to loss of spiral ganglion cells or an adverse tissue reaction (Clark et al., 1988). It was also found that a tear of the basilar membrane or a fracture of the spiral lamina only occurred if force was applied to the electrode array after resistance was felt. The insertion of the Cochlear electrode in the human temporal bone was also studied using surface preparation techniques (Clark et al., 1987b; Clifford and Gibson, 1987; Kennedy, 1987). The findings in these studies were similar to those obtained by Shepherd et al. (1985a) from histological sections, and they confirmed that the smooth, tapered, free-fitting array manufactured by Cochlear could be inserted with minimal trauma providing the insertion stopped when resistance was felt.

Further studies on the human temporal bone were also carried out to reduce the chance of the electrode tip perforating the basilar membrane. It was found that if the electrode array was rotated (anticlockwise for the right and clockwise for the left ear) this would direct the tip of the electrode down and away from the basilar membrane (Franz and Clark, 1987). This is a procedure that is now recommended to help ensure the atraumatic insertion of the Cochlear electrode array.

It has been shown that single electrodes made from wire with a diameter of 0.21 mm can cause trauma when inserted for a distance of about 20 mm (House and Edgerton, 1982; Johnsson, House and Linthicum, 1982). On the other hand, the multichannel Cochlear array is made of individual wires which have a diameter of only 0.025 mm. The array is also graded in stiffness as wires are added in sequence from the tip, where there is one, to the proximal end where there are 22. A comparative study of the Cochlear multielectrode array, and the thicker single wire has shown that the multielectrode array which is made from thinner wires is 10 times more flexible and will buckle with a force that is 25 times less than that required to make the single wire buckle (Patrick and MacFarlane, 1987).

Studies have also been undertaken to determine whether the spread of middle-ear infection to the inner ear is facilitated by the presence of an implant. This is especially important in the case of children who have a high incidence of otitis media. Although it has been shown by House and Luxford (1985) that the incidence of otitis media in children implanted with a single-channel intracochlear electrode was not higher than normal, and that none developed meningitis or other evidence of inner-ear infection, there is still a need to study the situation in the experimental animal to help ensure that there are no significant localised or long-term effects.

Studies on the experimental animal (Clark and Shepherd, 1984; Franz, Clark and Bloom, 1984, 1987a; Brennan and Clark, 1985; Cranswick et al., 1987) have shown that the spread of infection from *Staphylococcus aureus* or *Streptococcus pyogenes* is limited by the tissue at the electrode entry point and by the sheath that develops around the electrode. Further work is still necessary to ensure that *Streptococcus pneumoniae*, a common causal agent for otitis media in children, does not spread to the inner ear. The effect of different types of seals at the electrode entry point in preventing the spread of *Streptococcus pneumoniae* infection from the middle to the inner ear is presently being studied (Berkowitz et al., 1987; Shepherd et al., 1989).

In carrying out multielectrode intracochlear stimulation, it is very important that the electrical stimulus parameters do not lead to damage of nerve fibres or ganglion cells. Studies have shown that with pure platinum the charge density should be less than $50 \, \mu C/cm^2$ per phase (Agnew et al., 1981; Walsh and Leake-Jones, 1982). Furthermore, it is essential that there be no charge imbalance between pulses, otherwise there will be a direct current (d.c.) which can damage neurons. The Cochlear multichannel device has been engineered to ensure that the charge density is comfortably within the above limit, and charge imbalance has been eliminated down to 0.01% of the amplitude of the pulse. To ensure further that the parameters used by the Cochlear multielectrode implant are safe, long-term stimulation studies have been carried out on cats (Shepherd, Clark and Black, 1983; Shepherd et al., 1985b). These have shown that the stimulus parameters used do not damage the neural elements or electrodes for periods of up to 2000 hours of continuous stimulation. In addition, the temporal bone of a patient who died from cardiac disease has shown no adverse effects after 10 000 hours of stimulation (Clark et al., 1988).

Percutaneous Connector

A percutaneous connector was used by Simmons (1966) to carry out initial studies to obtain psychophysical data and evaluate speech-processing strategies. This connector had an outside cylinder of plastic (Kel-F) and the wires were embedded in its centre in resin. There was no report of tissue tolerance, infection or mechanical stability.

Subsequently, the Stanford group dispensed with the percutaneous connector, and used a transcutaneous ultrasonic link for transmitting information to an implanted receiver–stimulator which was joined to the electrode array via an interconnecting plug (Simmons et al., 1979).

In 1970, House and colleagues used a percutaneous connector to carry out initial studies on two patients (House et al., 1976). The percutaneous connector consisted of a metal stud screwed into the mastoid cortex and a disc containing sockets placed over the stud and passing through an opening in the skin. In one of the patients, the connector loosened in the bone after a few weeks and the experiment was terminated. In 1972, House et al. (1976) implanted a system using an induction coil for transcutaneous stimulation, and this continued to be the method for transmitting information.

A percutaneous plug of Teflon was used for the first 21 patients implanted by Pialoux et al. (1979), but skin infection necessitated the removal of the plugs and cutting of the electrodes. Subsequently, an implant system was developed where information could be transmitted transcutaneously through the intact skin by magnetic coupling.

The Utah/Ineraid device has been the main one where a percutaneous plug and socket arrangement has continued to be used. One reason for this is that it is very difficult to engineer an inductive transcutaneous link for the speech-processing strategy used with this device. The percutaneous pedestal is made from pyrolytic carbon, and is fixed to bone with self-tapping stainless steel screws. The pedestal has also been made of pyrolytic carbon as some studies have shown that this material can adhere to skin and fibrous tissue. It is not clear how effective this attachment is, but it is better than Teflon or stainless steel. Information from the clinical trial of the Ineraid cochlear implant has been reported by Medical Devices, Diagnostics and Instrumentation (MDDI) in 1989. This report indicated that there was 'a substantial amount of irritation and thickening around the pedestal'. There were also reports of skin regression and loosening of the bone screws used to fixate the pedestal.

More details of the complications with the Ineraid device have been reported to the NIH Consensus Conference in Bethesda (N.L. Cohen, 1988, personal communication). In 133 patients there were 9 major and 28 minor problems. Some of the nine major problems were due to the electrode, but in five cases significant infection occurred, and in one of these the pedestal had to be removed. The 28 minor problems were primarily due to inflammation around the pedestal. In 16 there was mild inflammation and in 12 minimal itching or crusting. These complications tended to abate over time. In addition, there were two cases where the pedestal sheared off due to external trauma.

Asepsis

The prevention of infection is important when implanting any foreign body in a patient, and this applies to single- and multichannel implants as well as to the pedestal or plug and socket for percutaneous stimulation. In the authors' own programme it ensured there are no pathogens on the skin in and around the ear, as well as in the upper respiratory tract. If present, treatment is instituted to remove them. The operating room should meet high standards of asepsis and this includes the use of an air filtration system. It is desirable to use a laminar flow unit providing filtered air in either a horizontal or vertical direction. The high level of sterility should extend to the management of instruments and drapes. There should be a limit to the number of people in the operating room and to traffic flow. In preparing the area, it is necessary to shave the scalp for at least two-thirds of the side involved (Figure 12.3). It is essential to leave a 6-cm margin between the wound edge and the hair. The area is prepared by the application of antiseptic solution and sterile plastic drapes are then applied. Antibiotics are given parenterally at the beginning of the operation and for one day postoperatively. They are continued parenterally or given orally if there is an infection. Amoxycillin and cloxacillin are used. In addition, the authors advocate irrigating the wound with a dilute solution of amoxycillin and cloxacillin.

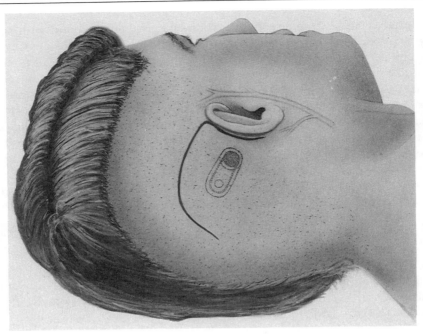

Figure 12.3. The inverted-U incision: this begins about one-third of the way up the postauricular sulcus and extends posteriorly for a distance of 6 mm, before curving inferiorly for 6 mm. (Reproduced with the permission of the Cochlear Corporation, from the *Surgical Procedure Manual*.)

Surgical Procedure

Incision

There are four flap incisions currently in use. These are postauricular inverted-U (Figure 12.3), extended endaural (Figure 12.4), C-shaped (Figure 12.5) and inverted-L (Figure 12.6). In each case the margins of the incisions should be at least 2 cm from the edge of the proposed implant. It is important to have a generous margin to provide the surgeon with flexibility in placing the implant in case he or she experiences unexpected problems or anatomical constraints in its siting. For this reason, it is desirable to examine plain X-rays and CT scans and look for mastoid emissary veins in particular before making the incision. Also assess the size of the mastoid air-cell system and the position of the dura.

The design and marking of the skin incision can be facilitated by resting a dummy package in an appropriate situation. It must be ensured that the anterior edge is at least 1 cm from the postauricular sulcus so that there is adequate room for spectacles to be worn. The incision is marked with methylene blue, and a vasoconstrictor agent injected to control bleeding.

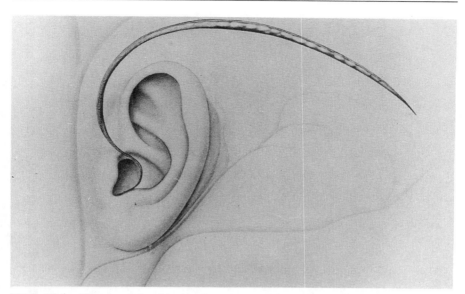

Figure 12.4. The extended endaural incision: this begins inferiorly in the external auditory canal and runs up the posterior wall just inside the bony cartilaginous junction to the incisura terminalis. It then curves posteriorly for about 8 cm. (Reproduced with permission of Professor E. Lehnhardt, Cochlear AG.)

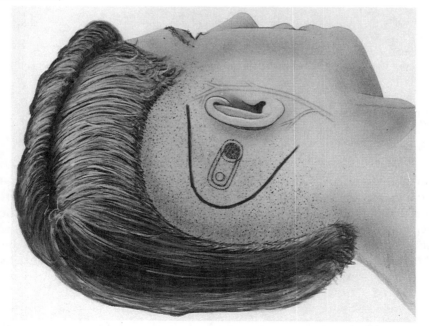

Figure 12.5. The C-incision: it is important to begin the superior limb of this incision 1–2 cm above the pinna and to continue posteriorly to a point 2 cm behind the dummy implant. The inferior limb runs forward to a point 1 cm below the lobule. (Reproduced with the permission of the Cochlear Corporation, from the *Surgical Procedure Manual*.)

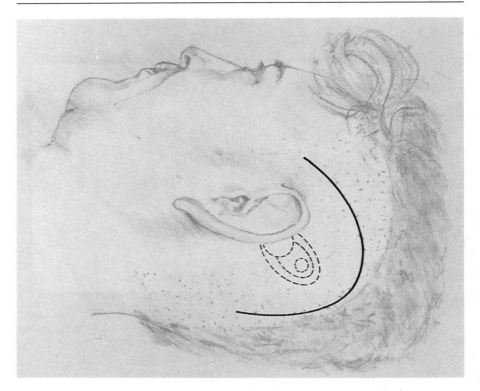

Figure 12.6. The inverted L-incision: this commences in front of the pinna, passes directly back 4 cm above the pinna and continues for a distance of 8 cm behind the pinna before turning inferiorly.

With the inverted-U incision, it is recommended that the skin and subcutaneous fascia are raised as a separate flap followed by an anteriorly based flap of deep fascia and periosteum. This helps ensure that the anterior limb of the incision does not lie directly over the package and that the anterior end of the package is always covered by viable tissue: this is illustrated in Figure 12.7a. The extended endaural incision is usually raised as a single flap, although a separate deep fascial flap may be constructed. The C-incision can be used to raise a single flap of skin, subcutaneous tissue and deep fascia, or alternatively the tissue can be separated into two flaps (Figure 12.7b). With the inverted-L incision the skin and fascia should be raised as a single flap. The upper limb should be well above the pinna to avoid cutting the posterior branch of the superficial temporal artery.

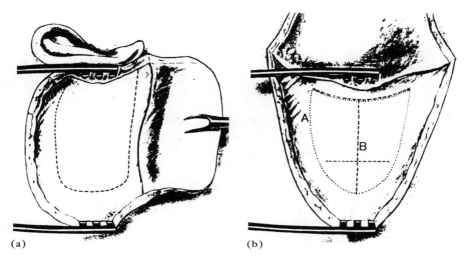

(a)   (b)

Figure 12.7. Deep fascial incisions: (a) the inverted-U flap of skin and superficial fascia has been raised. An incision is made through the deep fascia and periosteum 1 cm inside the margins of the skin incision, beginning superiorly and running posteriorly, then inferiorly and finally anteriorly. An anteriorly based deep fascial flap is raised. (b) The C-shaped flap of skin and superficial fascia has been raised: (A) an area of deep fascia and periosteum can be excised; (B) a cruciate incision is made in the deep fascia and periosteum, and joined to one placed anteriorly. The flaps are then raised. (Reproduced from Webb et al. (1991) with permission of the Cochlear Corporation, from the *Surgical Procedure Manual.*)

Mastoidectomy and posterior tympanotomy

A limited mastoidectomy is carried out to expose the mastoid antrum, the lateral semicircular canal and the short process of the incus (Figure 12.8). A bony overhang is created superiorly, or sometimes in the region of the mastoid tip to place holes for Dacron ties that will subsequently fix the lead wire in place (see Figure 12.12). With an anteriorly placed sigmoid sinus, it can sometimes be difficult to perform a posterior tympanotomy adequately. This can be facilitated by thinning the bone of the external auditory canal and reorienting the microscope. A posterior tympanotomy is then carried out to expose the round window and middle ear (Figure 12.9). In doing this it is necessary to be careful to identify the vertical section of the facial nerve, which can vary in its position. It is particularly important to look out for a sharp genu at the junction of the horizontal and vertical segments. It is also important to beware of a facial nerve that angles laterally in the lower section of the posterior tympanotomy (Figure 12.8). In exposing the round window it is often necessary to extend the posterior tympanotomy down quite a distance, to a point where the facial

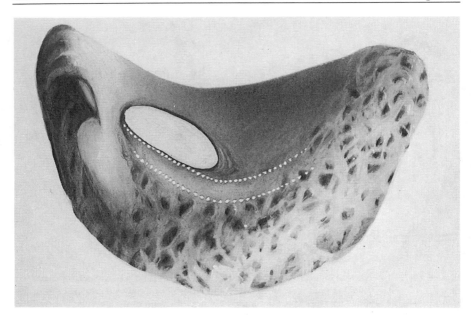

Figure 12.8.   The mastoidectomy: a limited mastoidectomy is carried out to expose the mastoid antrum, the lateral semicircular canal and the short process of the incus. The course of the facial nerve is shown by the dotted line. (Reproduced with the permission of the Cochlear Corporation, from the *Surgical Procedure Manual*.)

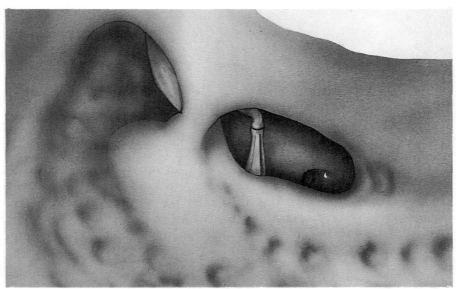

Figure 12.9.   The posterior tympanotomy: the round window has been exposed via the facial recess. The short process of the incus provides a guide to the vertical course of the facial nerve which, protected by a thin layer of bone, forms the posterior margin of the tympanotomy. The stapes provides a guide to the scala tympani if the round window is obliterated. (Reproduced with the permission of the Cochlear Corporation, from the *Surgical Procedure Manual*.)

nerve swings laterally and is at risk of injury. The identification of the facial nerve should be carried out with a diamond paste burr, and bone should be left over the nerve if possible. Entry into the middle ear can be facilitated if there is a sentinel cell lying beneath the floor of the antrum, and this can be followed forwards. It is often necessary to identify the chorda tympani, and if possible this should be preserved. Sometimes it can be quite difficult to find a round window which is directed more posteroinferiorly than normal. It can, however, usually be exposed by changing the angle of the microscope and drilling the bone anterior to the facial nerve. This should be performed carefully to avoid the heel of the burr damaging the nerve. After exposure of the round window, the posterior tympanotomy is then covered with a cottonoid to prevent dust entering the middle ear.

Preparation of package bed

The package bed is prepared after its placement has been reassessed. The position of the bed is marked by drilling around the template (Figure 12.10). The bone in the demarcated area is then drilled down to a depth that would prevent the package protruding significantly above the surface

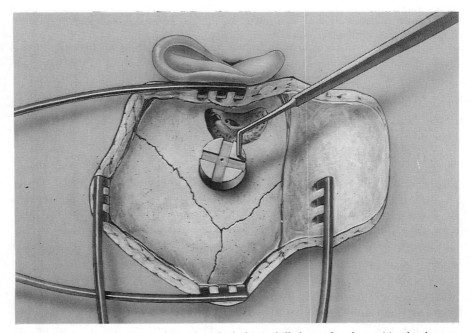

Figure 12.10. Preparation of the package bed: this is drilled out after the position has been marked around the template placed at least 1 cm behind the postauricular groove. (Reproduced with the permission of the Cochlear Corporation, from the *Surgical Procedure Manual.*)

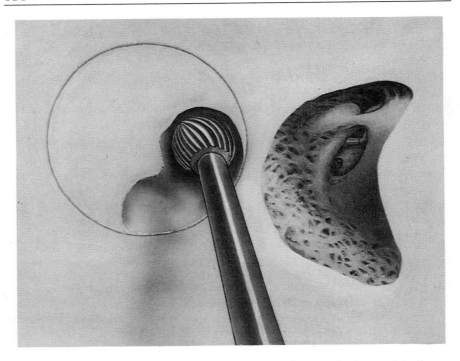

Figure 12.11. The package bed: the bed is created using a large cutting burr, and the floor smoothed with the diamond paste milling burr. (Reproduced with the permission of the Cochlear Corporation, from the *Surgical Procedure Manual.*)

of the bone (Figure 12.11). In bones that are thin it may be necessary to drill down to dura. In some cases the bone can be drilled down to dura around the edge of the bed to create an island of bone in the centre, and so allow the dura to be depressed without actually removing all the bone. Alternatively, the bone should be removed completely over the whole bed so that the package can be adequately placed, with the dura slightly depressed. On completion of the bed, it is necessary to create a groove from it to the mastoid cavity (Figure 12.12) – this contains the lead wire and is directed anteriorly and inferiorly. The edges of the groove are undercut and this helps in keeping the lead wire in place. At this stage of the operation, it is necessary to ensure that haemostasis is complete. Monopolar diathermy must not be used once the electrode has been inserted into the cochlea, because this can lead to electric current spreading inside the cochlea and damaging nerve tissue. The surgeons should at this stage regown and glove, check the drapes and cover wet areas if required.

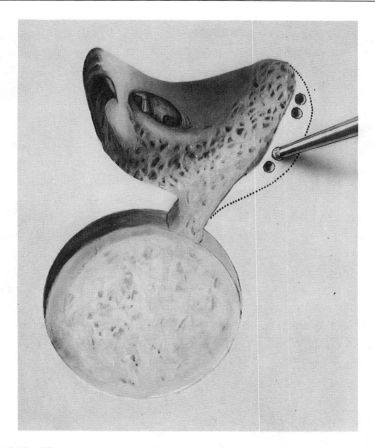

Figure 12.12. The mastoidectomy, package bed and interconnecting groove for the electrode lead wire. The holes for the Dacron ties have been drilled in bone overhanging the mastoid cavity. (Reproduced with the permission of the Cochlear Corporation, from the *Surgical Procedure Manual*.)

Electrode insertion

Attention is now directed to the round window. Exposure of the round window membrane may be facilitated by drilling the bony overhang anteroinferiorly (Figure 12.13). The lateral margin of the round window membrane is incised to provide entry to the scala tympani of the basal turn. Alternatively, it may be necessary or preferable to enter the basal turn by carrying out a cochleotomy anterolateral to the round window (Figure 12.14). Bone is thinned down with a diamond paste burr over an area at least 1 mm in diameter until a dark or blue line is observed. The bone is then picked out (Figure 12.15). In most cases no further drilling is

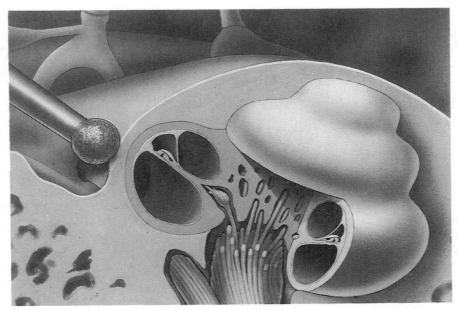

Figure 12.13. Enlarging the round window niche: the overhang over the round window membrane may need to be removed anteriorly and inferiorly with a fine drill to expose the membrane. (Reproduced with the permission of the Cochlear Corporation, from the *Surgical Procedure Manual.*)

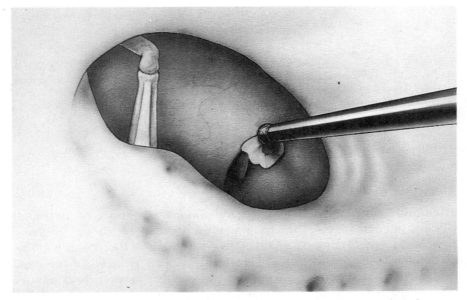

Figure 12.14. The anteroinferior fenestration: an alternative technique to round window reflection is to drill the bone away over the scala tympani anteroinferior to the round window until the underlying endosteum is seen as a blue-coloured area. (Reproduced with permission of the Cochlear Corporation, from the *Surgical Procedure Manual.*)

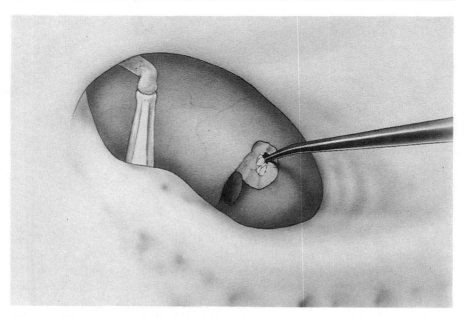

Figure 12.15.   Bone removal with a fine hook: the final entry into the scala media is best made with the removal of thin bone fragments using a fine hook.

required. Sometimes, with a round window insertion the crista fenestrae which lies anterolateral needs to be drilled away to obtain a good view along the line of the scala tympani (see Figure 12.2). Furthermore, when there is extensive fibrous tissue or bone within the first part of the scala tympani, this will need to be drilled or picked out to a point where the unimpeded scala tympani is seen (Figure 12.16). After preparation of the opening into the cochlea, it is then necessary to place the ties through the holes in the bone overhanging the mastoid cavity, and loop them so that the round window can be clearly seen (Figure 12.17). If a tie is also placed anteriorly around the floor of the antrum this should also be put into position. The receiver–stimulator package is then opened in front of a laminar flow of filtered air if this is being used. An insertion claw is selected and is used to direct the electrode tip to the opening into the cochlea. Holding the package in the other hand, the electrode is gently advanced into the basal turn. Its progress is facilitated by gently stroking the electrode (Figure 12.18). The insertion should be stopped when any significant resistance is felt or buckling commences. If the electrode insertion is not satisfactory this may be facilitated by withdrawing it slightly and then rotating it through 90 degrees. In the right ear the electrode is rotated anticlockwise (Figure 12.19) and in the left ear clockwise. This action brings the tip of the electrode down away from the basilar membrane and facilitates its further insertion.

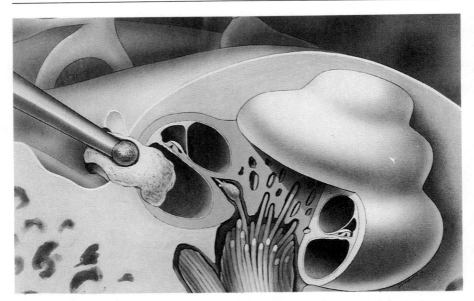

Figure 12.16. Drilling an obliterated basal turn: beginning at a site anteroinferior to the estimated round window position, bone is removed anteriorly and superiorly. The scala media is often filled with soft white bone. This is removed anteriorly until an open space is found. (Reproduced with permission of the Cochlear Corporation, from the *Surgical Procedure Manual.*)

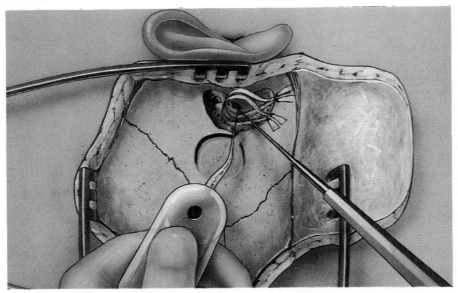

Figure 12.17. Placement of the ties: the Dacron ties have been placed in position, and are looped so that the electrode insertion is not impeded. The electrode is guided with the claw and at the same time the implant is advanced with the other hand so that the electrode tip enters the scala. (Reproduced with the permission of the Cochlear Corporation, from the *Surgical Procedure Manual.*)

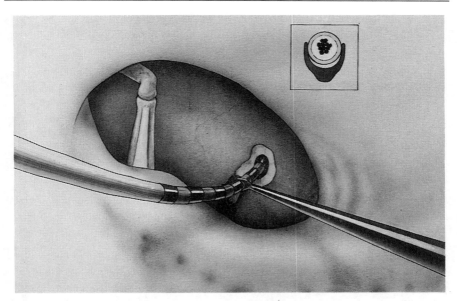

Figure 12.18. Electrode insertion: the claw is used to guide the electrode into the scala tympani. It can also help advance the electrode along the scala using gentle stroking movements. (Reproduced with permission of the Cochlear Corporation, from the *Surgical Procedure Manual*.)

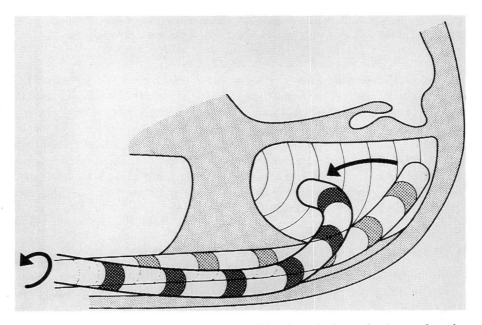

Figure 12.19. A diagram showing how rotation of the electrode directs the tip away from the basilar membrane and around the basal turn of the cochlea. (Reproduced from Franz and Clark (1987) with permission.)

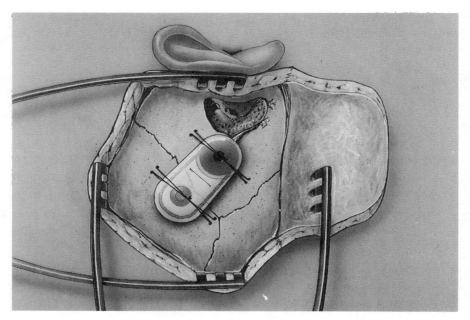

Figure 12.20. The secured package: the Dacron ties have secured the thick portion of the electrode lead wire, and the package is in its bed. Non-absorbable sutures are placed over the package and antenna. Holes for the sutures have been previously drilled in the cortical bone, or alternatively soft tissue can be used as the anchoring points. The sutures help to stabilise the implant and prevent the antenna protruding too much from the skull. (Reproduced with permission of the Cochlear Corporation, from the *Surgical Procedure Manual*.)

When the electrode insertion is complete the electrode is stabilised by pressing it against the edge of the posterior tympanotomy. The assistant surgeon then makes the Dacron ties. It is also desirable to fix the package in place by putting a suture over the section containing the coil as well as over the titanium capsule (Figure 12.20). The anteriorly based fascial flap when created is sutured over the package. It may be necessary to excise the deep fascia overlying the magnet if the skin and superficial fascia are more than 6 mm thick. If the flap thickness is greater than 6 mm, the external magnet may not be attached adequately.

Cochlear Implantation in Children

With children, the procedure is the same as for an adult when they are 10 years or older. In younger children some modifications are required as their skulls are smaller, thinner and skull growth is still occurring. The incision may be any of the ones described. It is, however, essential to ensure that there is a generous clearance beyond the edges of the proposed implant. The flap may look relatively large in a small child, but there is no

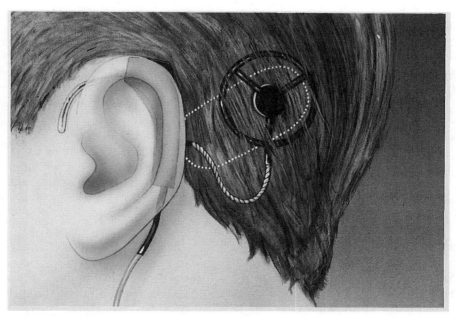

Figure 12.21. The postoperative result showing the microphone and transmitting coil in place. (Reproduced with permission of the Cochlear Corporation, from the *Surgical Procedure Manual.*)

real contraindication to a large generous flap. In fact, it is preferable to do so otherwise the package may come to lie close to a skin incision – this leads to wound breakdown. The package bed will need special attention. In many children it is necessary to drill down to dura and this should be carried out with care using a diamond paste burr. If there is any bleeding, this can be controlled with bipolar diathermy or applying compressed muscle or Gelfoam. If there is any extradural bleeding when the dura is separated from the surrounding bone, this may be controlled in a similar manner. A check should be made with a dummy package that it is sitting comfortably in place and that when it depresses dura it does not initiate bleeding. The techniques for electrode insertion are similar. In young children, it is recommended that there is an anteriorly placed tie not far from the round window so that any skull growth will not lead to the electrode array coming out. This is best placed around the floor of the antrum. The postoperative result in a child is shown in Figure 12.21.

Special Circumstances

Certain types of pathology and anatomical variations can lead to alterations in the surgical approach. This can usually be predetermined from clinical and radiological findings. Malformations such as the Mondini deformity, where the basal turn is dilated, may be accompanied by a perilymph 'gusher'. In this case the gusher is handled by suction and special attention given to sealing the scala tympani. If fibrosis or new bone is present in the basal turn, this can usually be removed for up to 6 mm to allow the electrode to be inserted around the remaining basal turn. If the basal turn is completely filled, a gutter may be created around the turn and the electrode placed in this. In this way some multichannel stimulation is still possible. Alternatively, an extracochlear multichannel device may be used, but in this case, because bone has a high impedance, multichannel stimulation will not be possible unless the bone overlying the cochlea and modiolus is drilled away.

Postoperative Care

Standard management should be given as for any otological operation. If a haematoma occurs then apply a pressure dressing and aspirate it if under tension. The sutures are best removed on the tenth day. A plain X-ray of the temporal bone is desirable at surgery or before going home to ensure that the electrode array is in a satisfactory position.

Complications

These may be due to any anaesthesia or otological operation. Haemorrhage from a mastoid emissary vein can be a major problem, but usually is well controlled with a diamond burr, bone wax or crushed muscle. If a perforation of the tympanic membrane occurs at the time of surgery, it should be repaired otherwise it may need to be grafted. If dura is injured it should be sealed with fascia or sutured to control any cerebrospinal fluid leak. If a facial nerve injury occurs this should be treated in the appropriate way. There were no permanent facial nerve injuries in 459 cases (Cohen, Hoffman and Strosthein, 1988), but there have been temporary ones in 8 or 1.7%. If signs of degeneration were to occur the facial nerve would need to be explored. A chorda tympani injury may lead to taste disturbance. A perilymph fistula has been reported in a small number of cases and is the cause of persistent postoperative vertigo. In this situation re-exploration and repair is necessary. As mentioned previously, a malpositioned electrode, particularly in a hypotympanic cell, may be an explanation for failure to induce a hearing sensation with electrical stimulation.

Wound breakdown is perhaps the most common and significant complication of cochlear implant surgery and it can be avoided by proper flap design and, in particular, the use of an adequately large flap. If there has been a postauricular incision, then a C-shaped flap is contraindicated (Harris and Cueva, 1987), and an inverted-U incision should be used. It may also be desirable to rotate a flap so that the wound edges are not under tension. If local infection is associated with a wound breakdown and is not corrected by antibiotic therapy and the installation of local antiseptic drops, then the package should be removed. In this case it is best to cut the electrode array close to the posterior tympanotomy as infection usually does not extend to the middle ear. Occasionally nose blowing will cause the skin flap to be lifted up with air. This is usually controlled by a pressure dressing until it stops and by avoiding the precipitating factor. If the skin flap is too thick for the magnet to hold the external antenna in position, it may need to be corrected. Usually it is temporary and due to postoperative oedema. If the skin flap is too thin, then the attraction between the magnets will be too strong and lead to skin irritation and even breakdown. This can be corrected by reducing the strength of the overlying magnet.

Occasionally the implant may be mobile in its bed and rock with pressure on it, or spectacles may press on its anterior section if there is inadequate space between the postauricular incision and the device. Stimulation of the facial or tympanic nerves can occur, and is most frequently seen in cases of otosclerosis. Usually the threshold is above that of the comfortable listening level and there is no problem. If the threshold is lower, then the electrodes concerned can be switched off. It is rare to find patients where the condition is so bad that all electrodes cannot be used. Tinnitus is usually unaffected or improved by implantation. The number of patients with an exacerbation of the tinnitus has been very small indeed. Vertigo is rarely a problem postoperatively and is usually temporary. If it persists a fistula should be suspected. The smaller mini-receiver–stimulator now manufactured by Cochlear is only 6 mm thick and does not lead to much protuberance even in the case of children. It was, however, quite often seen in the case of the clinical trial device which was mushroom-shaped and 10.5 mm thick.

Explantation and Reimplantation

An electrode for insertion into the cochlea should be designed so that it can be explanted and another reinserted with minimal trauma. In our own series of 100 operations it was necessary to remove the electrode and package in only one patient. This patient requested that the first receiver–stimulator used in the clinical trial be replaced by the improved device (see Figure 12.1) as this included a magnet for the easy attachment of the head set. In addition, the authors' first three patients, who had the University of Melbourne's prototype implanted, subsequently needed the Cochlear device. The explantation and reimplantation of arrays proved to be easy (Clark et al., 1987b) especially as the prototype array was similar in design to the one developed by Cochlear.

Furthermore, it was reported by Jackler, Leake and McKerrow (1989) that in the case of 1100 patients in North and South America who had received the Nucleus (Cochlear) device up to the end of 1988, 31 had undergone reimplantation (2.8%). The reasons for replacing the device included: device failure (12), skin flap complications (10), insertion in a hypotympanic air cell or buckling of the electrode due to insertion against resistance (7), trauma with haematoma at the receiver site (1) and accidental dislodgement of the array during revision surgery to place a magnet on the standard receiver–stimulator (1).

Details of the reimplantation operations were obtained in 21 out of the 31 procedures. In 20 an electrode was reinserted immediately after the other array had been removed, and the reinsertion was carried out without any difficulty. In one patient the reinsertion was performed 1 month after explantation and, although some resistance was experienced with the reintroduction of the array, a full insertion was obtained with a good functional result.

It was reported by Jackler, Leake and McKerrow (1989) that the Ineraid device had been implanted in 150 patients up to the end of 1988, with 5 patients requiring reimplantation (3.3%). The reasons for removing the devices were: device problems (2), shearing of the percutaneous pedestal (2) and infection (1). Four of the five reimplantations were with second Ineraid devices and one with a Cochlear device. An electrode array could only be reinserted for the same distance as the previous array in two out of the five patients. In one of the other three patients, reimplantation was difficult as explantation had resulted in the apical portion of the array along with three electrode balls remaining within the cochlea. This was presumably due to the fact that the Ineraid array has electrodes which are balls lying free or protruding beyond the surface of the carrier. As a result, when a fibrous or bony sheath forms around the array this prevents it from being easily extracted. In a second patient the array was removed because of infection, and reimplantation was attempted 3 months later with only two electrodes being placed within the cochlea. This lack of success was probably due to the development of dense fibrous tissue and/or bone which can occur 2 weeks after infection in the cochlea (Clark and Shepherd, 1984). In the third patient, there was no obvious reason why reimplantation resulted in less than full insertion, but this could have been due to the fact that the array does not have a smooth surface.

Reimplantation has been required for the University of California, San Francisco (UCSF) (Storz Corporation) patients (Jackler, Leake and McKerrow, 1989). Until December 1988, 30 patients had been implanted, and reimplantation was carried out in 2 for device failures (6.7%). In one patient a UCSF device was reimplanted, and in a second patient a Cochlear device used. In both cases explantation and reimplantation were uneventful.

Not only has reimplantation been required for multichannel devices, but single-channel devices have been replaced with other single-channel devices, and single-channel devices replaced with multichannel ones.

With the 3M House Alpha device (6 mm long), 294 children and 750 adults received implants up until December 1988 (Jackler, Leake and McKerrow, 1989). The total number of operations required to replace this device by the same type is not reported by Jackler, Leake and McKerrow, but in 25 cases obtained from a survey, difficulty with reimplantation occurred in one patient. In this patient, traction to remove the electrode caused the ball electrode to be removed from its lead wire – this occurred because the wire was enveloped by new bone. One case of the successful explantation and reimplantation of the 3M Vienna single-channel device (6 mm) has been reported.

In addition, 35 patients have had the 3M House Alpha single-channel device explanted, and the Cochlear multichannel prosthesis reimplanted. The longer electrode of the Cochlear device was successfully reimplanted in all cases. Furthermore, it has been reported that in 23 patients where the 3M House Alpha single-channel array was replaced by the Cochlear multielectrode array, the functional results after reimplantation were similar to those obtained in patients who had only had one operation to insert the Cochlear multichannel prosthesis (Lindeman, Mangham and Kuprewas, 1987; Brimacombe et al., 1988).

Experience with reimplanting the Cochlear device in patients has shown that the procedure can be made difficult if the tissue around the round window obscures the electrode entry point. In patients this was not due to granulation tissue as found in cats, but simply due to the retraction of tissue outside the round window. An electrode could then be reinserted extra-cochlearly between this tissue and bone. The problem can be avoided by incising the tissue around the electrode entry point, and making sure that there is a good view inside the sheath that surrounded the explanted electrode.

Studies have been undertaken on the experimental animal to examine the histopathological effects of explantation and reimplantation. Research by Jackler, Leake and McKerrow (1989) has shown that a short single-ball electrode (3 mm) can be removed and a long, smooth, shafted carrier (7 mm) reimplanted without loss of spiral ganglion cells in one out of four cats' ears. With the explantation and reimplantation of the long, smooth, shafted carrier, there was no loss of ganglion cells in two out of four cats. Overall, however, there was additional trauma associated with reinsertion.

Another experimental study on 10 cat cochleae has, however, shown that a banded multielectrode array (made according to the specification of Cochlear) can be explanted and another one reimplanted without significant overall loss of spiral ganglion cells (Department of Otolaryngology, University of Melbourne).

In summary, the explantation and reimplantation of electrodes can be carried out with minimal trauma, and with no adverse effects on speech perception results, provided a good view is obtained of the reimplantation site, and provided the multielectrode array possesses a smooth surface without protruding electrodes which may be dislodged during extraction (Jackler, Leake and McKerrow, 1989).

Summary

Surgery for multichannel cochlear implantation has become a well-established procedure. It has an acceptable morbidity rate, but this should be reduced to a minimum by attention to detail, adequate practice in a temporal bone laboratory, and attendance at workshops.

Acknowledgements

Research described in this chapter was funded by a programme grant from the National Health and Medical Research Council of Australia, a National Institutes of Health Contract NO1-NS-7-2342 Studies on Paediatric Auditory Prosthesis Implants, a Public Interest Grant from the Australian Government, the Deafness Foundation of Victoria, the Channel 10 Telethon and Lions Clubs International.

We would like to thank Mr R. West, Cochlear Corporation, for permission to publish figures drawn by Mr E. Zilberts for the Cochlear Corporation, *Surgical Procedure Manual*; and also Professor E. Lehnhardt and Dr M. Lehnhardt, Cochlear AG, for permission to publish the figure on the extended endaural incision. We would like to thank Mrs Margaret Gilmour for typing the manuscript and the Department of Photography, The Royal Victorian Eye and Ear Hospital, for assistance.

References

AGNEW, W.F., BULLARA, L., YUEN, G.H., McCREERY, D.B. and JACQUES, D.B. (1981). The effects of electrical stimulation on the central and peripheral nervous systems. *NIH Quarterly Progress Report* No. 1-NS-O-2319.

BANFAI, P., HORTMANN, G., KOBIK, S., KARCZAG, A., LUERS, P. and SURTH, W. (1985). Extracochlear eight-channel electrode system. *J. Laryngol. Otol.* 99, 549–553.

BANFAI, P., KARCZAG, A., KUBIK, S., LUERS, P., SURTH, W. and WEISKOPF, P. (1987). Cologne–Duren–Duisburg Research Group. In: Banfai, P. (ed.), *Proceedings of the International Cochlear Implant Symposium*, Düren.

BERKOWITZ, R.G., FRANZ, B.K-H.G, SHEPHERD, R.K., CLARK, G.M. and BLOOM, D.M. (1987). Pneumococcal middle ear infection and cochlear implantation. International Cochlear Implant Symposium and Workshop, Melbourne 1985. *Ann. Otol. Rhinol. Laryngol.* 96 (suppl. 128), 55–57.

BLACK, R.C. and CLARK, G.M. (1980). Differential excitation of the auditory nerve. *J. Acoust. Soc. Am.* 67, 868–874.

BLACK, R.C. and HANNAKER, P. (1979). Dissolution of smooth platinum electrodes in biological fluids. *Appl. Neurophysiol.* 42, 366–374.

BLACK, R.C., CLARK, G.M. and PATRICK, J.F. (1981). Current distribution measurements within the human cochlea. *IEEE Transact. Biomed. Eng.* **28**, 721–725.

BRENNAN, W.J. and CLARK, G.M. (1985). An animal model of acute otitis media and the histopathological assessment of a cochlear implant in the cat. *J. Laryngol. Otol.* **99**, 851–856.

BRIMACOMBE, J.A., BEITER, A.L., BARKET, M.J., MIKAMI, K.A. and STALLER, S.J. (1988). Comparative results of speech recognition testing with patients who have used both a single channel and multichannel cochlear implant system. *Proceedings of the American Auditory Society*. Boston, 17 November.

CLARK, G.M. (1973). A hearing prosthesis for severe perceptive deafness – experimental studies. *J. Laryngol. Otol.* **87**, 929–945.

CLARK, G.M. (1977). An evaluation of per-scalar cochlear electrode implantation techniques: a histopathological study. *J. Laryngol. Otol.* **91**, 185–199.

CLARK, G.M. and SHEPHERD, R.K. (1984). Cochlear implant round window sealing procedures in the cat: An investigation of autograft and heterograft materials. *Acta Oto-Laryngol. Suppl.* **410**, 5–16.

CLARK, G.M., FRANZ, B.K-H.G. and NATHAR, J.M. (1975). Histopathological findings in cochlear implants in cats. *J. Laryngol. Otol.* **89**, 945–504.

CLARK, G.M., PATRICK, J.F. and BAILEY, Q.R. (1979). A cochlear implant round window electrode array. *J. Laryngol. Otol.* **93**, 107–109.

CLARK, G.M., PYMAN, B.C. and BAILEY, Q.E. (1979). The surgery for multiple-electrode cochlear implantation. *J. Laryngol. Otol.* **93**, 215–223.

CLARK, G.M., BLACK, R.C., DEWHURST, D.J., FORSTER, I.C., PATRICK, J.F. and TONG, Y.C. (1977a). A multiple-electrode hearing prosthesis for cochlear implantation in deaf patients. *Med. Progr. Technol.* **5**, 127–140.

CLARK, G.M., TONG, Y.C., BLACK, R.C., FORSTER, I.C., PATRICK, J.F. and DEWHURST, D.J. (1977b). A multiple electrode cochlear implant. *J. Laryngol. Otol.* **91**, 935–945.

CLARK, G.M., PYMAN, B.C., WEBB, R.L., BAILEY, Q.E. and SHEPHERD R.K. (1984). Surgery for an improved multiple-channel cochlear implant. *Ann. Otol. Rhinol. Laryngol.* **93**, 204–207.

CLARK, G.M., BLAMEY, P.J., BROWN, A.M., BUSBY, P.A., DOWELL, R.C., FRANZ, B.K-H.G., PYMAN, B.C., SHEPHERD, R.K., TONG, Y.C. and WEBB, R.L. (1987a). The University of Melbourne–Nucleus multi-electrode cochlear implant. *Adv. Oto-Rhino-Laryngol.* **38**.

CLARK, G.M., PYMAN, B.C., WEBB, R.L., FRANZ, B.K-H.G., REDHEAD, T.J. and SHEPHERD, R.K. (1987b). Surgery for the safe insertion and reinsertion of the banded electrode array. International Cochlear Implant Symposium and Workshop, Melbourne 1985. *Ann. Otol. Rhinol. Laryngol.* **96** (suppl. 128), 10–12.

CLARK, G.M., SHEPHERD, R.K., FRANZ, B.K-H.G., DOWELL, R.C., TONG, Y.C., BLAMEY, P.J., WEBB, R.L., PYMAN, B.C., McNAUGHTAN, J., BLOOM, D.M., KAKULAS, B.A. and SIEJKA, S. (1988). The histopathology of the human temporal bone and auditory control nervous system following cochlear implantation in a patient: correlation with psychophysics and speech perception results. *Acta Oto-Laryngol. Suppl.* **448**, 5–65.

CLIFFORD, A.R. and GIBSON, W.P.R. (1987). Anatomy of the round window with respect to cochlear implant surgery. International Cochlear Implant Symposium and Workshop, Melbourne 1985. *Ann. Otol. Rhinol. Laryngol.* **96** (suppl. 128), 17–19.

COCHLEAR CORPORATION. Nucleus 22-channel cochlear implant system. *Surgical Procedure Manual.*

COHEN, N.L., HOFFMANN, R.A. and STROSTHEIN, M. (1988). Medical or surgical complications related to the Nucleus multichannel cochlear implant. *Ann. Otol. Rhinol. Laryngol.* **97**(suppl. 135), 8–13.

CRANSWICK, W.E., FRANZ, B.K-H.G., CLARK, G.M., SHEPHERD, R.K. and BLOOM, D.M. (1987). Middle ear infection post-implantation: the response of the round window membrane to *Streptococcus pyogenes*. International Cochlear Implant Symposium and Workshop, Melbourne 1985. *Ann. Otol. Rhinol. Laryngol.* 96 (suppl. 128), 53–54.

FOOD AND DRUG ADMINISTRATION (1985). Summary of Safety and Efficacy for the Nucleus Implantable Hearing Prosthesis. October 1985.

FRANZ, B.K.-H.G. and CLARK, G.M. (1987) Anatomy of the round window with respect to cochlear implant surgery. International Cochlear Implant Symposium and Workshop, Melbourne 1985. *Ann. Otol. Rhinol. Laryngol.* 96 (suppl. 128), 15–17.

FRANZ, B.K-H.G. and CLARK, G.M. (1988). The surgical anatomy for multiple-electrode extracochlear implant operations. *J. Laryngol. Otol.* 102, 685–688.

FRANZ, B.K-H.G., CLARK, G.M. and BLOOM, D.M. (1984). Permeability of the implanted round window membrane. *Acta Oto-Laryngol. Suppl.* 410, 17–23.

FRANZ, B.K-H.G., CLARK, G.M. and BLOOM, D.M. (1987a). Cochlear implants and otitis media: a comparison of cochlear implant electrode insertion techniques, and the effects of otitis media induced with group A streptococci. *Ann. Otol. Rhinol. Laryngol.* 96, 174–177.

FRANZ, B.K-H.G., CLARK, G.M. and BLOOM, D.M. (1987b). Surgical anatomy of the round window with special reference to cochlear implantation. *J. Laryngol. Otol.* 101, 97–102.

FRANZ, B.K-H.G., KUZMA, J.A., LEHNHARDT, E., CLARK, G.M., PATRICK, J.F. and LASZIG, R. (1990). Implantation of the Nucleus multiple-electrode extracochlear prostheses. *Ann. Otol. Rhinol. Laryngol.* in press.

HARRIS, J.P. and CUEVA, R.A. (1987). Flap design for cochlear implantations: avoidance of a potential complication. *Laryngoscope* 97, 755–757.

HINOJOSA, R. and MARION, M. (1983). Histopathology of profound sensorineural deafness. *Ann. N.Y. Acad. Sci.* 405, 459–484.

HINOJOSA, R., BLOUGH, R.R. and MHOON, E.E. (1987). Profound sensorineural deafness: a histopathological study. International Cochlear Implant Symposium and Workshop, Melbourne 1985. *Ann. Otol. Rhinol. Laryngol.* 96 (suppl. 128), 43–46.

HOUSE, W.F. and EDGERTON, B.J. (1982). A multiple-electrode cochlear implant. *Ann. Otol. Rhinol. Laryngol.* Suppl. 91, 104–116.

HOUSE, W.F. and LUXFORD, W.M. (1985). Otitis media in children following the cochlear implant. *Ear Hear* 6 (3) suppl., 245–265.

HOUSE, W.F., BERLINER, K., CRARY, W., GRAHAM, M., LUCKEY, R., NORTON, N., SELTERS, W., TOBIN, H., URBAN, J. and WEXLER, M. (1976). Cochlear Implants. *Ann. Otol. Rhinol. Laryngol.* 8 (suppl. 27), 2.

JACKLER, R.K., LEAKE, P.A. and McKERROW, W.S. (1989). Cochlear implant revision; the effects of reimplantation on the cochlea. *Proceedings of the American Otological Society Meeting*. San Francisco.

JOHNSSON, L.G., HOUSE, W.F. and LINTHICUM, I.H. (1982). Otopathological findings in a patient with bilateral cochlear implant. *Ann. Otol. Rhinol. Laryngol.* Suppl. 91, 74–90.

KENNEDY, D.N. (1987). Multichannel intracochlear electrodes: mechanism of insertion trauma. *Laryngoscope* 97, 42–49.

LINDEMAN, R.C., MANGHAM, C.A. and KUPREWAS, M.A. (1987). Single-channel and multichannel performance for reimplanted cochlear prosthesis patient. *Ann. Otol. Rhinol. Laryngol.* 96 (suppl. 128), 150–151.

MacLEOD, P., CHOUARD, C.H. and WEBER, J.P. (1985). French Device. In: Schindler, R.A. and Merzenich, M.M. (eds), *Cochlear Implants*, pp. 111–120. New York: Raven Press.

MERZENICH, M.M. (1974). Studies on electrical stimulation of the auditory nerve in animals and man: Cochlear implants. In: Tower, L. (ed.), *The Nervous System*, vol. 3, pp. 337–548. New York: Raven Press.

MERZENICH, M.M. (1985). UCSF Cochlear Implant Device. In: Schindler, R.A. and Merzenich, M.M. (eds), *Cochlear Implants*, pp. 121–129. New York: Raven Press.

MERZENICH, M.M., O'REILLY, B.F., VIVION, M.C. and LEAKE-JONES, P.A. (1979). Development of multichannel electrodes for an auditory prosthesis. *Eighth Quarterly Progress Report*, NIH Contract No. 1-NS-7-2367.

PARKIN, J.L., McCANDLESS, G.A. and YOUNGBLOOD, J. (1987). Utah design multichannel cochlear implant (Ineraid). In: Banfai, P. (ed.), *Proceedings of the International Cochlear Implant Symposium*, Düren.

PATRICK, J.F. and MacFARLANE, J.C. (1987). Comparative mechanical properties of single and multi-channel electrodes. International Cochlear Implant Symposium and Workshop Melbourne 1985. *Ann. Otol. Rhinol. Laryngol.* 96 (suppl. 128), 46–48.

PIALOUX, P., CHOUARD, C.H., MEYER, B. and FUGAIN, C. (1979). Indications and results of the multichannel cochlear implant. *Acta Otol-Laryngol.* 87, 185–189.

REBSCHER, S., MARKS, D., GREENBERG, S., HRADEK, G., JACKLER, R., LEAKE, P., MILCZUK, H., JONATHAN, D., SNYDER, R. and MERZENICH, M. (1988). Studies on pediatric auditory prosthesis implants. *Third Quarterly Progress Report*, January–March 1988, NIH Contract No. 1-NS-7-2391.

SCHINDLER, R.A., MERZENICH, M.M., WHITE, M.W. and BJORKROTH, B. (1977). Multi-electrode intracochlear implants: neural survival and stimulation patterns. *Arch. Otolaryngol.* 103, 691–699.

SHEPHERD, R.K. CLARK, G.M. and BLACK, R.C. (1983). Chronic electrical stimulation of the auditory nerve in cats: Physiological and histopathological results. *Acta Oto-Laryngol. Suppl.* 399, 19–31.

SHEPHERD, R.K., CLARK, G.M., PYMAN, B.C. and WEBB, R.L. (1985a). Banded intracochlear electrode array: evaluation of insertion trauma in human temporal bones. *Ann. Otol. Rhinol. Laryngol.* 94, 55–59.

SHEPHERD, R.K. MURRAY, M.T., HOUGHTON, N.E. and CLARK, G.M. (1985b). Scanning electron microscopy of chronically stimulated intracochlear electrodes. *Biomaterials* 6, 237–242.

SHEPHERD, R.K., XU, S.A., FRANZ, B.K-H.G., TONG, Y.C., CLARK, G.M., MILLARD, R.E., REDHEAD, J., BRIGGS, R. and PATRICK, J.F. (1987a). Studies on pediatric auditory prosthesis implants. *First Quarterly Progress Report*, May 1–July 31 1987, NIH Contract No.1-NS-7-2342.

SHEPHERD, R.K., XU, S.A., FRANZ, B.K-H.G., CHEN, Y., TONG, Y.C., CLARK, G.M., MILLARD, R.E., WILLS, R.A., KUZMA, J.A. and PATRICK, J.F. (1987b). Studies on pediatric auditory prosthesis implants. *Second Quarterly Progress Report*, August 1–October 31 1987, NIH Contract No.1-NS-7-2342.

SHEPHERD, R.K., XU, S.A., TONG, Y.C., MAFFI, C.L., CLARK, G.M., FRANZ, B.K-H.G., MILLARD, R.E., WILLS, R.A., KUZMA, J.A. and PATRICK, J.F. (1987c). Studies on pediatric auditory prosthesis implants. *Third Quarterly Progress Report*, November 1 1987–January 31 1988, NIH Contract No.1-NS-7-2342.

SHEPHERD, R.K., MAFFI, C.L., HATSUSHIKA, S., JAVEL, E., TONG, Y.C. and CLARK, G.M. (1989). Temporal and spatial coding in auditory prostheses. In: Aitkin, L.M. and Rowe, M.J. (eds), *Information Processing in the Mammalian Auditory and Tactile Systems.* New York: Alan R. Liss.

SIMMONS, F.B. (1966). Electrical stimulation of the auditory nerve in man. *Arch. Otolaryngol.* 84, 2–54.

SIMMONS, F.B. (1967). Permanent intracochlear electrodes in cats, tissue tolerance and cochlear microphonics. *Laryngoscope* **77**, 171–186.

SIMMONS, F.B., MATHEWS, R.G., WALKER, M.G. and WHITE, R.L. (1979). A functioning multichannel auditory nerve stimulator. *Acta Oto-Laryngol.* **87**, 170–175.

SUTTON, D., MILLAR, J.M. and PFINGST, B.E. (1980). Comparison of cochlear histopathology following two implant designs for use in scala tympani. *Ann. Otol. Rhinol. Laryngol.* Suppl. 89, 11–14.

WALSH, S.M. and LEAKE-JONES, P.A. (1982). Chronic electrical stimulation of the auditory nerve in cat: Physiological and histological results. *Hear. Res.* **7**, 281–304.

WEBB, R.L., CLARK, G.M., SHEPHERD, R.K., FRANZ, B.K-H.G. and PYMAN, B.C. (1988). The biological safety of the Cochlear Corporation multiple-electrode extracochlear implant. *Am. J. Otol.* **9**, 8–13.

WEBB, R.L., CLARK, G.M., PYMAN, B.C. and FRANZ, B.K-H.G. (1990). The surgery of cochlear implantation. In: Clark, G.M., Tong, Y.C. and Patrick, J.F. (eds), *Cochlear Prostheses.* London: Churchill-Livingstone.

WEBB, F.L., LEHNHARDT, E., PYMAN, B.C., LASZIG, R., FRANZ, B.K-H.G. and CLARK, G.M. (1991). Complications with the Cochlear multiple-channel cochlear implant: experience at Hannover and Melbourne. *Ann. Otol. Rhinol. Laryngol.* in press.

Chapter 13
Speech-processor Fitting for Cochlear Implants

SUE ROBERTS

Introduction

The basic function of the speech processor in any cochlear implant system is to change sound into electrical current in order to stimulate directly the remaining auditory nerve fibres of the profoundly deafened individual. The manner in which the speech processor, which is worn externally, converts the incoming sound patterns into electrical patterns will depend on the type of speech processing used by the particular implant system. As speech processing is discussed elsewhere in this book, suffice it to say that the speech processing can include feature extraction, frequency-dependent amplification and automatic gain control. Rather than focus on differences between cochlear implant systems, this chapter will draw on the similarities in fitting procedures across all systems.

The majority of devices available are multichannel, for example the Nucleus (Clark et al., 1987), the Implex (Hortmann et al., 1989), the Ineraid (Parkin and Stewart, 1988), the Laura (Peeters et al., 1989) and the Banfai devices (Banfai, 1985). There are also a few single-channel devices available. Two of these – the UCH/RNID (London) device (Conway and Boyle, 1989) and the Monosonic (Chouard et al., 1990) – are single-electrode systems whilst the single-channel device from Vienna (Hochmair-Desoyer, 1986) is a multielectrode, single-channel implant.

The fitting procedure common to all systems is the assessment of dynamic range. This requires the measurement of threshold and comfortable or uncomfortable loudness levels across the speech frequency range. The fitting of a multichannel device may also involve pitch ranking and channel selection.

Logistics and Preparation

Timing of the initial fitting

After the operation in which the internal package of the device is surgically implanted, the patient is required to wait for a period of time until the

Table 13.1 The variety of equipment used for the fitting of different cochlear implant systems

Device	Com- puter	Specialised equipment	Measurements made	Method of fitting	Recovery period
Nucleus 22	Yes	Diagnostic and programming interface unit	For each channel: threshold level maximum comfortable level loudness balance sweep channel selection	MAP into random access memory of processor	10 days– 3 weeks
Ineraid	No	Electrode analyser	For each channel: threshold level maximum comfortable level electrode impedance pitch placement channel selection	Adjustment of input gain controls Ear cabled according to channel selection	4–6 weeks
Implex Com 12	Yes	SAM interface Cochlear implant audiometer Cochlear Nerve Tester Syncom patient self-test unit	Medium range levels from promontory test results Comfortable level Sweep Electrode selection	Adjustment of gain controls to Vocoder	4 weeks
Laura	Yes	Interface unit	For each channel: threshold level comfort level loudness discomfort level channel selection	Program into processor memory	?

Banfai	Yes	Patient keyboard Battery-powered interface which can also be hooked up to a computer	For each channel: threshold level maximum comfortable level place pitch ranking	Program into processor memory	?
UCH (London)	Yes	Signal generator	For selected frequencies: threshold level comfort level uncomfortable loudness level loudness balance across frequency	Adjust graphic equaliser, centre frequencies so that it matches comfortable loudness curve	4 weeks
Vienna	Yes	Signal generator	For selected frequencies: threshold level uncomfortable loudness level frequency stepped sweep	Adjustment of gain controls to match comfortable loudness curve	10 days

wound has healed before the external part of the device can be fitted. The surgical procedure for different devices varies and thus so does the time required for healing of the implant wound. Suggested recovery periods for different systems range from 10 days to 6 weeks (Table 13.1).

Systems which use transcutaneous transmission of speech information have quite a finite tolerance for the distance between the transmitting coil and the internal receiver. The Nucleus device, for example, requires that the distance between the external transmitting coil and the internal coil is no more than 6 mm. Any greater distance than this can lead to some loss of power and data, and the transmission will not be as effective. With transcutaneous systems, it is therefore essential to wait until the postoperative swelling has subsided before attempting to fit the headset and speech processor.

Devices that employ a percutaneous connector may require a little more time to heal around the connecting plug or pedestal, and those which have the antennae situated in the ear canal may require 4–6 weeks.

It can be a very difficult waiting time for a patient before the processor is switched on. Some implant teams advocate an early fitting of the device to reassure the patient that the device is functioning. At an early stage, for example 1 week postoperatively, some preliminary measurements can be made where the patient can report sound sensations from their implant. The patient is not, however, able to take the processor outside the clinic until the device fitting is completed at a later date. At any initial fitting session, it is important to inform the patient and family that this is the first of many fittings in which the audiologist will progressively determine the optimum setting for the patient's speech processor.

Counselling and instructions

The patient will have received preoperative counselling about what to expect from his or her cochlear implant. Nevertheless, it is recommended that considerable time is spent during the first fitting session reconfirming that the sound which patients are about to hear from their implant will be quite strange to begin with and that speech may not sound the way they remember it; however, it should become more 'normal sounding' over time.

Clear instructions are also required at all stages of the testing session and it often helps to have prompt cards to ensure that the patient is really understanding what is required of him or her.

Equipment

Several of the implant systems available use personal computers which are connected with an interface unit (Table 13.1). With such systems the

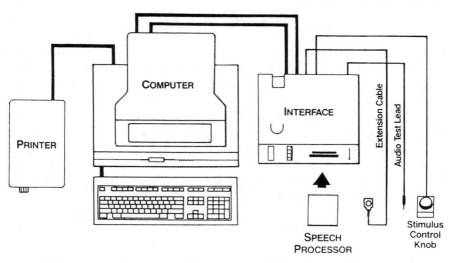

Figure 13.1. Block diagram showing a computer-controlled speech-processor interface unit for programming the speech processor.

patient's speech processor is placed into the interface unit and, using computer software, the clinician is able to drive the interface unit and deliver the necessary test signals through the speech processor to the patient. An example of this type of system can be seen in Figure 13.1.

Other implant systems use specially adapted test boxes to generate the type of signals required to test the functioning of the implant, whether it be sinusoidal or biphasic pulses of different frequency and duration. This type of equipment is manually switch operated or in some cases also controlled by a personal computer (PC).

Determining the Dynamic Range

The most critical step common to the fitting of all implant speech processors is the determination of the patient's dynamic range for electrical stimulation. The dynamic range is the difference between the amount of current that first induces an auditory sensation, or the threshold for electrical stimulation, and the maximum loudness level the patient will accept from the stimulating current. The recommended method for determining these levels is different for various implants. With the fitting of some devices, measurements of an uncomfortable loudness level are also made. The basic premise for obtaining the dynamic range is the same across all implant systems. Psychophysical measurements are made to enable the device to be set within the comfortable loudness range for the patient so that speech and other sounds will be delivered at a level that is audible but not too loud.

Threshold Measurements

In conventional pure-tone audiometry we begin to test a patient by delivering a stimulus which is above his or her threshold and then descending to a level which is nearer the threshold. In order to obtain a threshold for a cochlear implant, an ascending approach is used. This is because it is impossible to set a 'starting level' from which to descend due to the wide range in sensitivity to electrical stimulation across the patient population. Using an ascending approach avoids overstimulating the patient. The clinician instructs the patient to indicate when something is first heard, and gradually increases the amount of current delivered to the implant through the patient's speech processor until a response is recorded. First thresholds tend to be above the true threshold because patients are not sure what it is they are listening for. The audiologist can then descend to establish a more reliable or true threshold.

Threshold measurements may be made at different frequencies or different sites of stimulation in the cochlea. For example, single-channel devices, such as the UCH/RNID (London) and the Vienna (Hochmair-Desoyer, 1986; Conway and Boyle, 1989), require an estimation of thresholds across a broad frequency range whereas multichannel devices will require measurements made from electrodes located at different stimulating sites in or on the cochlea (Nucleus or Laura). In the case of the Monosonic device (Chouard et al., 1990), a single-threshold value is obtained to fit the device, whereas with the Nucleus device as many as 21 different threshold measurements may be obtained.

Comfort Level Measurements

All devices need to be set to have a maximum output level which is comfortable for the listener, and to do this may require testing for a comfortable level, a maximum comfort level or an uncomfortable loudness level. Whatever the definition, the determination of this particular setting is critical in providing a well-fitted device. If a patient experiences stimulation that exceeds this level, it can cause anxiety and reluctance to wear the device.

Loudness growth to electrical stimulation is not orderly and there is often a rapid increase in loudness at the top end of the dynamic range. Invariably, the patient will experience an uncomfortable level of stimulation before he or she is able to judge what is comfortable for him or her.

Again, an ascending approach is used to obtain comfort levels. The patient may be asked to point to a scale, or indicate by using some form of reference, how loud the sound is becoming as the clinician turns the current up (Figure 13.2). In the case of multichannel devices, it is essential

Loudness scale

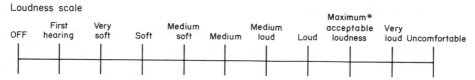

Figure 13.2.   An example of a loudness scale used with adults. *Matched to other electrodes.

to use an ascending approach to assess the comfort levels on each channel because adjacent electrodes may be stimulating areas of the cochlea with very different nerve survival. What is perceived as soft on one channel may be perceived as relatively uncomfortable on another stimulation channel. With analogue devices, this can be done by simply adjusting the gain compensation on each channel gradually upwards from a very low level, such as 5 μA, as recommended with the Ineraid. With devices which employ pulsatile stimulation, the stimulating test pulses are increased from a low to a higher level of stimulating current units.

With a single-channel, broad-band, analogue device, e.g. UCH/RNID, the comfort level will be obtained over the speech frequency range by presenting the patient with a sinusoidal signal at different frequencies and asking the patient to judge its loudness. When a comfortable loudness listening curve has been obtained across the frequency range, the frequency response of the patient's speech processor can be adjusted accordingly.

Dynamic Range Values

The true values of a dynamic range measurement are dependent upon a number of factors, including the stimulus waveform, repetition rate of the stimulus, electrode configuration and placement, and stimulus frequency, as well as neural density and distribution. However, generally it is said that the dynamic range for electrical stimulation is narrow, somewhere between the region of 2 and 15 dB throughout the receptive region (Miller and Pfingst, 1984).

The units in which the dynamic range is measured differ between systems. Some will express the range in terms of units of current, others will use an arbitrary set of number values and others will use electrical decibels. Regardless of the units used, suffice it to say that by measuring the dynamic range with any implant we are really assessing the electrode and electrode–nerve interface. Low thresholds and large dynamic ranges have been associated with a greater percentage of surviving neural elements (Pfingst, Spelman and Sutton, 1980).

Dynamic Range and Performance

Experience to date suggests that those patients who have achieved good results with their cochlear implants are typically those with a large dynamic range (Cooper et al., 1989).

When comparing different groups of patients, the House group have suggested that postlinguistically deafened adults will tolerate higher levels of current over time with their dynamic range widening considerably, whereas children show only a slight widening of dynamic range (Thielemeir et al., 1985). Other clinical observations have suggested that those patients who are recently deafened have a much wider dynamic range than those who have a long duration of deafness. Prelinguistically deafened patients, adults in particular, have been seen to have very small ranges for electrical stimulation (Busby, Tong and Clark, 1986). It seems therefore that previous auditory experience may play a large part in dynamic range values.

What is clear from experience so far is that threshold and comfort levels tend to vary considerably in the first few months following programming, but tend to settle with the patient's increased auditory experience and awareness.

There is no literature to suggest that neural responses to electrical stimulation deteriorate over time. In fact some patients have now had their implants for up to 10 years with no deterioration in performance.

Loudness Balance

The second critical step in the fitting of cochlear implant devices is to ensure that the perceived loudness of stimulation is balanced across the frequency range employed by the device.

The signals perceived on each electrode may sound different from one another because of the differences in their frequency components or their position in the cochlea. Loudness judgements are influenced by the pitch of the stimulus and, in turn, pitch judgements are influenced by the loudness of the signal (Hochmair-Desoyer, 1986). The patient needs to be able to confirm his or her loudness judgement by relating it to other adjacent electrodes (in the case of multichannel devices) or by relating judgements to a sound of a similar frequency (in the case of a single-channel device). When the presentation of sound across the frequency range is balanced in terms of loudness, better speech perception should result.

The Vienna and UCH (London) group use a frequency-stepped sweep to assess that sound is delivered at an equal loudness level across the electrode array. A continuous sinusoidal stimulus, increasing in frequency by small steps, is presented to the patient. The patient is then asked to judge if at any stage the sound has become too soft or too loud. Thus, the patient is able to give feedback as to the overall balance of loudness across the frequency range.

Multichannel fitting will involve having the patient make judgements about the comparative loudness of different channels along the electrode array. This can be done by presenting the established stimulus level to each electrode in turn along the array (sweeping) or presenting two adjacent electrodes for a same–different loudness judgement. The latter technique is often time consuming but more accurate.

Channel Selection

The concepts of establishing dynamic range and equal loudness signal presentation across the speech frequency range are common to both multi- and single-channel systems. In both cases, the entire speech signal will be presented to the implant wearer through their speech processor. Whereas the single-channel device will have all speech information presented at one site of stimulation, the underlying concept of a multichannel device is to divide speech more discretely into a number of channels and present it to different sites either in the cochlea or on the surface of the cochlea. Some sites of stimulation may be inherently better than others for stimulation because of factors such as neuronal survival. An added flexibility of a multichannel device is that there is a choice of different stimulation sites.

Channel selection takes place in three stages: first, electrodes must have an acceptable dynamic range. The rationale is that the range must be wide enough to provide an opportunity for amplitude distinctions to occur within the signal. If the dynamic range is too narrow, speech signals will be little more than on/off sensations with limited amplitude variation. Secondly, loudness percept and growth between electrodes should be comparable. Thirdly, the relationship of pitch and quality of a sound should be pleasing.

Pitch Ranking or Placement Evaluation

Intracochlear multichannel systems are designed to make use of the tonotopic nature of the cochlea so that the high frequency features of speech and other sounds will be presented to the basal end of the cochlea which is most sensitive to high frequency sounds, and the low frequency sounds to the apical end where low pitches are perceived.

The most simple pitch placement evaluation is to sweep through the electrodes in order either from the basal to the apical end of the cochlea or vice versa. The patient is then asked to judge whether the sounds are presented in increasing or decreasing pitch. With electrical stimulation, sometimes the percepts are best described by the terms of 'sharp' for high-pitched or 'dull' for low-pitched sounds. Sometimes judgement of pitch is very difficult for people with little experience with their implant. With intracochlear devices, it is inadvisable to change the order of the electrodes because of the tonotopic nature of the cochlea and auditory nerve. If any of the channels sound very different from the others, however, it may be advisable not to use it for stimulation rather than attempt to place it in another position in the stimulation order.

Extracochlear multichannel cochlear implants may require quite complex pitch ranking experiments (Banfai, 1985). As the electrode array of these devices is placed on the promontory, there is sometimes very little predictability of whether a channel should sound high or low in place pitch. In these types of experiments, patients may be asked to compare and rank different pairs of electrodes so that the sites of stimulation for high and low frequency sounds may be chosen appropriately.

Some multichannel devices require the selection of a finite number of channels. For example, the Ineraid device makes use of only four out of six possible electrodes. Qualitative judgements are made to select which channels are most pleasant for stimulation.

In some patients, it may not be possible to insert the full complement of electrodes into the cochlea as a result of ossification, for example with postmeningitic cases. The flexibility of being able to select a smaller number of channels for stimulation can be very valuable in these cases.

Performance Relative to Number of Stimulating Channels

Although some single-channel patients perform extremely well with their cochlear implants (Tyler, 1988), it is generally accepted that patients with multichannel systems have the potential to achieve greater speech understanding without lipreading. Results also tend to indicate that patients with multichannel intracochlear systems achieve a greater degree of speech understanding than those with extracochlear devices. Within the group of multichannel intracochlear devices there is a range of 4–22 channels used for stimulation.

Differences in results between different multichannel systems do not appear to be a function of the number of channels used by the particular device, but the coding strategy used. Patients with a 4-channel analogue device may show comparable performance to those with a 22-channel pulsatile device (Gantz et al., 1987).

However, it seems that with any one implant system the best performance will be achieved if the patient has the system operating as it was designed, i.e. the maximum number of channels are used for stimulation. In the author's experience with the Nucleus device, patients have been seen with as few as seven channels who obtain open-set speech recognition without lipreading.

Frequency Boundaries

Analogue devices which use a series of filter banks will deliver the whole speech signal in a particular band-pass frequency to the selected stimulating channel. Speech feature-extraction devices, however, have some flexibility in the frequency boundaries for delivering different speech frequencies to different sites of stimulation. The frequency boundaries may be made narrower or wider, for example, to enable better separation of confusing speech elements. Doering and Schneider (1989) have described a method of speech-processor fitting in which they looked at the formant output of the Nucleus devices in relation to German vowels. With the usual default boundaries of this device, they found that the patients were making some confusions in vowels with similar F_2 values. By making some frequency boundaries narrower in the F_2 range, they were able to improve the patients' vowel perception.

The fitting of some multichannel devices will therefore also include reassignment of frequency boundaries.

Adjusting the Speech Processor

Once all the necessary measurements have been made, the speech processor is adjusted and given to the patient.

The single-channel device will have had the gain control and frequency response adjusted so that sounds are at a comfortable loudness level for the patient across the frequency range. The multichannel analogue device will have had the gain adjusted for the selected channels of stimulation and the extracochlear multichannel device will have had the channels appropriately pitch ranked and adjusted accordingly. In a device which employs a memory and is computer programmed, such as the Nucleus device, the results of all the measurements which have been made are used to create a table (or MAP) to be stored in the memory of the processor for that particular patient (Table 13.2). When this is done the processor is ready to be tested and given to the patient.

Informal Testing

The first trial with the programmed speech processor within the clinic is usually to the sound of the clinician's voice or the voice of a family member. It is important that, if there are a few people in the room, only

Table 13.2 An example of a MAP which is programmed into the random access memory of the Nucleus speech processor

Summary of map 2 created on 18-Aug-90 at 13:44
The T stimulus level has been modified by 0%
The C stimulus level has been modified by 0%   Frequency spacing: Lin-Log
The Noise cut-out level = 1   Encoder Strategy: MPEAK
Electrode for Band 3 = 7 Band 4 = 4 Band 5 = 1

Elect.	Mode	T-level	C-level	Upper Freq. Bounds
20	BP+1	60	121	400
19	BP+1	62	125	500
18	BP+1	58	130	600
17	BP+1	67	131	700
16	BP+1	52	134	800
15	BP+1	53	135	900
14	BP+1	60	133	1000
13	BP+1	62	134	1112
12	BP+1	59	140	1237
11	BP+1	60	119	1377
10	BP+1	64	125	1531
9	BP+1	63	130	1704
8	BP+1	58	133	1896
7	BP+1	59	134	2109
6	BP+1	63	133	2346
5	BP+1	64	134	2611
4	BP+1	62	127	2904
3	BP+1	63	125	3231
2	BP+1	59	124	3595
1	BP+1	57	122	above 3595
				Sat Aug 18 13:44:54 1990

one person speaks at a time otherwise it will be quite confusing for the patient. The clinician will usually begin by turning the volume control or the microphone sensitivity to a low level and then gradually increase it while speaking to the patient.

This first moment of hearing can be exciting as well as very confusing for patients. It is important to give them time to sit and reflect on what they are hearing as well as to adjust to the concept of listening to their own voice which often sounds very loud to them.

After allowing the patient some time to speak with family members, the clinician should do some simple exercises to assess whether the patient is picking up speech across the frequency range. Exercises which also demonstrate to the patient that he or she is receiving information should also be used. This is most important as enthusiasm is sometimes dampened due to the different expectations patients have from the implant.

The Vienna group use a selection of German vowels: the patient is asked to indicate whether they are soft or loud. In this way the frequency response of the processor is assessed as well as providing the patient basic auditory experience with speech.

Exercises which involve time and intensity or suprasegmental information are often easy for the patient to begin with. For example, the patient can be asked to follow a passage from a book with his or her finger as the therapist reads the passage. This is called paragraph tracking. The aim is that the patient begins to follow the rhythm of speech. More details regarding this type of training can be found in Chapter 14.

Sometimes the clinician may develop a discrimination task between the names of two members of the family. It can be very meaningful for a patient to see that discrimination can be made at this level.

In some cases, some further minor adjustments may be made in the initial session. For example, sometimes the sound is described as being too loud when speech is first perceived through the implant. With multichannel systems this may be because each channel has been evaluated separately and, with the stimulation of multiple electrodes in response to the speech signal, the effect may be too overwhelming. It is important, however, not to spend too much time making fine adjustments in the first session because the patient is bound to be very tired from all the testing procedures.

Following the initial excitement of trying the device, the clinician should make sure that the patient is aware of all the controls and switches on the processor. A handbook is most useful for the patient to go over at home after the session and make sure that he or she has understood.

Further Adjustments

In the subsequent weeks following the initial fitting the device is often readjusted several times. Most implant teams agree that, with auditory experience, the patient is soon able to be quite accurate in his or her judgements and there is little need for more than minor adjustments.

It is important that patients are counselled to realise that the cochlear implant will never give them perfect hearing. Some patients will return repeatedly asking for another adjustment to their processor which may never give them the result they were expecting. Once the clinician is convinced that the optimal fitting has been achieved, the patient should be encouraged to focus on rehabilitation.

Device Fitting in Children

Initially there were some concerns that, due to the quite complex nature of some cochlear implant devices, it would not be feasible to fit the processors of these devices to children. There are at least 1000 children around the world who have been fitted with implants to date and, although there are some challenges in the fitting procedure, it can most often be accomplished successfully.

Most implant teams recommend that it is advisable for clinicians who are working with implants first to spend some time developing their programming skills with postlinguistically deafened adults. Adults are able to describe auditory percepts and have an auditory experience on which to base their judgements, whereas children may not have the memory or the linguistic competence necessary to communicate judgements about sound sensation to the clinician. Working with adults first will also allow the clinician to become aware of the capabilities and limitations of the device for speech and sound perception.

Children's initial reactions to electrical stimulation can vary from no apparent response, quieting, subtle changes in facial expressions to clear aversion responses. Even those children who are able to display a rapid clear response to either visual or tactile stimulation may not show any indication that they have heard any sound through their implant device.

The clinician who is fitting a speech processor to a child must be very acute at observing covert behavioural responses and must be able to use these responses to train the child to make conditioned responses to the stimuli.

Pre-programming training

Most teams will recommend that the younger child is given some pre-programming training. As well as learning to make a conditioned response, the child who is able to distinguish same/different and big/small may be able to make and convey better judgements of comfortable loudness and loudness balance.

Threshold testing

Traditional play audiometry may be used with most children to establish threshold responses. Once again, as with adults, to avoid overstimulation, an ascending technique has to be used, so that sometimes it may be difficult to condition a child to a stimulus initially. With younger children visual reinforcement techniques can be employed quite successfully.

Threshold is not the most critical measurement for fitting the processor, so that a rough estimation in the first session is often sufficient to use to program the device.

Comfort level

This is the most important level to establish. The sound must not be too loud or the child will reject wearing the speech processor. It is more judicious to set the processor too soft in the early stages than to spend tedious hours attempting to gain exact levels.

Children do not have sophisticated concepts for grading loudness or magnitude so that assessing the comfort level can often be difficult. However, the skilled clinician should be able to detect the first sign of aversion to a loud stimulus. Often a scale is developed which may be meaningful to the child to convey their experience of loudness percepts. For example, a picture of a bird making a soft sound (or 'little') vs the picture of a motor cycle making a loud (or 'big') sound may be meaningful to one child, whilst an older child may be able to scale on the basis of numbers where ten is loud and one soft.

As the test signals which are used for fitting the speech processor are often uninteresting to the child, one method was developed at the University of Melbourne where the fundamental frequency of a voice could be used on each separate channel to be assessed. Using this technique the child is encouraged to play as the clinician speaks to him or her. The level of voice input is gradually increased until the first sign of aversion is seen. Often the child will tell the clinician that he or she is speaking too loud when the stimulation has reached uncomfortable level (L.C. Rowland, P.W. Dawson, S.J. Dettman, A.M. Brown, R.C. Dowell and G.M. Clark, 1990, unpublished data).

Objective measurements

Due to the challenge of developing fitting techniques for children, several groups have been researching more objective measurement techniques.

Research into the use of auditory brain-stem responses to help determine thresholds looks promising. With young children it is possible to confirm questionable threshold responses if a definite wave V response is seen. There are still some problems to overcome with this technique, but many researchers believe that evoked potentials may be successfully used for device fitting in the near future (Game, Thomson and Gibson, 1990; Allum et al., 1990).

Another method currently under investigation is the use of stapedial reflexes. Jerger, Oliver and Chmiel (1988) investigated the relationship between reflex measurements and behavioural measurements in seven postlinguistically deafened adults using the Nucleus device. They found that the range from the reflex threshold to the reflex saturation level was within the subject's dynamic range. Battmer (1989) concurred that the stapedius reflex in adults occurs at about 70% of the dynamic range. No doubt future investigations will yield information which may be useful for setting comfort levels in children.

Loudness balance

With many children, it is difficult to balance loudness levels across the electrode array so that the child may not be receiving the optimal speech signal. However, it has been suggested that the neural plasticity of children appears to allow them to compensate for any imbalance in the signal. Some children with very questionable fittings begin to display good early responses to sound (Rowland et al., 1990).

Electrode selection

With multichannel devices, it may not always be possible to assess and program the device to include all channels in the first session. Experience with the Nucleus devices shows that the average number of channels programmed in the devices after 3 months is 17. With children it is often a very gradual process of fine tuning the device over time.

Summary

The fitting procedure and equipment used vary from one implant system to another but there are some common principles involved. Psychophysical measurements must first be made to establish the dynamic range so that the processor may be adjusted to deliver speech and sound at a level that is comfortable for the patient. The processor must also be adjusted so that sound is delivered at an equal loudness level across the frequency range. With multichannel devices, further adjustments may be made with the selection of channels to be stimulated and their designated frequency boundaries. Speech-processor fitting is a process that occurs over a period of time. At each step, the patient must be carefully counselled to ensure that he or she has understood the nature of the task and what to expect. Young children have been successfully fitted with cochlear implant devices using behavioural techniques. Research now focuses on more objective measurements for setting device parameters. As future devices become more flexible in the number of parameters available for adjustment, these objective measures will become invaluable to the clinician working with cochlear implants.

Acknowledgements

The author wishes to thank Dr D.J. Mecklenburg and Miss C.E. Kovesi for their valuable comments and input into this chapter.

References

ALLUM, J.H.J., SHALLOP, J.K., HOTZ, M.A. and PFALTZ, C.R. (1990). Relationship of electrically evoked 'Auditory' brainstem responses to electrode position, and psychophysically determined threshold and maximum comfortable levels, for the Nucleus intracochlear implant. Paper presented at the Second International Cochlear Implant Symposium. Iowa City, Iowa, USA June 4–9.

BANFAI, P. (1985). *Das Cochlear Implant der Koln-Durener Forschunsgruppe Erfahrungen and Ergebnisse.* Heidelberg, Julius Groos Verlag.

BATTMER, R.D. (1989). Electrically elicited stapedius reflex in cochlear implant patients. In: Fraysse, B.H. (ed.), *Cochlear Implants: Acquisitions and Controversies*, pp.65–68. Toulouse: Paragraphic.

BUSBY, P.A., TONG, Y.C. and CLARK, G.M. (1986). Speech perception studies in the first year of usage of a multiple-electrode cochlear implant by prelingual patients. *J. Acoust. Soc. Am.* suppl. 1, 530.

CHOUARD, C.H., GENIN, J., MEYER, B. and FUGAIN, C. (1990). The Monosonic – a digitalised single channel system. Paper presented at the Second International Cochlear Implants Symposium, Iowa City, Iowa, USA June 4–9.

CLARK, G.M., BLAMEY, P.J., BROWN, A.M., BUSBY, P.A., DOWELL, R.C., FRANZ, B.K-H.G. et al. (1987). The University of Melbourne-Nucleus Multi-electrode Cochlear Implant. *Adv. Oto-Rhino-Laryngol.* **38**.

CONWAY, M.J. and BOYLE, P. (1989). Design of the UCH/RNID cochlear implant system. *J. Laryngol. Otol.* suppl. 18, 4–10.

COOPER, H.R., CARPENTER, L., ALEKSY, W., BOOTH, C.L., READ, T.E., GRAHAM, J.M. and FRASER, J.G. (1989). UCH/RNID single channel extracochlear implant; results in thirty profoundly deafened adults. *J. Laryngol. Otol.* suppl. 18, 22–38.

DOERING, W.H. and SCHNEIDER, L. (1989). Electrical vs acoustical speech patterns of German phonemes using the Nucleus CI-system. In: Fraysse, B.H. (ed.), *Cochlear Implants: Acquisitions and Controversies*, pp. 243–253. Toulouse: Paragraphic.

EDDINGTON, D.K. (1980). Speech discrimination in deaf subjects with cochlear implants. *J. Acoust. Soc. Am.* **82**, 1503–1511.

GAME, C.J.A., THOMSON, D.R. and GIBSON, W.P.R. (1990). Measurement of auditory brainstem responses evoked by electrical stimulation with a cochlear implant. *Br. J. Audiol.* **24**, 145–149.

GANTZ, B.J., McCABE, B.F., TYLER, R.S. and PREECE, J.P. (1987). Evaluation of four cochlear implant designs. *Ann. Otol. Rhinol. Laryngol.* suppl. 128, 145–147.

HOCHMAIR, E.S. and HOCHMAIR-DESOYER, I.J. (1985). Aspects of sound signal processing using the Vienna intra- and extra cochlear implants. In: Schindler, R.A. and Merzenich, M.M. (eds), *Cochlear Implants*, pp. 101–110. New York: Raven Press.

HOCHMAIR-DESOYER, I.J. (1986). Fitting of an analogue cochlear-prosthesis: Introduction of a new method and preliminary findings. *Br. J. Audiol.* **20**, 45–53.

HORTMANN, G., PULEC, J.L., CAUSSE, J., BRIAND, C., FONTAINE, J.P., TETY, F. and AZEMA, B. (1989). Experience with the extracochlear multi-channel Implex system. In: Fraysse, B.H. (ed.) *Cochlear Implants: Acquisitions and Controversies.* Toulouse: Paragraphic.

JERGER, J., OLIVER, T.A. and CHMIEL, R.A. (1988). Prediction of dynamic range for stapedius reflex in cochlear implant patients. *Ear Hear.* **9**, 4–8.

MILLER, J. and PFINGST, B.E. (1984). Cochlear implants. In: Berlin, C.J. (ed.), *Hearing Science: Recent Advances*, pp. 309–339. San Diego: College-Hill Press.

PARKIN, J. and STEWART, B.E. (1988). Multi channel cochlear implantation: Utah design. *Laryngoscope* **98**, 491–502.

PEETERS, S., OFFECIERS, F.E., MARQUET, J. and VAN CAMP, K. (1989). The Laura Cochlear prosthesis: technical aspects. In Fraysse, B.H. (ed.), *Cochlear Implants: Acquisitions and Controversies*. Toulouse: Paragraphic.

PFINGST, B.E., SPELMAN, F.A. and SUTTON, D. (1980). Operating ranges for cochlear implants. *Ann. Otol. Rhinol. Laryngol.* **89**(suppl. 66), 1–4.

THIELEMEIR, M.A., TONOKAWA, L.L., PETERSEN, B. and EISENBERG, L.S. (1985). Audiological results in children with a cochlear implant. *Ear Hear.* **6**, suppl. 3.

TYLER, R.S. (1988). Open set word recognition with the 3M Vienna single channel cochlear implant. *Arch. Otolaryngol.* **114**, 1123–1126.

TYLER, R.S., MOORE, B.C. and KUK, F.K. (1989). Performance of some of the better cochlear-implant patients: *J. Speech Hear. Res.* **32**, 887–911.

Chapter 14
Training and Rehabilitation for Cochlear Implant Users

HUW COOPER

Introduction

It is now generally accepted that, for most cochlear implant users, some form of training process is necessary in order for them to obtain the maximum possible benefit from their devices. In most cases, the provision of the implant hardware following surgery, without an accompanying training programme, would be likely to markedly limit, or at least delay, the benefit received and so reduce the 'success rate' among implantees. In view of this, nearly all active implant programmes include an element of training, often with specialist personnel employed exclusively for this purpose. The degree, type and intensity of the training provided does, however, vary considerably from centre to centre. In some cases the basic minimum is provided, amounting to little more than instructions on how to operate the controls of the sound processor. In others a comprehensive, intensive, long-term training process is entered by each patient going through implant surgery.

At least one manufacturer of the implant hardware (Nucleus/Cochlear) acknowledges the value of training to the extent that they make strong recommendations concerning the training which should accompany the use of their device, and provide a comprehensive, detailed manual for this purpose.

Before discussing in more detail methods and approaches to training of this sort, it is important to put the subject into context. Providers of cochlear implants are not merely issuing a particular piece of hardware to carefully selected individuals who have met stringent criteria. They should also be deeply involved in the rehabilitation of profoundly or totally deaf people. Cochlear implantation is just one option that is available in a range of treatments and approaches, from which professionals in the rehabilitation team select that which is most appropriate for each individual, based on the results of detailed evaluation for each case. Training programmes

are needed by all the patients receiving rehabilitation, whether the
hardware they are fitted with is a cochlear implant, a hearing aid or a
vibrotactile aid. The general approach used will be broadly similar in each
case, although there will be some differences related to the differences in
the nature of the information provided by different prostheses.

There is a huge literature on 'aural rehabilitation' in the hearing impaired
and many of the techniques developed in this area are applicable equally
to cochlear implantation. Some of the controversies concerning the
relative effectiveness of different techniques are also not new. It is
surprising, however, how little has been written on the training of cochlear
implant users. Even large international conferences on implants frequently
include only a handful of papers on the topic.

What follows is an overview of some of the issues involved, with the
emphasis on practical guidelines and methodology. Chapter 15 is an
example of a real programme that has been enormously successful and
which should stand as a model of how rehabilitation of the hearing
impaired can be done in a carefully thought out, scientific way.

Personnel

There are no hard-and-fast rules concerning the qualifications of the
personnel involved with rehabilitation in profound deafness. There are,
however, clear areas of skill and knowledge which are prerequisites. All
those working in this field, regardless of their particular specialisation,
need a sound knowledge of acoustics, particularly the acoustics of speech,
some understanding of the principles of psychological testing, the basics
of phonetics and linguistics and (very importantly) an understanding of
the functioning of the cochlear implant and of the sounds which an implant
user is likely to be receiving. It is clearly also essential to have good
communication skills with deaf people, to have a patient and caring
approach, and preferably to have some knowledge of counselling techniques.

This may seem to be asking a lot from each person. In fact, each member
of the rehabilitation team brings different skills and knowledge and so one
complements the other, as already described in Chapter 5. When put
together, a good all-round approach is achieved which might not be
possible if one professional were working in isolation. A team approach is
therefore vital for this reason and also because it avoids placing all the
responsibility (and workload) for training on one person's shoulders.

Training of professionals in this field varies from country to country. In
the UK, there has been somewhat more specialisation, with speech
therapists, audiologists, hearing therapists and teachers of the deaf all
undergoing distinct training. These four professions ideally form the core
of the rehabilitation team. In other countries, where hearing therapists do

not exist as such, these functions may be served by speech pathologists, audiologists or 'aural rehabilitationalists'. Beyond this central core there are certain other key professions with which collaboration is beneficial. The clinical psychologist with specialised knowledge of hearing impairment has a valuable contribution to make. In some cases the involvement of the social worker for the deaf is also called for. Technical support from the hospital's medical physics department is also crucial when dealing with complex technology.

Equipment

A large proportion of this type of work requires only the simplest of equipment: a room, two chairs and the live voice of the therapist.* Many therapists also utilise a variety of other pieces of hardware which are helpful to the training process.

Visual speech displays

Computer-based visual displays of speech have been used extensively in the rehabilitation of cochlear implant users. There are two types of display: those that analyse a signal representing changing electrical resistance across the larynx via electrode input and those that analyse an acoustic signal via microphone input. The visual display enables the trainer to provide immediate or delayed visual feedback of the speech signal to the cochlear implant user. Visual feedback is withdrawn as soon as the implant user is able to discriminate the contrast being worked on by auditory input alone. It also enables the trainers to monitor their own speech to ensure that they are providing consistent stimuli. In addition to their use as a training device, the visual display can be used to provide a record (on disk or hard copy) of the implant user's speech production in both histogram and statistical form. These characteristics can be found in most of the available models. There are inevitably advantages and disadvantages to different types of display. Table 14.1 gives details of some of the most commonly used computer-based displays of speech.

The choice of a particular model is usually guided by personal preference of the trainer, financial constraints and whether or not the equipment has already been provided in the unit. Some people find the models using an acoustic signal via microphone input more 'user friendly', as some patients find the throat electrodes uncomfortable and getting a good contact can sometimes be difficult. However, the wave-by-wave analysis available from the throat electrodes is extremely useful for

---

*'Therapist' will be used throughout to denote the professional providing the training.

Table 14.1 Some currently available systems for visual speech display

Model name (manufacturer)	Electrode (E) or microphone (M) input	Pitch/time display	Intensity/ energy time display	Wave- form analysis	Vowel quality
Laryngograph (Laryngograph Ltd)	E	*		*	
Soundtrack (Jessops)	M	*	*		
Speech Viewer (IBM)	M	*	*		*
Visipitch (Kay)	M	*	*		*
Visispeech (SCI Instruments)	M	*	*		
Voiscope (Laryngograph Ltd)	E	*		*	

*Indicates that the facility is available.

research purposes. Some models have additional features (such as automatic intensity analyser, overwrite facility or games) which may influence choice of display.

Recorded materials

A system for playback of audio or audiovisual recorded materials is often used. It must be emphasised, however, that recorded material cannot be a substitute for live speech or environmental sounds; it can be used within a training programme to supplement the 'live' sound input, but should not replace it entirely. This will comprise either audio-tape, video tape, or video disc. A good quality audio-cassette recorder is the simplest of these, and random access, as described in Chapter 15, greatly increases the flexibility, although access times on conventional audio tape are slow. For presentation of audiovisual material, video disc has now become widely available at an affordable cost and again has the great advantage of very rapid random access, as well as picture quality superior to video tape. Interactive video systems are now used extensively and software and materials have been developed in several centres for audiovisual training (described in more detail below). For self-administered training exercises, domestic-standard (VHS) video is often used, as a majority of households now have video machines, or can be loaned a VHS recorder for the duration of the training period. For sound-only self-training, simple exercises can be recorded on tape for the Dixon's Language Master which patients can then practise with on their own at home.

It is obviously necessary to avoid using any test materials in training. If sentence or word lists are used, careful note must be taken of which lists are used so that these do not form part of tests at a later stage. Materials for training are often recorded 'in house' and selected carefully to fit in with the training programme. Exercises graded in a hierarchy of difficulty can be developed so that patients can proceed at their own pace.

Video

Video is used to record patients' communication abilities, social skills, listening tactics etc., in controlled situations in the hospital or even in the home. A permanent video set-up is the ideal, preferably using a one-way mirror so that patients are unaware of the filming. Subtle changes in behaviour and performance over time can then be monitored using repeated recordings.

Musical instruments

These are used by some therapists in training on listening skills. An electronic keyboard/synthesiser is particularly effective as such a wide range of sounds can be produced. At a simpler level, instruments more normally used in the auditory training of deaf children, such as tone bars, tambourines etc., can also be used. Whatever instrument is used, the musical sounds cannot be used as a substitute for speech. Patients do enjoy listening to musical instruments, particularly at the beginning of the training programme, but their use should be restricted to a limited number of sessions interspersed with training using speech.

Goals in Rehabilitation

There is considerable evidence that performance with an implant as assessed (mainly) by measures of speech perception generally improves over time. For example, Tye-Murray and Tyler (1990) showed that for nearly all of a set of audio-only speech perception tests, performance of 16 multichannel implant users improved significantly between 1 month and 9 months postoperatively, but not between 9 and 18 months. In other words, the full potential benefit of a cochlear implant is not apparent immediately, but patients learn to make use of the new auditory input over time (even in multichannel implants as were used in the aforementioned study). Most workers agree that a systematic training programme can enhance and accelerate this learning process.

Lansing and Davis (1988) describe the rehabilitation process as having three main goals:

1. Development of realistic expectations concerning the outcome of cochlear implantation.
2. Provision of systematic auditory and audiovisual training.
3. Provision of training in communication skills.

This definition emphasises the wide scope of the rehabilitative process as a whole. Many other writers on the subject take a somewhat narrower view, concentrating on the second of these goals: auditory training. For example, Abberton et al. (1985) stated: 'The rehabilitative task in electrical hearing is to teach the listener to relate the new sensations provided by cochlear stimulation to auditory patterns which were familiar before his total deafness.' This definition is based on a highly speech-centred, analytical approach to training and does not, therefore, take into account the wider goals of rehabilitation of which auditory training is just one element.

Bamford (1981) provided a useful consensus definition of the aims of auditory training. He was concerned with the rehabilitation of the hearing impaired as a whole, not specifically the cochlear implant user, but the definition can be applied to the latter case equally well: 'to encourage an allocation of cognitive resources to the residual hearing in such a way as to improve the encoding and decoding processes basic to auditory learning.' In this context, the words 'auditory sensations provided by the implant' need to be substituted for 'residual hearing'. He goes on to describe auditory training as 'learning to attend' and points out that it cannot be expected to improve peripheral sensitivity. Instead, it is discrimination that can be improved with training. In other words, even if an implant user's basic psychophysical abilities do not improve over time, his or her ability to attend to and make use of cues can improve and training is aimed at directing attention to these cues by maximising exposure to them in a controlled way. For example, even if a patient's gap-detection threshold remains constant over time, his or her ability to make use of an awareness of the presence and duration of gaps in speech sounds can improve, leading to enhanced recognition of voiced/voiceless contrasts.

Methods

As described by Rubinstein and Boothroyd (1987), there are three main approaches to 'aural rehabilitation' in the hearing impaired in general:

1. Counselling, discussion and support without any specific 'drill work' or training.
2. 'Synthetic' or 'global' training, where systematic instruction is given using sentence-level speech materials.
3. 'Analytical' training where the emphasis is on the recognition and discrimination of particular components of speech such as consonants, vowels and suprasegmental aspects (intonation, syllable number etc.).

These three basic approaches are equally applicable to the training of cochlear implant recipients. A balanced, carefully planned training programme will include all three of these elements as all three approaches give different benefits and are complementary.

Counselling

All cochlear implant recipients will benefit from the first of the approaches described above: ongoing support, encouragement and counselling throughout a very disorienting and emotional period. Much of this will focus on: discussion of the new sounds being experienced following acquisition of the implant; expectations regarding achievable goals; and ways to use the implant most effectively in differing communicative situations. More in-depth, non-directive counselling may also be appropriate to allow patients to talk about their feelings, hopes and fears regarding their deafness and the new possibilities available to them with the implant. The 'client-centred' approach developed by Rogers (1951) is specifically adhered to by some groups (e.g. Eisenwort, Brauneis and Burian, 1985). Therapists may feel in need of additional training in counselling techniques to have the confidence to carry out this work. Some group work, allowing interaction with other implant users, can be beneficial and most patients find this a valuable source of reassurance. Where possible, the patient's family should also participate in at least some counselling sessions. They have an important role to play in the development of the patient's communication skills with the implant and as providers of continuing support at home, particularly in cases where the patient's attendance for professional help is limited.

Auditory/audiovisual training

One of the controversies that has raged in the field of aural rehabilitation has concerned the relative merits of analytical and synthetic or 'global' training. Several attempts have been made to compare the effectiveness of the two approaches in cochlear implant users, but no clear evidence of superiority of one over the other has emerged (Boothroyd et al., 1987; Rubinstein and Boothroyd, 1987). A balanced programme incorporating both types of training is therefore probably most effective, e.g. the one described by Lansing and Davis (1988), and the one developed at University College Hospital, London (Aleksy et al., 1990). As already mentioned, the two approaches are complementary. Skills learned during analytical training can then be integrated into more life-like communication in synthetic-type training. A breakdown of the types of task involved in each approach is shown in Figure 14.1.

Analytical training

This level of training concentrates on the development of skills in the discrimination and recognition of particular features of speech. In all

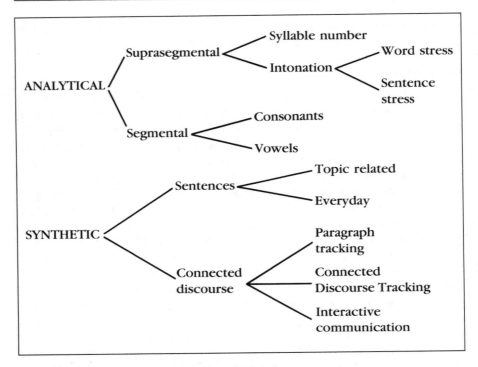

Figure 14.1. A breakdown of typical tasks in analytical and synthetic training.

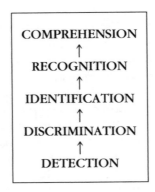

Figure 14.2. Hierarchy of processes in speech perceptual training.

analytical training, a hierarchy of difficulty is used so that the patient is allowed to progress at his or her own pace from easy to more difficult tasks. A skilled therapist will ensure that at each point the patient is achieving an encouraging level of success whilst at the same time gently pushing him or her forward.

As mentioned above, a visual speech display can provide both therapist and patient with a visual representation of the particular contrast being worked on. The contrast is then presented first with sound, lipreading and visual display; then with sound only and visual display; and finally with sound alone. Training can be given at both segmental and suprasegmental levels of speech.

Development of speech perceptual skills and the training aimed at enhancing them progress through five main stages as shown in Figure 14.2.

Detection

The very first stage involves the awareness of the presence or absence of sounds and the gross temporal pattern of speech segments. Training at this level is given at the beginning of the training programme, following first acquisition of the implant during basic 'tuning in'.

Discrimination

The next step in training on any particular speech feature is aimed at developing awareness of the difference between two sounds using a same/different task. A minimal pair is selected to emphasise the feature being worked on, e.g. voiced vs voiceless consonant. First, three from one of the minimal pair are presented followed by a change to the other, e.g. 'AMA', 'AMA', 'AMA', 'APA'. This makes clear to the patient the difference between the two sounds. Next sounds are presented in pairs and the patient is asked to state whether they are the same or different. They are not required to identify which sound is which, only whether there is a difference or not.

Identification

Tasks at this level require the patient to select the correct response from a closed set, starting with a minimal pair as described above and progressing to larger sets. To do this they need not only to detect the sounds and discriminate between them, but to identify correctly which is which. One sound is presented at a time. As the size of the response set is increased, the task becomes more difficult and is nearer to the next step – recognition.

Recognition

At this level, no response set is given to the patient and the task is open-set. A sound is presented and the patient must identify it. Direct or indirect clues can be given to help make the task less difficult. Even with these, this sort of task is significantly harder for most patients and some may not be able to carry it out at all.

Comprehension

At this, the highest level, sounds must not only be identified and recognised, but their meaning understood. Patients are required to give more than repetition or imitation of sounds. They must demonstrate that they are able to make use of the sounds heard in an interactive way in natural communication.

Some of the tasks involved in analytical training will now be outlined in brief. Further detail and suitable materials will be found in the manuals listed at the end of the chapter.

Suprasegmental level

Syllable number

One of the very first discriminations a new cochlear implant user is able to make concerns the gross temporal structure of speech segments. At the simplest level, this will mean counting the number of sounds heard in each segment. The next step is to identify the number of sounds within shorter segments, i.e. words. Training on the number of syllables in a word can begin with nonsense syllables, such as /ba//ba//ba/. Varying numbers of sounds are presented, without lipreading, and the patient's task is to report how many sounds they have heard. Following this, real words can be introduced, selected to give clear syllable boundaries.

Intonation

Intonation carries important information concerning meaning and emotional tone in both single words and sentences. The concept of the fluctuations in voice pitch is a difficult one even for normally hearing people and the visual speech display is essential for patients to understand the nature of the feature they are working on. Initially single vowels are presented with either flat, falling or rising pitch; a prolonged duration is used at first, moving on to a more natural duration once the patient is able to make the discrimination. The next step is to move on to single real words, selected to contain mainly voiced sounds (e.g. moon, around etc.) again presented with a flat, falling or rising contour. Single words in which stress placement is variable and changes meaning are then introduced, e.g. object, contract etc. The relevance of intonation in sentence meaning can then be clarified by tasks using sentences. The same sentence is presented repeatedly with variable stress pattern; the patient's task is to identify the nucleus, or 'the most important word', e.g. my OLD car vs MY old car etc. Another task is to present a sentence in which the final word could have either a falling or rising pitch contour, thus changing it from a statement to a question, e.g. 'She drove the car!' vs 'She drove the car?'.

Segmental level

Consonants

Much analytical work will concentrate on discrimination and recognition of consonants, as they carry the most information in speech whilst at the same time presenting the lipreader with the most difficult problems. Nonsense syllables consisting of intervocalic consonants (e.g. 'AMA', 'ADA', 'AGA' etc.) may be used and have the advantage that they allow the patient to concentrate on the particular contrast being worked on without the distraction of differing adjacent phonemes.

Intervocalic nonsense syllables are presented initially in pairs (in the way described above) that, for example, differ only in voicing but have the same place and manner of articulation (homorganic), e.g. 'ADA' vs 'ATA'; 'AZA' vs 'ASA'. Once two different pairs have been worked on and the therapist is satisfied that the patient is able to make each discrimination (achieving 8 out of 10 correct or better), all four consonants are presented at random as a closed-set task. As more pairs are mastered, the size of the set is increased, to 6, 8 and finally 12 consonants. Initial or final consonants in real words can then be introduced, with a similar progression from minimal pairs to larger closed sets. Eventually, sentence pairs incorporating a consonant contrast are brought in (e.g. 'I want a new FAN' vs 'I want a new VAN').

Vowels

A similar progression from simple to more complex tasks is used. Vowels can be presented initially in isolation, in minimal pairs, first with a flat intonation and prolonged duration, moving on to natural intonation and duration, e.g. /a/ vs /i/ or /o/ vs /e/. Vowels in real words, in pairs and then in closed sets are introduced, e.g. heed vs hard etc. As above, words in sentences would then be the next step.

Synthetic training

'Synthetic' speech perceptual training involves mainly sentence-level materials or connected discourse (running speech). The aim is to make use of the skills acquired by the patient in analytical training in tasks that are more 'natural' and closer to real life communication. Conversation is the most natural of these tasks and provides valuable training in itself. The remaining tasks break speech down into smaller segments and are more structured. Brief mention of each of the commonly used methods will follow, but for more detail and suitable materials readers should again refer to the manuals listed at the end of the chapter.

Paragraph tracking

This exercise, also known as text-following, is often one of the first that is introduced to new implant users. Therapist and patient each have identical copies of the same text, which is selected to contain a level of vocabulary and syntax appropriate for each patient's abilities, and in some cases a particular balance of monosyllables, spondees or multisyllabic words. The therapist reads the text and the patient follows it (without lipreading) using a pointer or finger. This allows the trainer to observe that the patient is keeping up. The task makes use of skills developed in analytical training at the suprasegmental level (syllable number, word number etc.) and provides practice in recognising the gross temporal structure of speech.

Sentence length/pattern recognition (sound alone)

A closed set of sentences or phrases of varying length and pattern are used. The task can be done as a discrimination exercise (two sentences are presented and the patient states whether they are the same or different) or as an identification task (the patient identifies which sentence has been read from a closed set of two or more). The aim is to give further practice on the recognition of prosodic (duration and pattern) cues.

Topic-related sentences

These are widely used in synthetic speech perceptual training. A list of sentences is presented, all about the same topic. This provides strong contextual information which makes the task far less daunting to patients than truly open-set sentences, and they often enjoy it for that reason. The sentences can be presented with lipreading in most cases, or in the sound-alone condition for patients who are able to discriminate some speech without lipreading. Lists of suitable sentences are found in the manuals listed at the end of the chapter.

Everyday sentences

These are one step on from topic-related sentences. There is no context and the task is truly open set. The only constraining factor is that the sentences are 'everyday' and so do not contain complex or unusual vocabulary or syntax, and are intended to have a high probability of occurrence in real life, e.g. 'What's the time please?', 'Please pass the salt'. Again, these will be presented with lipreading in most cases.

As this is a more difficult task, a smaller proportion of patients will be capable of performing it in the sound-alone condition.

Connected Discourse Tracking (CDT)

This procedure, developed by deFillipo and Scott (1978), is the most frequently used and well-known form of synthetic training. Text is read to the patient segment by segment and the task is to repeat back every word. A verbatim repetition must be achieved and the therapist uses a set of strategies and tactics to help the patient do this. The choice of which tactic or strategy to use may be made by the therapist, or by the patient; the latter approach has the advantage that the patient receives excellent training in controlling the communication situation. This approach has been particularly advocated by the team based at the University of California at San Francisco (Owens and Telleen, 1981). A clear description of the methods that can be used in CDT is available on video (Cochlear Corporation, 1985).

Typical strategies that are used are:

1. Repetition of a word, phrase or sentence.
2. Emphasis of a particular word or phrase.
3. Change in the rate of presentation.
4. Change in the length of the segment: it may be shortened, or a difficult word isolated, or lengthened to provide more contextual information.
5. 'Aside': a clue can sometimes be given to help with a particularly difficult word, e.g. 'I'm talking about something you sit on – a CHAIR'.
6. Reaffirm.

Once a word has been correctly repeated using one of the above strategies, it can be put back in the sentence: 'That's right – CHAIR. He put the book on the CHAIR.'

Tactics which are used include the following:

1. Prompters, e.g. 'That's right!', 'What was the last word?' etc.
2. Hand signals: these are not used by all therapists, and some may feel their use is inappropriate. Examples are: one hand raised to tell the patient to wait; one finger used to 'underline' a word in the air; 'bracketing' of a word using two hands to clarify which parts of a sentence the patient has correctly identified. More complex signals such as meaningful gestures or actual signs should not be used.

The text used must be carefully selected to be appropriate to each patient's lipreading and language ability. Some patients are able to perform the task in the sound-alone condition for which simpler texts will probably be required. The procedure can be timed to give a words/minute score. This allows therapist and patient to keep track of progress over time. Allowances must clearly be made for changes in speaker, text, and conditions, such as lighting etc., all of which can have a significant effect on the rate achieved.

CDT is one of the closest tasks to real conversation and most patients find it rewarding. If the 'San Francisco' method is used, and the listener has control over the choice of strategies or tactics used, it gives valuable practice in assertiveness and communication skills. It is also an exercise which the patient's family or friends can learn to carry out at home, after some training from the therapist. It can also be used as a measure of performance. A score can be obtained for each condition (sound + vision, vision alone and sound alone) to give a measure of the contribution of the sound input to lipreading. The difficulty with its application as a numerical measure of performance in this way is the variety of factors which affect the score, as mentioned above. The problems of standardisation of CDT scores have led some groups (e.g. the University of Iowa) to abandon it as a performance measure. Despite this, it clearly has a major role to play in synthetic training and will continue to be used by many therapists.

Interactive Communication Training (ICT)

This method is similar in approach to CDT in that text is read to the patient. The difference is that instead of simply repeating back every word, the listener must not only discriminate the speech but demonstrate comprehension of it. A passage, selected to contain appropriate vocabulary and syntax, is read. The patient requests the speaker to repeat a word or sentence if necessary. Once the whole passage has been read and the listener reports that they have received all of it satisfactorily, his or her comprehension of it is assessed with a set of questions. For example, following a piece about the price of food in supermarkets, one question might be: 'Which foods are cheap and which are expensive in supermarkets?' Along with quite specific questions based on the content of the passage, more general conversation can follow on the same topic, e.g. 'Do you shop in a supermarket or in the corner shop?'. This technique is the closest so far described to 'real' communication. The listener is encouraged to control the situation as they would do in a genuine interaction. It gives practice at all the levels of speech perception: detection, discrimination, recognition and comprehension. Thus it is the most complete communication exercise and has great value.

Communication Skills Training

Understandably, most deafened adults find interaction and spoken communication with others difficult. The limited information afforded by a cochlear implant should help to make the understanding of speech less taxing, but the communicative situation may still be daunting, tiring and difficult. Effective communication strategies can help to overcome some of these difficulties. Deafened adults often develop unhelpful strategies such as speaking constantly in order to avoid the problems of receiving speech, or failing to maintain eye contact and pay attention to facial expression.

In addition to the perceptual training described above, training in communication skills is beneficial for cochlear implant users as much as for other hearing-impaired people, and should therefore be part of the rehabilitation programme.

The techniques of communication skills training are well known among those involved in the rehabilitation of the hearing impaired and are well documented (e.g. see Brooks and Cleaver, 1989, for a concise review). Counselling, role-play and group work are used to develop effective strategies. The term 'hearing tactics' is used widely to denote the strategies that are used to facilitate communication. These are concerned with two main aims:

1. The optimisation of the acoustic and visual environment for reception of auditory and visual (facial) information. This refers to the organisation of the speaker, listener and lighting in such a way as to give the clearest possible view of the speaker's face and the best possible signal-to-noise ratio of the speech signal.
2. Conversational techniques: effective two-way spoken communication requires complex listening skills. These include paying attention to facial expression and non-verbal cues to meaning, appropriate turn-taking in conversation, providing appropriate feedback, having the confidence to say when something has been missed and ask for it to be repeated, and so on. These skills are of course needed by both members of the conversational pair. The implant user's spouse or partner may require just as much help with his or her communication technique and should be offered advice on this where necessary.

Environmental Sounds

Cochlear implant users gain significant benefit from the awareness of environmental (non-speech) sounds that their devices can provide. Many new implant users find that environmental sounds are confusing, or even in some cases unpleasant at first. There is clearly a period of learning involved in the perception of these sounds as there is for speech. Although the implant gives nearly continuous exposure to non-speech sounds in everyday life, some therapists believe that systematic training with recorded or live material is useful to enhance the process of learning to discriminate and identify sounds. This training can take three main forms: first, the presentation of 'live' sounds within the therapist's room, such as running water, drawers opening etc.; secondly, the use of sounds on audio tape; and thirdly, environmental sound 'walks' outside in the street or elsewhere.

Automation of Training

As seen above, speech perceptual training is very labour intensive and time consuming. For this reason, there have been various attempts over recent years to develop systems for automated training, whereby patients can give themselves practice on simple speech perceptual exercises without a therapist being present.

One of the simplest methods for achieving this is Dixon's Language Master. In this, stimuli such as single words are recorded on short segments of audio tape stuck to cards. Patients can play back each stimulus, as many times as they wish, by passing the tape-card through the machine. This method has the advantages that it is simple and cheap, but is limited by the fact that only an audio recording is used and the length of the stimuli is restricted to short segments.

A more advanced system using digital audio tape is the one described by Birgit Cook in Chapter 15, in which the tape-recorder is brought under computer control.

The great step forward in this area has been the development of video/ computer-based training systems. In early 1979, the Data Analysis Video Interactive Device (DAVID) developed at NTID was described (Sims et al., 1979). The implant programme at the University of California, San Francisco used a video recorder interfaced with an Apple computer (Owens, 1983). The team at Stockholm have developed their own system using computer-controlled video tape, again described by Birgit Cook in Chapter 15. Another computer-controlled interactive video system has been developed at the City University, New York (Boothroyd, 1987). These systems demonstrated that automated, computer-controlled systems were a valuable contribution to the training process. Their main limitation was that video tape does not permit very rapid random access to recorded materials. The advent of video disc has meant that such access is now possible and has opened up exciting new possibilities for training systems. Perhaps the best example of the use of video disc for this purpose is the system which has been developed at the University of Iowa. In this, an IBM personal computer with touch-screen monitor controls a Pioneer laser video disc player. A graded series of training exercises is available, mainly aimed at the development of communication skills in children, but equally applicable in parts to adults. These exercises range from quite analytical tasks on consonant discrimination in words through to sentences presented in simulated real-life communication situations such as, for example, a receptionist in a doctor's surgery. The listener is given a set of options to choose from in order to improve the intelligibility of each sentence. These are strategies such as moving closer to the speaker, asking the speakers to remove their hands from their mouths etc. The chosen strategy is selected by touching the screen in the appropriate place.

The touch-sensitive screen is probably the optimal method for patient response as it makes no requirement of the patient for keyboard skills. Patients enjoy the immediate control they can have over the video. One limitation of this method is that only closed-set responses can be made. The input of open-set responses poses a special problem for computer-controlled training systems. Electronic speech recognition is not yet sufficiently advanced to be applicable and patients cannot be expected to have typing skills good enough to type in their own responses. This makes the prospect of a completely automated version of Connected Discourse Tracking seem unlikely. A partial solution is the semi-automated version used at the City University, New York (Boothroyd, 1987). In this, patients give their spoken responses to an experimenter who then enters them on the computer using a code-system.

Computer-assisted training programmes such as those described clearly have a role to play as a supplement to 'live' training provided by the therapist, although they cannot be used as a substitute for it. Interactive video-disc systems are now widely used and offer the greatest potential for development of advanced training programmes. There will, however, be a need to pool resources. The production of a new video-disc master is a very lengthy and expensive process. For example, the University of Iowa system has taken 3 years and six computer programmers to complete. Hopefully, those without the resources available to carry out this sort of development will be able to make use of systems produced at centres who do have access to the skills and personpower required.

Manuals

A number of written manuals have been produced with the aim of providing therapists with detailed guidelines and materials for training of cochlear implant users. *Commtram*, written by Geoff Plant in Sydney, is one of the most comprehensive of these and is intended for use with profoundly deafened adults, including cochlear implant, vibrotactile aid and hearing aid users. It includes considerable discussion of the theoretical bases of the training, as well as a good quantity of materials organised into exercise format. The *Nucleus/Cochlear Rehabilitation Manual* is intended specifically for the Nucleus multichannel implant and contains rather less on the theory behind the training, but it does give a wide selection of materials and exercises graded into four levels of difficulty. These levels follow the hierarchy of performance as described above, progressing from detection to discrimination and then to identification, recognition and finally comprehension.

Both these manuals have a broadly similar approach. All of the training uses real words and sentences, with a strong emphasis on synthetic tasks. They differ in that *Commtram* has an extra section on speech production which is absent from the *Nucleus Manual*, whilst the latter has a useful section on telephone training which does not feature in *Commtram*. They are both a very useful source of training materials and most therapists will find access to them very valuable.

A manual with a slightly different approach has been produced by the rehabilitation team at University College Hospital, London. This is intended for use with single-channel implants and has much more of a balance between analytical and synthetic tasks.

Full details for each of the manuals are given in the references (Plant, 1984; Mecklenburg, Dowell and Jenison, 1989; Aleksy et al., 1990).

Evaluation

Although most professionals involved in the rehabilitation of cochlear implant recipients believe that systematic training is worth while and can lead to a significantly better outcome, and can frequently give anecdotal evidence to support this view, there are disappointingly few hard data available from properly conducted studies to back up their opinion. There are others in the field of rehabilitation of the hearing impaired who have expressed great scepticism about the value of auditory training. For example, Ross (1987) said: 'What I am questioning is whether therapeutic intervention for the specific purpose of improving speech perception, either visually or auditorily, can be supported by the evidence.' He was mainly referring to so-called 'lipreading classes' rather than the specific training given to cochlear implant users as described in this chapter, but his remarks do reflect a feeling among some professionals that the evidence to justify the time and effort invested in training is not yet available. It is important to be clear about which aspects of an implant user's abilities can be expected to be improved through training. There is no clear evidence to suggest that lipreading ability, for example, can be significantly improved by formal instruction. This has led some to question the value of the 'lipreading class' (e.g. Brooks, 1989). These classes can give the hearing impaired very real benefits in terms of increased confidence and communication skills but are unlikely to enhance lipreading skills per se. As already mentioned, peripheral sensitivity cannot be expected to be improved through training although discrimination and recognition can.

However, there have been some attempts to measure the benefit provided by training, with various conclusions. Unfortunately, as pointed out by Bamford (1981), many of the reported studies did not use adequate control groups, if at all. The experimental design of studies of this type is inherently difficult because of the huge variability between patients on motivational level, intelligence, communication ability etc. For this reason a single-subject experimental design is often used. Some studies have produced discouraging results. For example, Boothroyd et al. (1987) found that the biggest improvements in performance resulted simply in the acquisition of the implant, with training only having a small effect. In another report, Boothroyd et al. (1987) examined the effects of training on six patients and concluded that for the combined lipreading and implant condition, formal training was unnecessary for successful implantees, and 'ineffective' for unsuccessful ones. Differences between successful and unsuccessful patients were apparently seen immediately following implantation. They went on to suggest that formal training was only helpful in the audio-alone condition and that sufficient practice in the implant/lipreading combination was usually to be had in everyday life. These conclusions must be treated with caution. Only speech–perceptual performance was assessed, without a proper measure of overall benefit. Although there is no doubt that some very successful patients can achieve their full potential rapidly without formal training, such cases are probably in a minority and they will still benefit from ongoing counselling and support. Also, many patients may not receive very much practice in communication in everyday life, if they live alone and lead solitary lives. The key point is that every patient is different and training programmes must be flexible and tailored individually for each patient. A recent report by Gagne et al. (1990) also purported to demonstrate a 'negligible' effect of training on speech perception performance in a small group ($n=4$) of implant users. The onset of the training programme was staggered between patients over a 5-month period. It would clearly not be advisable to draw profound conclusions from such a small patient group. The training might well have had a more positive benefit if provided earlier, as this has been demonstrated to be an advantage. Lansing and Davis (1988) demonstrated that early (1 month post 'tune up') training generally had a more beneficial effect on speech perception performance than delayed (9 months) training. The effect was clearest for consonant recognition and less so for a vowel recognition task; there was also considerable variability between patients. However, they did demonstrate the clear benefit of training over and above experience alone. Lansing and Davis (1990) followed up a group of 17 patients after 18 months and found the advantage for the group receiving early training was still maintained. This study has provided some of the strongest evidence so far of the value of a systematic training programme in cochlear implantation.

It is to be hoped that more evidence of the benefit of training will be forthcoming from studies conducted with the thoroughness and scientific approach exemplified by the work of Charissa Lansing and her colleagues. It is clearly important to consider carefully what is the most appropriate measure of outcome in studies of this kind. Performance on a limited set of speech–perceptual tests is probably not sufficient to give a full picture of the benefits of training programmes. As discussed in Chapter 16, there is also a need for an assessment of the functional benefit being provided by the implant. This would include measures of communication ability in 'real life' as well as some measure of changes in the quality of life brought about by the implant. A measure of the degree to which a particular training method can give benefits that generalise to other types of task is also required. For example, analytical training on the discrimination of consonants may well lead to improved performance on a consonant recognition test, but has limited value if it does not also have a carry-over effect to other tasks such as those involving connected speech. This is the basis of one of the strongest arguments in favour of more synthetic or 'global' types of training. It will also be necessary to examine more fully the longer-term benefits of training as well as the immediate effects; to be worth while, training must lead to improvements in performance which are robust and last for some considerable time after the end of the training period.

It must be remembered that the ultimate aim of the rehabilitation process is to enhance the communication ability and quality of life of the implant user over and above that which simple provision of the implant can give. The training methods that have been described are highly time-consuming and labour-intensive. The author believes that convincing evidence to show that they can achieve these aims, which justifies the investment of time and resources that they involve, has already begun to emerge and more will be forthcoming in the very near future.

References

ABBERTON, E., FOURCIN, A.J., ROSEN, S., WALLIKER, J.R., HOWARD, D.M., MOORE, B.C.J., DOUEK, E.E. and FRAMPTON, S. (1985). Speech perceptual and productive rehabilitation in electro-cochlear stimulation. In: Schindler, R.A. and Merzenich, M.M. (eds), *Cochlear Implants*, pp. 527–538. New York: Raven Press.

ALEKSY, W., BOOTH, C.L., COOPER, H.R. and READ, T.E. (1990). *A Training Manual for use with the UCH/RNID Single Channel Cochlear Implant*. University College Hospital, London.

BAMFORD, J. (1981). Auditory training. What is it, what is it supposed to do and does it do it? *Br. J. Audiol.* **15**, 75–78.

BOOTHROYD, A. (1987). CASPER: Computer assisted speech perception evaluation and training. RESNA 10th Annual Conference, San José, California.

BOOTHROYD, A., HANIN, L., HNATH-CHISOLM, T. and WALTZMAN, S. (1987). Response of cochlear implantees to speech perception training. Presentation to Annual Convention of American Speech, Language and Hearing Association, New Orleans.

BROOKS, D.N. (1989). Lip-reading instruction and hearing aid use. *Br. J. Audiol.* **23**, 275–278.

BROOKS, D.N. and CLEAVER, V. (1989). Communication training. In: Brooks, D.N. (ed.), *Adult Aural Rehabilitation*, pp. 170–186. London: Chapman & Hall.

COCHLEAR CORPORATION (1985). 22 Channel implant and speech training (video).

DEFILIPPO, C.L. and SCOTT, B.L. (1978). A method for training and evaluating the reception of ongoing speech. *J. Acoust. Soc. Am.* **63**, 1186–1192.

EISENWORT, B., BRAUNEIS, K. and BURIAN, K. (1985). Rehabilitation of the cochlear implant patient. In: Gray, R. (ed.), *Cochlear Implants*, pp. 194–210. New York: Croom Helm.

GAGNE, J.P., PARNES, L., LaROCQUE, M. and HASSAN, R. (1990). Effect of aural rehabilitation programs for cochlear implant patients. Paper presented at 2nd International Cochlear Implant Symposium, Iowa.

LANSING, C.R. and DAVIS, J.M. (1988). Early versus delayed speech perception training for adult cochlear implant users: initial results. *J. Acad. Rehabil. Audiol.* **21**, 29–41.

LANSING, C.R. and DAVIS, J.M. (1990). Evaluating the relative contribution of aural rehabilitation and experience to the communication performance of adult cochlear implant users: preliminary data. In: Olswang, L.B., Thompson, C.K. and Warren, I.S. (eds), *Treatment Efficacy Research in Communication Disorders*, in press.

MECKLENBURG, D.J., DOWELL, R.C. and JENISON, W.W. (1989). *Nucleus 22-Channel Cochlear Implant System Rehabilitation Manual.*

OWENS, T.E. (1983). An overview of cochlear implants in relation to aural rehabilitation and habilitation. *J. Acad. Rehabil. Audiol.* **16**, 68–86.

OWENS, T.E. and TELLEEN, C.C. (1981). Tracking as an aural rehabilitative process. *J. Acad. Rehabil. Audiol.* **14**, 259–273.

PLANT, G. (1984). *Commtram: A communication training program for profoundly deafened adults.* National Acoustical Laboratories, Sydney.

ROGERS, C. (1951). *Client Centred Counselling.* Boston, MA: Houghton Mifflin.

ROSS, M. (1987). Aural rehabilitation revisited. *J. Acad. Rehabil. Audiol.* **20**, 13–23.

RUBINSTEIN, A. and BOOTHROYD, A. (1987). Effect of two approaches to auditory training on speech recognition by hearing-impaired adults. *J. Speech Hear. Res.* **30**, 153–160.

SIMS, D., VON FELDT, J., DOWALIBY, F., HUTCHINSON, K. and MEYERS, T. (1979). A pilot experiment in computer assisted speech reading instruction utilizing the Data Analysis Video Interface Device (DAVID). *Am. Ann. Deaf* **124**, 618–624.

TYE-MURRAY, N. and TYLER, R. (1990). Performance over time. Paper presented at the 2nd International Cochlear Implant Symposium, Iowa.

Chapter 15
Testing and Rehabilitation of Cochlear Implant Patients at the Department of Audiology, Södersjukhuset, Stockholm

BIRGIT O. COOK

Background

As the outcome of a conference on the subject of cochlear implants arranged by the Swedish Medical Research Council in 1983, a reference group was formed which recommended that the Department of Audiology at Södersjukhuset, Stockholm, in cooperation with the Department of Speech Communication and Music Acoustics at the Royal Institute of Technology (KTH), should undertake a cochlear implant programme. The programme was to be limited to 10 postlingually deafened adults as shown in Table 15.1. The Vienna/3M implant (an extracochlear, single-channel device) was to be used.

Regular detailed testing and a systematic postoperative training programme was to be undertaken and a thorough evaluation made of all the patients 2 years after the last patient had been implanted. The result of this evaluation was intended to be used as a direction for a future implant programme. The initial cochlear implant programme was duly completed and evaluated in March 1988. The decision was then taken to continue to use the operation in Sweden and, in those cases where it was considered appropriate, also to use intracochlear implants. By April 1989, a further six patients had been given intracochlear implants (the 22-channel Nucleus device, in all cases) (Table 15.2).

Pre- and Postoperative Testing Procedure

All patients were tested with a battery of pre- and postoperative tests. The battery consisted of a number of tests developed for other groups of

Table 15.1 Ten patients with Vienna/3M extracochlear single channel implant

Patient no.	Age at surgery (years)	Duration of deafness (years)	Aetiology
1	28	3	Progressive
2	53	37	Meningitis
3	52	7	Gentamicin
4	41	20	Skull fracture
5	54	46	Meningitis
6	25	16	Progressive
7	49	10	Progressive
8	22	2	Meningitis
9	55	4–5	Streptomycin
10	50	7	Otosclerosis

Table 15.2 Six patients with Nucleus 22-channel intracochlear implant

Patient no.	Age at surgery (years)	Duration of deafness (years)	Aetiology
11	63	10	Progressive
12	58	37	Meningitis
13	63	24	Skull fracture
14	65	3	Progressive
15	53	10	Progressive
16	36	1	Meningitis

hearing-impaired patients or developed by the manufacturer of the implant.

Preoperative testing was as follows:

1. Audiological tests with both headphones and hearing aid.
2. Psychoacoustic tests.
3. Speech perception tests: auditory, visual and audiovisual.
4. Recording of speech.
5. Promontory stimulation test.
6. Other medical tests (X-ray, balance etc.).
7. Psychological tests.

The pre- and postoperative speech–perceptual testing and all of the postoperative rehabilitation training of implant patients are undertaken by the rehabilitation unit which forms part of the Audiological Clinic and in this initial programme the following tests were used:

1. Three-digits test.
2. Consonant confusions (aCa).
3. Vowel confusions (bVb).
4. Everyday sentences.
5. Spondee test and speech-tracking.

The psychological tests used for implant patients are the following:

1. Raven's Progressive Matrices (Raven, Court and Raven, 1986): through this non-verbal test an idea is obtained of the patients' intellectual resources and the extent of their capacity to handle the new auditory stimuli that they will receive as a result of the cochlear implant.
2. WIT III (Westrin Intelligence Test III: Westrin, 1966): to measure the patients' verbal capability.
3. CMPS (Cesarec–Marke Personality Scale: Cesarec and Marke, 1967): this is a personality test used to give an indication of the patients' likely ability to make use of the implant and to benefit from the training programme.

Clinical interviews between a psychologist and the patient and, where possible, the patient's closest relative formed an integral part of the psychological assessment.

All the information gathered about the patient up to this stage was then thoroughly examined and discussed before a decision was taken as to whether or not the patient was a suitable candidate for the operation.

General Outline of Training Programme

1. Three days' training.
2. Home training programme.
3. Three days' training (intensive).
4. Home training programme.
5. One day's training per month (up to 1 year if necessary).
6. Tests at 6 months.
7. Tests at 1 year.
8. Tests at 2 years.

The postoperative rehabilitation training programme starts 4–5 weeks after the operation when the signal processor has been adjusted for the individual patient. At the outset, the programme started with a whole week of intensive training but this was found to be too much for the patients to undertake. Accordingly, the programme now starts with 3 days of exploratory tests involving discussion about the new sounds that will be experienced, the rules to be followed in speech-tracking, which forms an important part of the global training, and explanation of the two different computer programs used in the training. Experience has shown that the psychological tests carried out prior to the operation are of value in designing the rehabilitation programme for individual patients.

Preliminary Test and Training Period (3 Days)

1. Adjustment of speech processor by the technician.
2. Instructions on how to use the controls on the processor.
3. Discussion about the new sounds.
4. Information about the training programme and how to use the computers and tape-recorders.
5. Global training involving speech-tracking.
6. Assessment of voice and speech quality.
7. Assessment of whether a relaxation programme is needed.

Both the voice and the speech quality are checked to see whether voice and speech exercises and role-play ought to be included for individual patients in the programme during the training that follows. An endeavour is made to estimate each patient's degree of muscular tension to see whether relaxation exercises should be included in the programme as well. Some of the sessions are recorded on video. The patients then go home, returning the following week for intensive training, which is the first stage of an extended period based on each individual patient's need.

Intensive Training Period

1. Global and analytical training.
2. Computer-assisted training.
3. Preparation of home training material.
4. Voice, speech and relaxation training.
5. Telephone training

The training programme follows a general pattern, although adapted to suit the individual patient's needs, depending on the results of the preoperative tests and progress during the period of training. A typical day's activity during the intensive training always includes speech-tracking, and might also include voice modulation exercises, relaxation exercises, practice with the speech processor, preparation of home training material, computer-assisted training etc. A number of different computer-assisted programmes are available for auditory and audiovisual training. These programmes have been developed together with Professor Arne Risberg, KTH, Stockholm (Mizuno and Risberg, 1984). The equipment is a personal

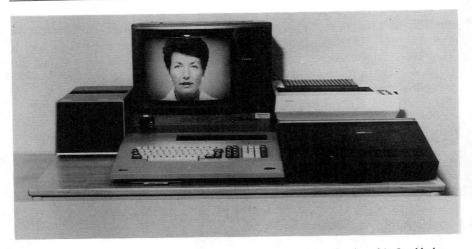

Figure 15.1. Computer-controlled system for audiovisual training developed in Stockholm, Sweden.

computer that controls a random access audio-cassette tape recorder (Figure 15.1). This computer equipment can be extended so that a video recorder can be linked to the computer, permitting the patients to exercise their audiovisual capability as well.

The program most commonly used involves the patient listening to separate tapes of environmental sounds, words, sentences, syllables etc. and choosing the correct answer from a list of up to 12 alternatives presented on the screen. The stimulus is randomly selected by the computer. Before answering, the patient can repeat the stimulus any number of times. If the correct answer is given, the image on the screen will confirm this and the next stimulus will be given. If the answer is wrong, the correct answer will be displayed on the screen and the tape recorder will repeat the stimulus to give the patient feedback of the answer. To add a further dimension to the training, the patients can practise with open lists of stimuli from the tape recorder only, and type in the answers without getting any prior guidance from the screen. As soon as the patients become fully accustomed to using the computer, they can continue on their own as the operating instructions are built into the programs. At the end of every program a printout is obtained in the form of a confusion matrix which gives valuable information as to whether the patient experienced any difficulties. The patients quickly become used to computer work, and it is obvious that they find it reassuring to be able to work with the computer on their own and to repeat the task as many times as they wish. They also appear to like the computer's quick response and its ability to score their results as a percentage.

Home training

As the subsequent training programme will increasingly consist of homework undertaken by the patient at home without direct guidance, the systematic preparation of the home training material forms an important part of the routine. The home training material consists of audio-cassette tapes made up of a range of different environmental sounds, syllables, words, phrases or stories etc. which the patients listen to while following a written text. An alert signal is recorded on the tape to keep the patient in synchrony with the text.

The therapist plays a very important role, of course, in the setting up of new home training material, but checking of the home training can mostly be done on a computer by the patients, working on their own. This checking always forms the first part of each session in order to see whether a move can be made to the next exercises or further exercises on the same level should be continued. Home training and computer-assisted training are mainly on the analytical level – to train the patients to detect differences between sounds, words etc. Training by the therapist to a large extent concentrates on global training with, for instance, Connected Discourse Tracking (CDT) (DeFilippo and Scott, 1978; Mecklenburg, 1983).

CDT has proved to be a very good exercise in increasing the patients' audiovisual and auditory comprehension and also as a good means of measuring the patients' ability to communicate. A text is read to the patient phrase by phrase, which has to be correctly repeated. The result is measured in words per minute. For comparison, the speech-tracking is performed at regular intervals without the audio signal.

Telephone training

This has been increasingly included in the programme because of the good results obtained by a number of the intracochlear-implanted patients. Such training, when necessary, starts with closed lists and develops in due course to a full conversation in those cases where this is possible.

Where a full conversational level is not achievable, the patients are encouraged to use the telephone; development of a telephone procedure among family and friends with all affirmative responses being restricted to a 'yes' and all negative responses containing such phrases as 'No, I can't', 'No, I haven't', 'No, it isn't', creates a means by which the patient can differentiate between the two forms of response.

Group Sessions

Patients who have suffered from progressive or sudden loss of hearing tend to become very isolated and so it has been found to be beneficial to arrange regular group meetings for all of the implant patients, with therapists in attendance if needed, in addition to the individual training programme. At these meetings, the patients seem to gain encouragement from each other and learn from each other's difficulties. Meetings are also arranged for patients' relatives to attend, in order for them to learn about the programmes and to be given the opportunity for discussion.

Continued Contact with Patients

One of the problems to be faced is what happens after the formal training period is over. Tests have shown that the patients continue to improve and some feel a need for further training and social contact with the unit. It is, of course, not possible to continue to include them in the on-going programme but they continue to be invited to the group sessions and are always at liberty to make use of the computer-training facilities.

Organisation of the Analytical Training Material

A training manual has been developed which is divided into seven different blocks.

Block 1

The material consists of different recorded tapes, e.g. very easy tasks involving discrimination of noise vs silence, identifying when an individual person is talking, discrimination between high and low tones with different gaps, discrimination between simple sounds, up to the difficult exercise of identifying 20 different common environmental sounds.

Block 2

This consists of 60 exercises to train the patient to learn discrimination of temporal aspects of speech, e.g. word length, sentence length, prosodic aspects of speech intonation, accent etc.

Block 3

This consists of about 100 different exercises designed to train the patient to discriminate, identify and recognise all the consonants and phonetic discrimination of sounds in the initial, medial and final position of words.

Block 4

This consists of vowel discrimination, using both real words and nonsense syllables, such as 'BAB', 'BOB', 'BIB' etc.

Block 5

This consists mostly of open lists, exercises and training in telephone usage, the latter being particularly necessary in the case of patients fitted with the 22-channel implant.

Block 6

This consists of exercises for voice and speech training and a relaxation programme.

Block 7

This includes all the testing material.

Discussion

The members of the author's group have asked themselves whether the described rehabilitation training of cochlear implant patients is essential or merely desirable, basing their judgement on experience to date. If those few patients are considered who, for a variety of reasons, have been unable to pursue the training offered to the full, the author's group has found that progress towards improved responses has reached a virtual standstill since formal training ended. Turning to those patients who remained in the course throughout, with regular attendance, a steady improvement is seen over the period of training, which will vary considerably between individual patients. However, improvement in perception and understanding of spoken language using the auditory signal alone or the auditory/ visual signals, is present to a greater or lesser degree as a result of the rehabilitation programme.

In order to demonstrate this conclusion, the case histories of two of the patients are described below.

Subject S2

Subject S2 is a male patient, 58 years of age, who was deafened as a result of meningitis as a teenager. He was totally deaf for 35 years and a very poor lipreader. He has been working as a skilled engineer, communicating mostly in writing and, together with his hearing-impaired wife and similarly handicapped friends, by Swedish sign language.

The patient has been actively participating in the rehabilitation programme since his first cochlear implant operation in 1984. Figure 15.2 shows that during the 5.5 years' period of training, using the Vienna/3M extracochlear implant, the patient doubled his pure lipreading visual perception of spoken language – but only added a few words per minute audiovisually after 12 months of training. After the patient's reoperation,

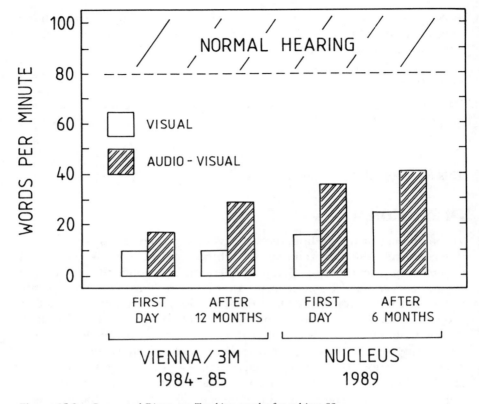

Figure 15.2. Connected Discourse Tracking results for subject S2.

with a Nucleus 22-channel intracochlear device, his audiovisual speech-tracking speed has increased in his 6 months' usage of the implant to double the speed, compared with 5.5 years ago.

The patient is still attending twice a month for training which will continue for another 6 months, but it is unlikely that any further significant improvement will be achieved.

Subject S16

Subject S16 is a female patient, 52 years of age, who, through a head injury, became hearing impaired as an 8-year-old child. She passed through the ordinary school system without having any hearing aids and became a very skilled lipreader. As an adult she evidently experimented with various conventional hearing aids, but after another accident in 1977 she became totally deaf.

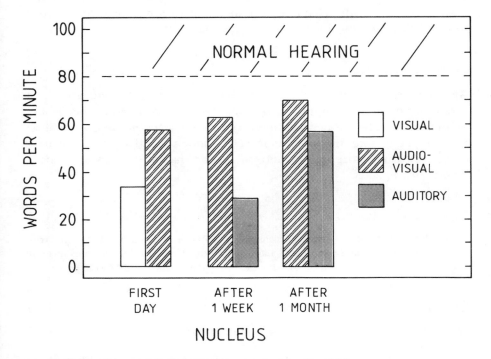

Figure 15.3. Connected Discourse Tracking results for subject S16.

Figure 15.3 shows that from the first day of training this patient demonstrated an ability to coordinate the audiovisual signals.

After the first week of training, she showed about a 10% improvement in audiovisual speech-tracking. A month later, with only home training, her speed improved nearly to the level of a normally hearing person. Performance in pure auditory perception in speech-tracking form was already better than her former lipreading understanding.

She could hold a conversation on the telephone without hesitation and with only a few mistakes. Her good progress led to a much shorter programme than originally planned and it is now just a question of time before she achieves the same level of hearing as a slightly hearing-impaired person.

The battery of tests and procedures that have been designed enables the author's group to determine the extent of the rehabilitation training required in each case. The aim is to retain the patient within the unit only for as long as it is felt that benefit will be derived from further training. Once the unit and the patient are fully satisfied that no further benefit will result from continued training, the course of instruction is terminated but, as stated earlier in the chapter, patients are always welcome to return if they feel the need for further training and support.

Conclusions

The conclusions, based on the experience of this group to date, are that a period of formal training individually tailored to each patient's needs and abilities, in combination with monitored practical usage, helps cochlear implant patients to increase their self-confidence, adapt to their new artificial hearing more rapidly and obtain the maximum possible benefit from their implants.

Acknowledgements

I would like to thank Eva Agelfors, Ferens Albert, Göran Bredberg, Bo Lindström, Arne Risberg, and also I would particularly like to mention those of my colleagues directly involved in the rehabilitation programme: Kerstin Klason and Birgitta Rollvén

References

CESAREC, Z. and MARKE, S. (1967). *Cesarec–Marke Personality Scale*. The Pedagogic Institution, Lund University, Lund, Sweden.

DeFILIPPO, C.L. and SCOTT, B.L. (1978). A method for training and evaluating the reception of ongoing speech. *J. Acoust. Soc. Am.* **63**, 1186–1192.

MECKLENBURG, D.J. (1983). *Speech Tracking: Instructions Only*. Englewood CO: Cochlear Corporation.

MIZUNO, C. and RISBERG, A. (1984). Computer-aided testing and training of the hearing impaired. STL-QPSR 2-3/1984, 109–118. Department of Speech Communication and Music Acoustics, The Royal Institute of Technology, Stockholm, Sweden.

RAVEN, J.C., COURT, J. and RAVEN, J. (1986). *Progressive Matrices*. Pasadena, CA: The Psychological Center.

WESTRIN, P.A. (1966). *Westrin Intelligence Test III*. The Pedagogic Institution, Lund University, Lund, Sweden.

Chapter 16
Speech Perception and Its Assessment

ANDREW FAULKNER and THEODORA READ

The ultimate aim of speech receptive assessment is to measure the ability to receive information through speech in a way which reflects the most important aspects of speech perception, and is related to real-world performance. In this chapter, an attempt is made to consider the goals and needs of both clinical and research practitioners. The emphasis will be on methods which are appropriate for postlingually deafened adult and older child patients. Reference will be made to procedures used in the studies reviewed in other chapters of this book and, particularly, to analytical assessment methods developed within the External Pattern Input Group at University College London, and commonly used in the UK and elsewhere. A forward-looking clinical approach to assessment is suggested which includes analytical elements together with assessments that closely approximate real-world speech communication. Particular emphasis is placed on an understanding of the acoustic phonetic factors underlying speech perception.

The Functions of Assessment

Speech receptive assessment has a role at a number of stages in the provision of a cochlear implant. At the preoperative stage, it is an essential indicator of the benefit the patient derives from a hearing aid and from visual information in lipreading. During the course of postoperative rehabilitation, speech assessment can play an important clinical role in guiding training, and may indicate beneficial adjustments to a patient's speech processor. In a wider sense, in both scientific and service-oriented research, speech receptive assessment is central to the evaluation of existing implant devices and, most importantly, during the next few years, in the development of novel speech-processing strategies.

One of the purposes of this chapter is to define a selection of 'core' tests suited to clinical assessment. A common core of tests is an appealing prospect, from which we might hope for a degree of comparability between clinics and research groups, at least within one country, which has only been available from a few multicentre studies (Gantz et al., 1988; Rosen et al., 1988). In defining such a core, an attempt is made to select those tests which it is believed will predict, with the maximum possible efficiency, the speech receptive abilities of the patient in the real world. Unfortunately, there is no certain basis for this prediction, because there is no agreed means of assessing overall speech receptive ability. However, the disciplines of experimental phonetics and experimental psychology provide a theoretical basis which can be adopted in setting targets for the core tests.

Patient performance depends on a wide range of factors, some of which are not directly related to the performance of the prosthesis, but rather to the extent to which the patient's cognitive system can make sense of the limited input data provided by the implant and, often, also from the speaker's facial and oral movements. These levels can be illustrated, in respect of the functions carried out and the information represented, as in Table 16.1, which is based loosely on the classification of Risberg and Agelfors (1986).

Table 16.1   Levels of processing in speech perception

Transformation	From acoustic signal to auditory response
Auditory analysis	Extraction of auditory patterns related to speech contrasts
Phonetic classification	Interpretation (where possible) of auditory patterns in terms of phonological contrasts, e.g. voiced/voiceless, plosive/fricative, rising/falling intonation
Linguistic processing	Identification of phonemes, words and grammatical structure; extraction of meaning

Whilst all of these levels are of importance, it is only possible for the use of a cochlear implant to affect the first two levels directly. The relationship between the device and the first level of transformation depends upon the implant system's response to the various acoustic components of speech and its effectiveness in stimulating one or more cochlear sites. The relationship between the implant and the second level is more subtle. Here, we refer to the extent to which the implant provides stimulation matched to the user's receptive abilities. This may be achieved by the use of simplification in the speech processor (Fourcin et al., 1979), whereby the detection of important auditory patterns may be made easier for the user through the removal of extraneous acoustic information. Speech processors with this capability include the UCL Microstim device, which extracts simply the voice fundamental frequency component of speech (Walliker, Rosen and Fourcin, 1986), and the Nucleus multichannel device (Clark et al., 1987), which extracts several patterns, including fundamental frequency and formant information. Beyond this second level, rehabilitation may have an important role in improving performance, but the ultimate achievement in terms of understanding speech will largely depend upon the patient's cognitive abilities. Much of the interest in assessment, therefore, is centred upon the factors which are more amenable to external influence.

Speech perceptual tests can be of two broad classes: one class of test is primarily analytical in nature, and can indicate which phonological contrasts the listener is able to utilise in the identification of test items that are presented without linguistic context. The second, more holistic, class of test is concerned with speech as language, where the test material is meaningful and the evidence which accumulates during the course of hearing (and seeing) a sentence or a longer section of prose can contribute to the perception of speech by the provision of higher-order cues to likely candidate words. Both classes of test represent essential components of a balanced assessment strategy, and examples of each will be considered later in the chapter.

The Acoustic Patterns of Speech

First, a brief review is given of some basic aspects of acoustic phonetics, so that some of the elements of speech that are likely to be available to users of cochlear implants can be identified, and also to illustrate the conceptual basis of analytical assessment. For fuller discussions of acoustic phonetics, the reader can consult Rosen and Fourcin (1986) for an audiological perspective, or Pickett (1980) for a more general basic text. Here the emphasis will be on consonants rather than vowels, although not exclusively, because it is the consonants which bear the greater information load in speech. Furthermore, in unaided lipreading, important consonantal contrasts of voicing and manner are hard to see (Summerfield, 1985), whilst vowels are relatively distinct. Throughout the chapter, substantial importance is placed upon aided lipreading. This is not because the ability of many patients to communicate without lipreading is not valued, but rather that such tests allow an informative assessment to be made in most implant users, and because aided lipreading is of very real communicative importance for even the most accomplished implant users, especially when noise or reverberation occur in the acoustic environment.

The acoustic basis of speech can simply be thought of as comprising two components: an acoustic source and a filter which shapes the acoustic spectrum of the source. This source–filter model is illustrated in Figure 16.1. The primary acoustic source arises from the approximately periodic opening and closing of the vocal folds, which occurs at

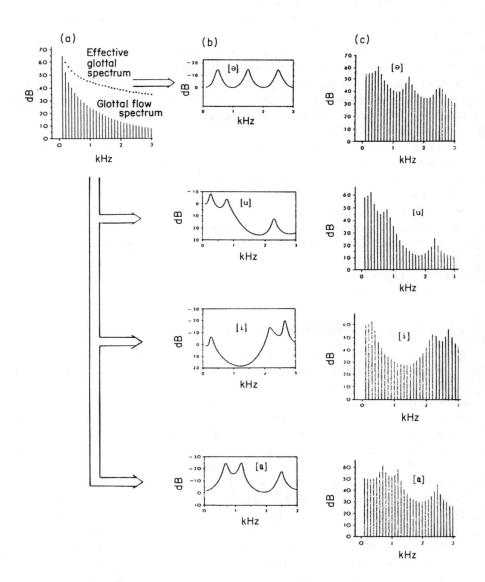

Figure 16.1. The source–filter model of speech production. (a) The effective source spectrum has a spectral envelope which decreases by 6 dB/octave. This reflects the true source spectrum, which decreases by about 12 dB/octave, and the effect of lip radiation, which imposes a response that rises by about 6 dB/octave. (b) This shows the idealised frequency response of the vocal tract for the four vowels /ə/, as in the British English word 'herd' or the American English 'bud', /u/ as in 'food', /i/, as in 'heed', and /ɑ/, as in the British English word 'hard', or the American English 'hod'. (c) The final acoustic spectra of these vowels, resulting from the source spectrum, the vocal tract response and the effects of lip radiation. (Reproduced with permission from Pickett, 1980.)

a rate typically between 80 and 150 Hz in adult male speakers, and 160 and 240 Hz in adult females (Troughear and Davis, 1979). This repeated closure of the vocal folds generates a train of acoustic impulses whose basic spectrum is composed of a series of discrete frequency components at frequencies corresponding to the rate of vocal fold closure, i.e., the fundamental frequency (f_0), and at integer multiples of f_0: $2f_0$, $3f_0$ etc. Periodic vocal fold closure leads to the perception of voicing in speech, and the fundamental frequency determines the sense of pitch produced by the speaker's voice*. The filter is provided by the acoustic resonances of the vocal tract, which depend upon the configuration of the articulating elements, the tongue, the hard palate, the teeth and lips, and the velum, or soft palate, which closes or opens the nasal passages. These resonances, known as formants, cause the vocal tract to pass acoustic energy in the region of the resonant frequencies, and to absorb energy at other frequencies. The formants are numbered from one upwards; the first two formants, F_1 and F_2, which may take values in the approximate frequency ranges 150–850 Hz and 500–2500 Hz respectively in a male speaker (Fant, 1956), are of more importance than higher formants in the identification of speech sounds, although F_3 is also of some significance. The formants thus determine the frequencies of the stronger spectral components, and hence the subjective sense of timbre, of the speech sound. The patterns of vocal tract resonance for four different vowels are shown in the central column of Figure 16.1. The final acoustic signal, shown in the third column of Figure 16.1 contains the same series of harmonics as the source, but the overall spectrum is now shaped according to the formant structure.

In addition to vocal fold activity, a second acoustic source is significant. Aperiodic sound arises from turbulence generated as air flows either through the open vocal folds, as in the sound /h/, or through a constriction of the vocal tract, for example, when the tongue is raised near to the alveolar ridge in the sound /s/. The perceptual correlate of aperiodic excitation can be called friction. Aperiodic excitation produces no sense of pitch, but because its spectrum is shaped by the vocal tract, it does produce a percept of timbre related to the vocal tract resonances.

Figure 16.2 shows the phrase 'a deeper table', which is illustrated acoustically by the speech pressure waveform, the amplitude envelope, the pattern and rate of vocal fold closure, which corresponds to the

---

*Both voicing and pitch strictly refer to perceptual events, and not to physical properties of sound. Here, the phrase *vocal fold activity* is used to refer to the physical correlate of voicing, and fundamental frequency for the physical correlate of pitch. These terms are, however often used rather indiscriminately.

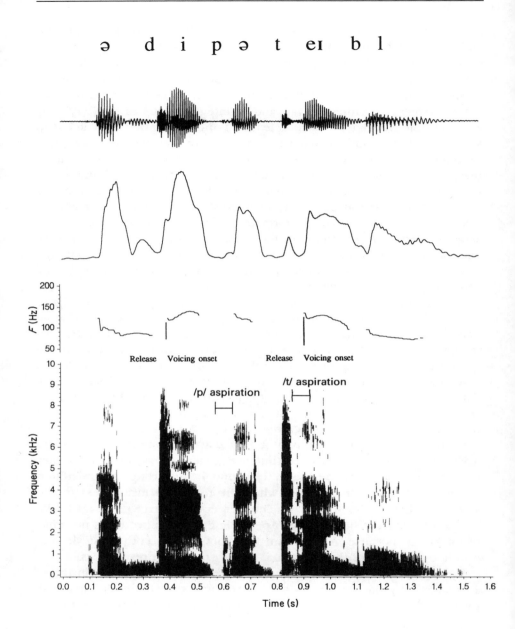

Figure 16.2. Representations of the phrase 'a deeper table' produced by a low-pitched male speaker of British English. Underneath the phonetic annotation appears the speech pressure waveform, the speech amplitude envelope, the voice fundamental frequency pattern and the spectrogram. The amplitude envelope was produced from the speech pressure waveform by full-wave rectification and low-pass filtering at 30 Hz. The fundamental frequency pattern was derived from an electrolaryngograph recording which indicated the time of occurrence of each vocal fold closure (Fourcin, 1981). The spectrogram used a filter bandwidth of 200 Hz.

perceived pattern of voicing and voice pitch, and the speech spectrogram*. The gross amplitude envelope of the speech pressure waveform contains a variety of cues. First, consonants, and hence many syllable boundaries, correspond to relatively rapid changes in amplitude, whilst vowels show a relatively steady amplitude. For example, a reduction of amplitude to a very low level is seen when the oral tract is closed during the [d] of 'deeper'. The amplitude envelope is also somewhat correlated with the fundamental frequency pattern, in that stressed syllables, e.g. the first syllable of '*deep*er', are produced with a higher fundamental frequency and with higher amplitude. The fundamental frequency pattern corresponds to the presence and rate of the quasi-periodic oscillations in the speech pressure waveform, whilst in the spectrogram the effects of this activity are seen in the presence of lower frequency energy and in the vertical striations, which occur at the rate of vocal fold closure. The spectrogram also shows clearly the presence of aperiodic excitation between the release and the voicing onset of the [t] of 'table', as high frequency energy which does not exhibit the periodic striations seen during vocal fold activity. The vocal tract resonances can be seen in the spectrogram as the formant patterns which are visible, although not always clearly, as denser areas. For example, from the release of the [d] of 'deeper', F_1 initially has a very low value and rises to about 300 Hz during the course of the [i] vowel, while F_2 begins around 1800 Hz, and rises slightly to about 2200 Hz in the following vowel.

The range of auditory abilities in cochlear implant users

For the purposes of this chapter, it will be useful to consider the acoustic speech cues which will be available to different classes of cochlear implant user. For users of single-channel devices and multichannel devices which are functionally only single channel, only temporal information is available. The temporal information in speech has been classified by Rosen (1989) in terms of rate. The slowest temporal changes, those that occur at up to about 50 Hz, are related to the speech amplitude envelope. Temporal factors at rates between about 50 and 500 Hz are related to the occurrence and rate of vocal fold closure and to the lower frequency components of aperiodic voiceless speech sounds, whilst, above 500 Hz, temporal fine-structure is determined by the resonances of the vocal tract and by the presence of aperiodic excitation. Most patients are sensitive to gross amplitude envelope changes (Fourcin et al., 1979; Shannon and Muller, 1990), and to fundamental frequency information (Fourcin et al., 1979).

---

*The spectrogram shows the distribution of energy over both time and frequency. The illustrated spectrograms use a frequency analysis bandwidth of 200 Hz.

Few single-channel patients are sensitive to the faster temporal patterns related to the spectrum of aperiodic speech sounds, since temporal rate coding is rarely observed above 1000 Hz. Nor is there strong evidence that temporal information can provide implant users with formant frequency information, although there are suggestive results from some adult patients using the Vienna single-channel extracochlear implant (Agelfors and Risberg, 1987).

In users of multichannel implants, a proportion, perhaps 40%, appear to be able to make use of the distribution of stimulation over electrodes to receive spectral speech information. Since the remainder of these, and all users of single-channel implants are only sensitive to temporal information at rates up to perhaps 500 or 1000 Hz, a discussion of temporal factors and their role in consonant perception will come first. Consonants are contrasted on a temporal basis in two important ways, with respect to voicing and to manner of articulation.

Voicing information

The annotations [d] and [t] at the top of Figure 16.2 indicate the location of a pair of *plosive* consonants which differ only with respect to voicing. Both of these sounds are formed in the vocal tract by a closure between the tongue and alveolar ridge and its subsequent release. Consequently, they look very similar to the lipreader. The voicing contrast is, however, clearly evident in the different patterns of vocal fold activity. Vocal fold activity ceases during both of these consonants, but for the voiced [d] the interval between the release of the oral closure and the resumption of vocal fold activity is relatively short – about 25 ms. A VOT of around 25–30 ms is typical for an English voiced plosive, but in some cases vocal fold activity can begin at, or even before, the release of the closure. This interval is generally called the voice-onset time or VOT. In the voiceless [t], there is a substantially longer VOT of about 80 ms. The periodic source thus ceases for a relatively short period during the voiced plosive and for a longer period during the voiceless one. The detection of VOT differences in implant users may be due to the cessation of periodic stimulation or simply to the different temporal amplitude patterns.

An additional potential cue to the voicing contrast in plosives for those patients who are able to detect high frequency speech energy is illustrated by the extended presence of high frequency aperiodic excitation following the release of the voiceless [t]. Only a very brief burst of aperiodic excitation occurs with the voiced [d]. Figure 16.2 also shows a second voicing contrast between the bilabial plosives [b] and [p]. Here, a comparable pattern of vocal fold activity can be seen to that in [d] and [t]. As in the [d], vocal fold closure begins very soon, about 25 ms after the release of the [b] closure, but is delayed by about 40 ms in the [p]. The [p], like the [t], contains a period of aperiodic excitation prior to the onset of vocal fold activity, but here this is lower in amplitude, and concentrated at much lower frequencies than in the [t].

Intonation information

Apart from consonantal voicing contrasts, vocal fold activity has another basic role in speech, through the contrastive function of voice pitch. In speech, we use variations in the rate of vocal fold closure in several ways. Stressed syllables are usually uttered with a rise and then a fall in the rate of vocal fold closure and, hence, heard with a rise then a fall in pitch. Semantic information such as irony, and the declarative/interrogative (statement/question) contrast is also conveyed by the pattern of intonation running through a sentence. Figure 16.3 shows an example of three

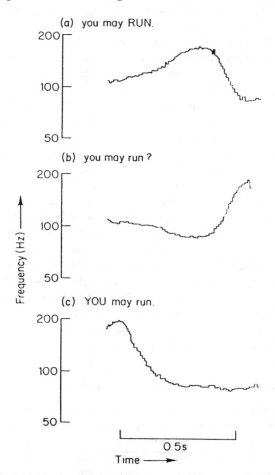

Figure 16.3. Contrastive fundamental frequency contours from an adult male speaker. The phrase 'you may run' was produced with the stress place (a) in 'run', (b) using an interrogative form, and (c) with stress placed on 'you'. (Reproduced with permission from Moore, 1986.)

alternative contrastive uses of voice pitch for the phrase 'you may run', in which the intonation pattern changes with the location of the stressed syllable, and between declarative and interrogative forms. Contrasts of this sort are most likely to be perceived from the rate of vocal fold closure, although limited stress placement information may also be available from the amplitude envelope due to its partial correlation with fundamental frequency.

Vocal fold activity is thus of basic communicative importance both for the transmission of consonantal voicing contrasts and for intonation. Since it is invisible, and carries such a significant communicative load, acoustic information related to vocal fold activity provides the most important auditory supplement to the visual speech information gained from lipreading (Rosen, Moore and Fourcin, 1979; Breeuwer and Plomp, 1985; Summerfield, 1985). We might, therefore, hope that a cochlear implant would ensure the effective reception of voicing and intonation patterns. Certainly, the auditory abilities required to perceive voicing contrasts, as measured by gap detection tasks, are available to most cochlear implant users (Fourcin et al., 1979; Hochmair-Desoyer, Hochmair and Stiglbrunner, 1985) and indeed, with an acoustic input from an appropriate hearing aid, to many of the profoundly hearing-impaired population (Faulkner, Fourcin and Moore, 1990). However, it is important to realise that a patient's basic auditory abilities can only be utilised in the perception of speech with an appropriate prosthesis, and that cochlear implants, and indeed hearing aids, often fail to make the best use of a patient's abilities. For example, patients using single-channel implants which provide an analogue 'whole-speech' signal may receive less voicing information than when they receive a simpler electrical signal that represents only voicing and voice pitch information (see Figure 16.7 and Rosen and Ball, 1986). Conversely, users of the early Nucleus device with the F_0F_2 coding strategy appeared to receive less voicing information than users of the House/3M single-channel whole-speech device (Rosen et al., 1988), despite receiving what seems to be a simpler signal in which the voice pitch pattern is explicitly extracted (the newer Nucleus $F_0F_1F_2$ strategy appears much superior to the F_0F_2 strategy) (Blamey et al., 1987b).

Manner contrasts I: friction and voicing cues

Friction is normally a major factor in the perception of consonantal manner contrasts; however, for many single-channel cochlear implant users (Rosen and Ball, 1987; Rosen et al., 1988) and profoundly hearing-impaired hearing aid users (Faulkner, Fourcin and Moore, 1990), this information is inaudible unless it is matched to the listener's receptive abilities, for example by recoding aperiodic excitation as a lower frequency aperiodic stimulus (Summerfield, 1985; Faulkner, Ball and Fourcin, 1990; Faulkner,

Fourcin and Moore, 1990). The upper panel of Figure 16.4 shows three alveolar consonants /z,s,t/ which differ with respect to manner and voicing. The [s] and [t] are both characterised by the absence of vocal fold activity and the presence of high frequency aperiodic excitation. In the voiceless fricative [s], the aperiodic energy is relatively long lasting and stable. In the voiceless plosive [t], however, there is a shorter burst of aperiodic excitation which decays in amplitude. The [z] exhibits both periodic vocal fold activity and aperiodic excitation, although vocal fold closure is often absent at the peak of the oral constriction. The ability to detect both voicing and friction together is present in at least some users of the Nucleus device (Blamey et al., 1987b) and the Ineraid device (Dorman et al., 1988). There is little evidence of such an ability in single-channel patients using the House/3M device (Rosen et al., 1988).

Manner contrasts II: amplitude envelope and spectral cues

The lower panel of Figure 16.4 shows examples of three voiced alveolar sounds /d,n,l/. The nasal [n] differs from the voiced plosive [d] in several ways. First, vocal fold activity continues throughout the oral closure in the nasal, whilst it generally ceases briefly during the voiced plosive. The mouth is closed during both the plosive and the nasal, but during the nasal consonant sound is produced through the open nasal passages. Hence the speech pressure waveform does not show the low amplitude or silent interval which is evident in the [d]. Whilst amplitude envelope information is likely to be a useful cue in distinguishing [d] and [n], it will not, however, provide a basis for the contrasts between [n], [z] and [l]. These contrasts are likely to require some degree of sensitivity to spectral information or temporal fine-structure. In the [n], and in other nasals, the energy present during the period of oral closure is predominantly below 500 Hz, in contrast to the [l], in which energy extends beyond 4000 Hz, and where the spectrum is contrasted from the surrounding vowel by the greater strength of the higher formants. The voiced fricative [z] is similar to [n] and [l], except for the presence of high-frequency aperiodic excitation during the oral constriction. If, as is likely in users of single-channel devices, this factor cannot be distinguished in the presence of lower frequency periodic energy, then sounds like [z] and [n] will be highly confusable, since their vocal fold activity and amplitude patterns are essentially similar.

Place of articulation I: vowels

Finally, there are the speech contrasts arising from different places of articulation, which are transmitted principally through spectral contrasts. In vowels, where the spectral structure is relatively stable, the formants are principally related to the configuration of the tongue. The tongue can form constrictions of the vocal tract of varying degree between the front

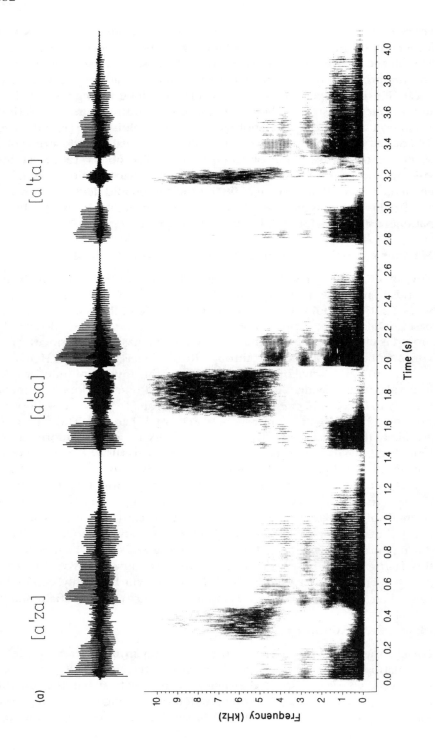

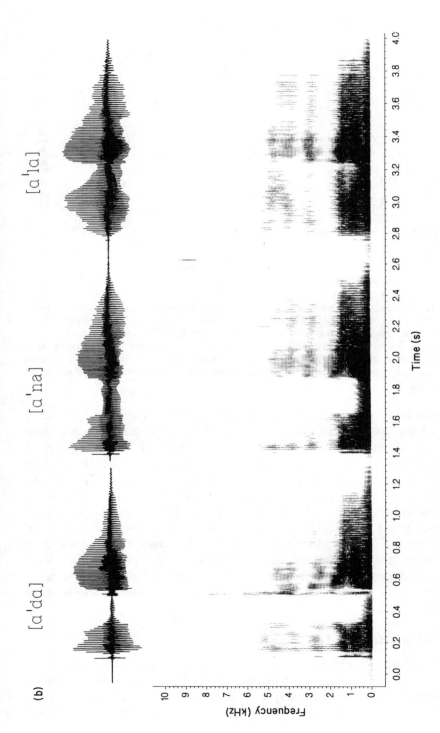

Figure 16.4. Six alveolar intervocalic consonants representing contrasts of manner and voicing, produced by a low-pitched male speaker of British English. The upper panel shows speech pressure waveforms and spectrograms for [z], [s], and [t], and the lower panel for [d], [n], and [l].

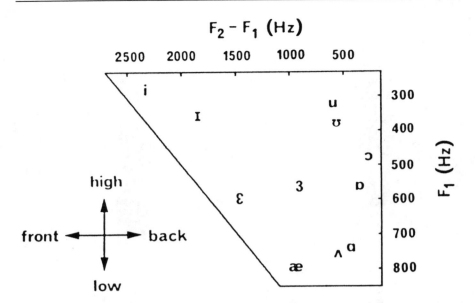

Figure 16.5. Formant frequency values for vowels of British English received pronunciation (RP) (Gimson, 1962). The second formant value is shown as the difference between F_2 and F_1, since this corresponds more closely with the front/back position of the tongue. The vowels represented are /i/ as in 'heed', /ɪ/ as in 'hid', /ɛ/ as in 'head', /æ/ as in 'had', /ʌ/ as in 'Hudd', /ɑ/ as in RP 'hard' (or American 'hod'), /ɒ/ as in RP 'hod', /ɔ/ as in 'hawed', /ʊ/ as in 'hood', and /u/ as in 'who'd'. The central vowel /ɜ/ occurs in RP 'her'. (Reproduced with permission from Rosen and Fourcin, 1986.)

and back of the mouth. A narrow constriction, where the tongue is said to be in a high position, produces a lower first formant frequency than a more open vocal tract. The second formant is related to the place of constrictions; a constriction near the back of the mouth produces lower second formant frequencies than those towards the front. The formant frequencies corresponding to a range of British English vowels are illustrated in Figure 16.5. Other acoustic differences are also significant for vowels, particularly duration, as, for example between the otherwise quite similar vowels in 'hid' and 'heed', or 'hod' and 'hoard'. The acoustic cues for vowels are substantially affected by stress placement. Unstressed vowels will generally be shorter, and will tend to be articulated more centrally, with correspondingly less contrasting formant patterns than stressed vowels.

Place of articulation II: consonants

Vowel place of articulation has fairly simple spectral correlates. Consonants, however, are formed by rapid changes in the configuration of the articulators and, consequently, have rapidly changing spectral correlates which are likely to be more difficult for the cochlear implant user to extract. Figure

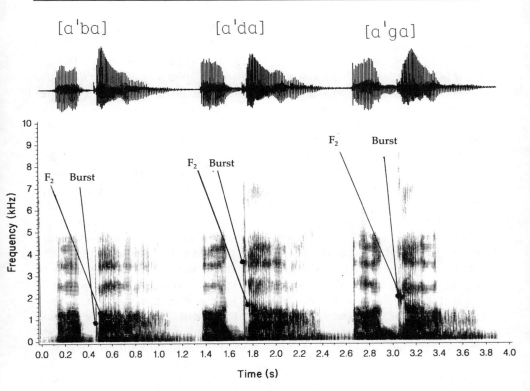

Figure 16.6. Three voiced intervocalic plosives illustrating place of articulation contrasts, produced by a low-pitched male speaker of British English. The F₂ frequencies and the dominant frequency region of the release burst are indicated in each spectrogram.

16.6 shows the speech pressure waveform and spectrogram for the nonsense sounds [ɑ'bɑ], [ɑ'dɑ], [ɑ'gɑ], and illustrates the place of articulation contrasts between the bilabial, alveolar and velar voiced plosives. The spectral patterning has two distinct aspects. One is the movement of the second formant frequency, which in these examples starts, at the closure release, at a relatively low frequency for the [b], at an intermediate frequency for the [d], and rather higher frequency for the [g]. The direction and terminal value of the second formant transition is determined by the following vowel. For example, with a /d/ followed by an /i/ vowel, whose F_2 is high, the transition will rise (see Figure 16.1), whereas a vowel with a lower F_2 such as /ɑ/, as in Figure 16.6, would lead to a falling F_2. Although formant transitions are dominant in normal listeners' perception of plosive place of articulation (Walley and Carrell, 1983), there is little evidence that cochlear implant users are able to make use of these cues, at least with the Ineraid device (Dorman et al., 1988, 1991). This may be due in part to the complex interaction between the consonant and vowel, but it is also likely that these cues are too slight and too rapid to be detected by the relatively crude resolution of spectral detail available to users of the Ineraid device. There are no clear published data relating to the ability of users of the Nucleus device to use F_2 transition cues. However, with very simple stimuli, some users are known to be able to discriminate rapid temporal variations in the position of the stimulating electrode (Tong et al., 1982), which could, in principle, encode F_2 transitions.

The second aspect of place in plosives is the spectrum of the initial burst of the plosive and, in voiceless plosives, of the aperiodic excitation which typically occurs between the release burst and the onset of vocal fold activity. It is the burst spectrum that users of the Ineraid implant appear able to use in identifying the place of articulation of voiced plosives (Dorman et al., 1988, 1991). The spectral shape of the release burst persists for about 10–20 ms in voiced plosives. In voiceless plosives, the aperiodic excitation which often follows the burst maintains the same general spectral shape as the burst, so that this spectral cue may be present for 50 ms or more. The burst spectra of the voiced plosives are visible in Figure 16.6; in the bilabial plosives /b/ and /p/, burst spectrum energy is typically concentrated below 1000 Hz; in the alveolars, /d/ and /t/, it is mainly high in frequency (above 3000 Hz), whilst in the velars, /g/ and /k/, burst energy is concentrated in an intermediate frequency range, and tends to occur around the first and second formant of the following vowel.

In fricatives, the spectrum imposed upon the aperiodic excitation is also related to place of articulation, and this too has been shown to be a useful cue for users of the Ineraid device in distinguishing /s/ from /ʃ/, as in the contrast between 'sip' and 'ship' (Dorman et al., 1988, 1991).

The perception of consonantal place information from sound-only presentation is likely to be essential if patients are to have any substantial ability to understand speech without lipreading, and it seems unlikely that this would be available from a single-channel system. However, there are reports of substantial speech understanding without lipreading in some adults using the Vienna single-channel extracochlear device (Hochmair-Desoyer, Hochmair and Stiglbrunner, 1985) and children using the House/3M device (Berliner et al., 1989). For the lipreader, place of articulation contrasts between consonants are, like many vowel contrasts, largely visible, although alveolar and velar consonants are only visually distinct in ideal viewing conditions. Some acoustically based place of articulation information is undoubtedly available to many multichannel patients where spectral aspects are coded by site of stimulation, although it remains possible that these abilities may in part be mediated by temporal fine-structure.

Co-articulation

The phenomenon of co-articulation has already been met in the context of F_2 transitions, which depend upon the place of articulation of both a consonant and the following vowel. Similar interdependencies are common in speech, so that the acoustic characteristics of successive speech sounds are almost never independent of their immediate context. For this reason, there are no simple invariant acoustic cues to phoneme identity, rather, perception is always dependent on the dynamic acoustic structure of the speech signal.

Normalisation

Another complexity of speech perception is that the resonances of the vocal tract depend not only on the configuration of the articulators, but also on the length of the vocal tract. Typically, an adult female speaker will have a shorter and narrower vocal tract than an adult male, and a child will have an even smaller vocal tract. Since F_1 and F_2 are related to vocal tract length, the range of formant resonances will be highest in a child, and lowest in a man. Similarly, the voice pitch ranges of men, women and children differ. These individual variations have substantial effects upon the acoustic speech signal, but not upon our phonological categorisation of speech. Our ability to adjust to acoustic variations of this sort is known as normalisation.

Many of the approaches adopted in cochlear implant design exploit normalisation. For example, voice pitch patterns can be effectively presented in a variety of pitch registers without impairing the patient's ability to perceive voicing and intonation information (Fourcin et al., 1984). In another case, the Nucleus device presents formant frequency information by stimulation of cochlear sites which, in the normal ear, would be acoustically stimulated by frequencies approximately twice the true formant frequencies (Blamey et al., 1987a).

Use of an analytical consonant test

As discussed below, a range of analytical tests is required at the level of phonetic classification (see Table 16.1), to cover the perception of consonants, vowels and intonation. The first of these, a consonant recognition test, is discussed to illustrate how an analytical speech test can give important information regarding the factors of voicing, place and manner. Figure 16.7 shows sets of results in a consonant identification task from single- and multichannel patients. The scoring of the test results is both in terms of the number of correct responses and also in terms of information transfer (Miller and Nicely, 1955) for phonological contrasts of voicing, manner and place. The information transfer score is attractive as a measure of the patient's accuracy in assigning stimuli to phonological classes, because, unlike an error score, it does not depend upon the number of alternative classes, and random guessing will always result in a

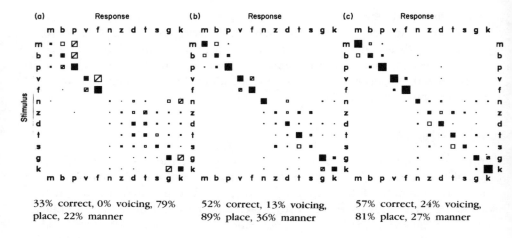

33% correct, 0% voicing, 79% place, 22% manner

52% correct, 13% voicing, 89% place, 36% manner

57% correct, 24% voicing, 81% place, 27% manner

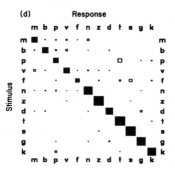

Overall correct: 71.4%.
Place information: 38.7%.
Voicing information: 74.2%.
Manner information: 56.0%.

Figure 16.7. Consonant confusion matrices obtained from an analytical test based on 12 intervocalic consonants (Rosen, Moore and Fourcin, 1979). For each stimulus item, the distribution of responses is represented by the size of the squares comprising the matrix. Correct responses are shown as filled squares, and errors as empty squares; errors of voicing are indicated by a diagonal line through an empty square. (a–c) Audiovisual data from a patient using the Vienna single-channel extracochlear device. The test conditions include (a) unaided lipreading, (b) lipreading with the compressed and equalised whole-speech signal provided by this device, and (c) lipreading with a constant amplitude voice fundamental frequency signal (Rosen and Ball, 1986). The overall percentage of correct responses, and information transmission scores (Miller and Nicely, 1955) relating to the reception of voicing, place and manner information are shown in the figures. (d) Auditory-only data from three of the better performing users of the Nucleus device (Blamey et al., 1987b). Whereas the patient in (a–c) would obtain essentially no place information from auditory-only presentation, these three patients are receiving useful place of articulation information from their implants.

score close to zero. As a result of this, the relative contributions of different phonological features can be compared more readily.

The unaided lipreading results from the single-channel patient are typical of both implant users (Rosen, Moore and Fourcin, 1979) and the normally hearing (Faulkner et al., 1989); homorganic consonants (consonants having the same place of articulation) are confused with each other. For this single-channel patient, the main effect of auditory information is to improve discrimination between the homorganic consonants, primarily through a marked decrease in errors of voicing, and also, more modestly, through fewer manner errors. By comparing the scores with speech and with voice fundamental frequency information, it can be seen that the speech signal is not providing this patient with any more information than that which is available simply from the voice fundamental frequency pattern. The place scores are, of course, dominated by visual information.

The other patients represented in Figure 16.7 are three of the better performing users from a group of 28 users of the Nucleus device whose speech perceptual abilities were described by Blamey et al. (1987b). These data are for auditory-only presentation and it should be noted that these three patients showed rather better performance than the group as a whole. Of the 25 patients who would attempt this test without lipreading, the average overall score was 37% correct; the average place information score was 37% and the average voicing score was, perhaps surprisingly, only 35%, which is substantially lower than the score of 74% seen in the best three patients. One important aspect of a test such as this is that it can usefully be applied to patients with a wide range of receptive abilities through the use of both audiovisual and auditory-only presentation.

Before consideration is given to a wider variety of assessment approaches, it is worth touching on the use of analytical assessment in the context of speech-processor development. Figure 16.8 shows audiovisual consonant identification results obtained with an experimental speech processor which explicitly presents speech pattern information representing the three temporal factors used in the preceding discussion of speech perceptual factors: vocal fold activity, aperiodic excitation and amplitude envelope. The patient in this case was profoundly deaf (average hearing loss at 500, 1000 and 2000 Hz was 114 db), and was receiving low frequency acoustic stimulation (Faulkner, Ball and Fourcin, 1990). With voice fundamental frequency information alone, there is the expected benefit in respect of voicing information. When amplitude envelope information is added, an increase can be seen in this patient's reception of manner information from 27% to 56%, mainly because the amplitude information is making the voiced nasals distinct from the voiced plosives (/m/ from /b/, /n/ from /d/). When a temporal cue to aperiodic excitation is added to fundamental frequency information, as in the lower left panel,

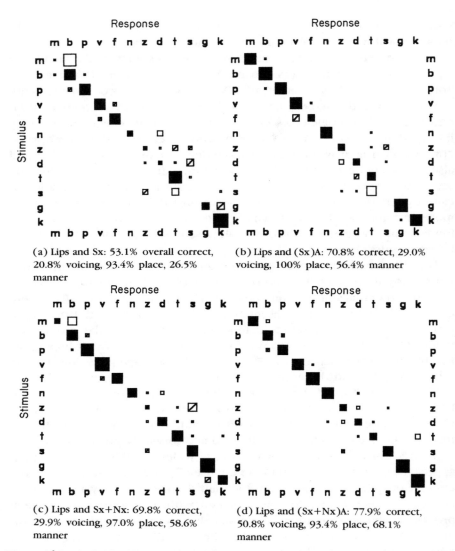

(a) Lips and Sx: 53.1% overall correct, 20.8% voicing, 93.4% place, 26.5% manner

(b) Lips and (Sx)A: 70.8% correct, 29.0% voicing, 100% place, 56.4% manner

(c) Lips and Sx+Nx: 69.8% correct, 29.9% voicing, 97.0% place, 58.6% manner

(d) Lips and (Sx+Nx)A: 77.9% correct, 50.8% voicing, 93.4% place, 68.1% manner

Figure 16.8. Audiovisual consonant confusion matrices obtained with simple and compound speech pattern information (Faulkner, Ball and Fourcin, 1990). (a) Data for lipreading with fundamental frequency information; (b) lipreading fundamental frequency and amplitude envelope information; (c) the auditory signal consists of fundamental frequency information during voiced speech and an aperiodic sound during voiceless speech sounds; (d) the combination of this third condition with amplitude envelope information. The subject was a profoundly deaf adult and in this instance, auditory stimulation was acoustic rather than electrical.

there is also a marked increase in the reception of manner information compared to the first condition. This gain in manner information arises because the voiceless /s/ and /t/ can now be distinguished, and because /z/ is classified as a fricative, i.e. either as /z/ or /s/, whilst it was confused with the visually similar /d/ and /t/ when the voiceless cue was absent. Finally, when all three speech patterns are combined, each component continues to contribute useful information.

Through analytical tests of this sort, and others based on the perception of intonation and vowel contrasts, it is possible to discover how much of the range of information potentially available from the implant is in fact received by the user, and to indicate specific improvements that can be made in speech processing or the fitting of the device.

Holistic and Functional Assessment

When we hear meaningful spoken language, many higher-order linguistic and other cognitive processes are operating to aid our perception, so that the sounds we believe we have heard do not always derive solely from the acoustic speech signal. One compelling example of this is the phonemic induction effect (Warren, 1970). Warren took a tape-recorded sentence, and substituted non-speech sounds such as a cough for speech sounds. As long as the non-speech sound was roughly similar in its spectral content to the deleted sound, listeners typically reported hearing both the deleted speech sound and its substitute. Clearly, the listeners' expectations from linguistic context can override the acoustic evidence. Whilst analytical tests use materials which contain no linguistic message, so as to give a relatively pure measure of the extent to which the implant user is able to perceive basic acoustic patterns in speech, holistic tests have a very different function. Here the need is to reflect the combined activities of auditory (and visual) perceptual processing together with linguistic and other cognitive operations. Thus, such tests give a more realistic picture of the patient's ability to use speech perception in everyday communication.

In addition to specific tests of speech perception at the phoneme level and tests of ability to understand connected speech, it is also important to evaluate the functional performance of the implant user in real life situations*. For most implant centres, a test procedure involving investigation of an implant user in a variety of different real life situations would be impractical (although the rehabilitation programmes in most centres include exposure of the user to different situations). One way of obtaining information on this wider aspect of an implant user's performance is to use one of the already available questionnaires devised to examine an individual's communication function. Not only should this provide

---

*In the authors' experience, there are some implant users who perform well in test procedures but who fail in real-life situations and, conversely, some patients may show little benefit from the implant in speech perception tests but perform more confidently in situations outside the clinic with their implant. Some measure of this benefit should be made.

information on an individual's performance, but it should also take into account communication difficulties encountered in the user's environment. One such test is the Denver Scale of Communication Function (Alpiner et al., 1974) which was designed 'to make a subjective assessment of communication attitudes of adults with acquired hearing loss', and is therefore suitable for use with a population of adult cochlear implant users with acquired hearing losses.

Standard Test Batteries

Several of the centres which have been providing cochlear implants for some years have assembled batteries of tests. Table 16.2 lists the most commonly used batteries and the centres where they were developed.

Table 16.2   Standard test batteries

Test	Reference/Source	Location
MAC Battery (Minimal Audiotory Capabilities)	Owens et al. (1981)	San Francisco
SPAC Battery (Speech Pattern Contrast Test)	Boothroyd (1986)	New York
Iowa Test Battery	Tyler, Tye-Murray	Iowa City
HIPPS Profile	Cooper et al. (1990)	London
NAL Lipreading Tests	Plant and Macrae (1987)	Sydney
Sound Pattern Tests	King (1987)	London
Five Linguistic Levels Profile	Risberg and Agelfors (1986)	Stockholm

Appendices I–VII outline the subtests for each test battery. There is some overlap and some similarities between certain test batteries. As the cochlear implant becomes an accepted clinical procedure, rather than an experimental approach, a balance needs to be found in assessment between gross evaluation and more analytical inquiry. There will be a continuing need for research with cochlear implants but clinical centres will have very different assessment needs. A clinical assessment tool which is accurate, comprehensive but not excessively time-consuming or tedious for the implant user needs to be available for the majority of implant centres.

Suggested Components of a Core Test Battery

A complete assessment profile would address each of the four levels of processing outlined in Table 16.1. The first level, that of transformation, does not specifically refer to speech and should be covered during the setting up of the speech processor. The second level, that of auditory analysis, requires the application of sound pattern tests of the sort proposed by Fourcin et al. (1979), and King (1987). The MAC battery provides only one such test, the Noise/Voice test, which in itself will not provide sufficient information. In clinical practice, tests of this sort may not be required unless a user is showing difficulties in phonological processing, in which case sound pattern tests should aid the team to identify the specific areas of difficulty.

At the third level, that of phonological processing, a set of analytical tests is required, to cover the perception of vowels, of consonants and of intonation. The consonant and vowel tests would be administered in auditory, audiovisual and visual conditions. The intonation test, for example, a question/statement or stress location test (e.g. the 'Important word in a sentence test'), should be presented only in the auditory condition, since facial expression can also give cues to intonation. The vowel test in particular must be based upon a dialect that is familiar to the patient; American vowels will not generally be appropriate for patients accustomed to Australian or British English. We would propose the use of a vowel test covering a range of both F_1 and F_2.

The authors have preferred to use consonant tests rather than closed-set word identification tests for a number of reasons. First, word tests are less efficient. The limited number of phonologically similar alternatives limits the response set to 4 or at most 6 alternatives, whilst a consonant test may have 12 or 16 alternative responses, so that more information will be obtained from each response in the consonant test. Secondly, word tests require careful standardisation so that alternative lists are of equal difficulty, and this must be carried out for both auditory and audiovisual presentation. Finally, word tests always consist of a finite pool of test items, which, if repeated, will become familiar to the patient, and thus no longer representative. A consonant test, however, is an exhaustive set, and can be endlessly reused as long as different item orders are employed. From the alternative forms of consonant test, based on syllable-initial (CV), intervocalic (VCV) and syllable-final (VC) consonants, the authors would select intervocalic materials as most essential because, in natural running speech, most consonants occur intervocalically and not in isolation.

At the fourth level, the range of suitable tests include open-set sentence tests, and Connected Discourse Tracking (CDT; DeFilippo and Scott, 1978), where the patient must repeat, phrase by phrase, a passage of connected prose. CDT can give very useful information when administered by an appropriately skilled speaker; in particular, unlike sentence materials, CDT performance reflects the contribution of suprasegmental factors such as intonation. There are, however, difficulties in its practical application as a core assessment item. The most serious of these is that, as it is an interactive procedure, the material is necessarily not repeatable and, furthermore, the speaker may be led, perhaps unconsciously, to speak with more or less care in different conditions or with different patients. Work is now in progress to develop video-based techniques for a CDT type assessment using repeatable material, but, for the present, a video-based sentence test will be most appropriate, backed up by an intonation reception test. The specific test used will depend upon the availability of materials that have been appropriately standardised. The BKB sentences (Bench and Bamford, 1979) have been carefully constructed, and have been used in both the UK and Australia. One strength of the BKB sentence materials is that 21 lists are available, substantially more than some other sentence tests, so that these materials may be used to test patients in a number of alternative conditions without repeating lists.

Presentation of Tests

The establishment of a standard battery of tests does not ensure that accurate and appropriate results are obtained from all patients. The nature and quality of the test material, the situation in which the tests are carried out, the conditions under which the patient is tested and the order of conditions are important factors to be considered. To ensure consistency of presentation, test material should be pre-recorded and the recording should be of a high standard. The equipment on which the material is played to the patient must be of high enough quality to ensure that the speech signal is accurately reproduced. The domestic VHS system is unacceptable unless the so-called 'HiFi' sound facility, available on a minority of machines, is used. Testing needs to be carried out in an audiometric sound-treated test suite to eliminate competing noise from elsewhere. It is suggested in the MAC battery manual that, within the audiometric sound-treated test-room, there should be one loudspeaker in the sound field and the listener should be one metre from the loudspeaker. The listener's device should be set to the most comfortable listening level. Perhaps it is most important to ensure that the patient has a thorough understanding of the task. In consonant identification and intonation tests, for example, the authors have found it essential with many patients to provide specific training based on visual display of the voicing and voice fundamental frequency pattern (Fourcin and Abberton, 1971).

Increasingly, assessment will make use of speech presented in noise; standard methods of calibrating speech-to-noise levels are discussed by Fuller (1987). In some centres, laser video disc systems are being used to administer test material. These systems provide high quality visual stimuli and have the added advantage of random access to the test material so that customised tests may be constructed and appropriate feedback provided.

Consistency and precision of measurement

One vital aspect of assessment is that the results should, within reasonable limits, be repeatable. There are two main factors involved here. First, the stimulus materials must be presented in a controlled way. This means, for example, using video-recorded material rather than a live speaker for audiovisual testing. Secondly, sufficient data must be collected to ensure reasonable precision of measurement. If a patient should score, say, 75% correct out of 50 test items, what is the likely range of scores if the same test were given to the same patient again? Standard statistical methods can be employed to indicate this range for item-based tests such as consonant and vowel tests, where the precision of measurement is theoretically limited by the binomial distribution. In this instance, the binomial distribution indicates that the test score is likely to lie between 66.5% and 83.5% on 95 occasions out of 100. The precision of these scores will increase in proportion to the square root of the number of presentations, so that, if we doubled the number of trials, this 95% confidence interval would then be between 69% and 81%. Test administration must also allow for other factors too. For example, the patient may become more familiar with the task over time, or may tire during an afternoon's testing, or perhaps his or her tinnitus is aggravated by stimulation or by the stress of the test situation. All these factors will make measurements less precise than the limit determined by the binomial distribution. A simple moral is that tests based on much fewer than 100 observations give only a very rough indication of the patient's receptive ability. Further discussion of this and related issues is given by Lyregaard (1987).

Concluding Remarks

The authors have tried to convey to the reader the purpose behind speech assessment, and its relation to the auditory abilities of different patients and the abilities which they show in speech perception. Much remains to be done in the definition of a set of efficient test procedures which give the best indication of a patient's overall receptive abilities outside of the clinic, but the authors believe that the phonological, linguistic and functional assessments suggested will provide a fair representation. The appendices list some test batteries; more complete descriptions will be found at source. The task of specifying a detailed test procedure must be left to the group responsible for testing, although, increasingly, national standards are emerging, and it is hoped that these will be adhered to as far as possible.

Appendix I: MAC (Minimal Auditory Capabilities) Battery*

1. Question/statement test	Rising vs falling inflection
2. Vowel test	Fifteen phonemes (including diphthongs); four-choice alternative
3. Spondee recognition	
4. Noise/voice test	Speech/low buzz/high buzz/low-pass noise
5. Accent test	Identify stressed word in given sentences
6. Everyday sentences (CID)	Forty sentences, 200 key words
7. Initial consonant test	(Voicing/nasality/glides); four-choice alternatives
8. Spondee same/different test	Same four spondees used in different combinations
9. Words in context	High predictability items of SPIN test
10. Everyday sound	Fifteen common sounds
11. Monosyllabic word test	NU6 (North Western University Auditory Test No. 6) – discontinued after 10 items if subject is failing to respond
12. Four-choice spondee test	Four alternative choice – pool of 48 words
13. Final consonant test	(Voice/nasality); four-choice alternative
14. Visual enhancement	Lipreading test. Everyday sentences CID – avoiding items used in (6)

*From Owens et al. (1981).

Appendix II: Iowa Test Battery

	Conditions
1. Sentence test without context	A V AV
2. Medial consonant test	A V AV
3. MAC item 12 spondee four-choice in quiet	A
4. MAC item 12 spondee four-choice in noise	A
5. Vowel test	A
6. Iowa NU6	A
7. Minimal pairs in quiet	A
8. Minimal pairs in noise	A
9. Environmental sounds	A
10. Sentence test with context	A
11. Accent test	A
12. MAC item 4 noise/voice	A
13. Soundfield thresholds	
14. Speech detection threshold	

A = auditory input alone.
V = visual input alone.
AV = auditory and visual input.

Appendix III: HIPPS Profile of Perceptual Skills*

Name: ....

Date: ....

Months since 'switched on': ....

Aid(s) used: ....

Symbols: ○ = Lipreading alone (LA)
× = Implant alone (SP)
⊗ = Implant and Lipreading (LSP)
★ = FX/SIVO alone (FX)
✦ = FX and lipreading (LFX)
+ = Hearing aid alone (HA)
⊕ = Aid and lipreading (LHA)

CONDITION

	LA	SP	LSP	FX	LFX	HA	LHA
1. Syllable number							
2. Male/female speaker							
3. Word stress							
4. Sentence stress							
5. Vowels							
6. VCV							
7. BKB							
8. CDT							
9. Environmental sounds							

10. Subjective questionnaire ....
11. Denver scale ....
12. Speech recording and histogram ....

COMMENTS: ....

*From Cooper et al. (1990).

Appendix IV: Speech Pattern Contrast Test (SPAC)*

SPAC is a forced-choice procedure to measure perception of phonologically significant contrasts. Subtests are administered in three modes: auditory alone, visual alone and auditory plus visual.

Test materials

a. Consonant confusion test (VCV).
b. Vowel confusion test (CVC).
c. Open-set sentences, topic related (10 questions, 10 statements).

Specific contrasts investigated

Segmental contrasts

1. Location of stress.
2. Direction of pitch change (statement/question).
3. Male/female speaker.
4. Pitch variation (monotone/natural intonation).

Segmental contrasts

5. Vowel height.
6. Vowel place.
7. Initial consonant voicing.
8. Initial consonant continuance.
9. Final consonant voicing.
10. Final consonant continuance.
11. Initial consonant place.
12. Final consonant place.

---

* From Boothroyd, 1986.

Appendix V: NAL Test Battery*

Subtests are presented in auditory alone, visual alone and auditory visual modes.
    Tests are also presented in the audiovisual mode in quiet and in noise.

Test materials

a. Consonant test: VCV 20 consonants in /ɑCɑ/frame.
b. Sentence test: an English translation of the first four lists of the Helen test (Ludwigson, 1974).

---

*From Plant and Macrae (1987).

Appendix VI: Psychoacoustic Sound Pattern Tests*

Using microcomputer presentation:

1. Gap detection.
2. Detection of amplitude dip.
3. Discrimination of aperiodic/periodic sound.
4. Discrimination of vowel-like sounds.
5. Perception of pitch contour (flat/fall).

*From King (1987).

Appendix VII: Battery of Tests used in Sweden*

A battery of tests used in Stockholm is described with subtests at five linguistic levels.

1. *Transformation* from an acoustic signal to signals in the auditory sustem. Audiometric tests are made across a range of frequencies up to 135 dB SPL. Detection threshold, most comfortable level and uncomfortable level are measured. Preoperatively, headphones are used; postoperatively measurements are made with electronic stimulation.

2. *Signal analysis* This level of tests investigates the ability to detect changes in amplitude, duration and frequency:
   (a) Duration discrimination
   (b) frequency discrimination with sinusoidal signal
   (c) frequency discrimination with band-pass filtered pulse trains
   (d) gap-detection with band-pass filtered white noise
   (e) identification time for periodic and non-periodic signals
   (f) pitch scaling

3. *Phonetic interpretation* investigates the ability to extract basic linguistic information from an acoustic signal:
   (a) number of syllables
   (b) vowel length
   (c) voiced–unvoiced plosives
   (d) male/female voices
   (e) word stress (three-word sentences)
   (f) differences between /s/–/st/–/t/ in initial position
   (g) vowel test 1 /u:/–/o:/ or /o:/–/ɑ:/ (difference in F_1)
   (h) vowel test 2 /i:/–/u:/ or /e:/–/o:/ (difference in F_2)

4. *Linguistic interpretation*:
   (a) tests with a forced choice between a closed-set of words, e.g. 12 spondee words and sentences (auditory alone)
   (b) tests with unknown words and sentences (auditory and lipreading)
   (c) tests are carried out with and without the implant

*From Risberg and Agelfors (1986).

Acknowledgements

Thanks are extended to colleagues in the EPI group at UCL, particularly Stuart Rosen and Ginny Ball, and to Huw Cooper for his patience.

References

ALPINER, J., CHEVRETTE, W., GLASCOE, G., METZ, M. and OLSEN, B. (1974). *The Denver Scale of Communication Function.* University of Denver.

AGELFORS, E. and RISBERG, A. (1987). The identification of synthetic vowels by patients using a single-channel cochlear implant. *STL-OPSR 2-3/1987*, 31–38.

BENCH, J. and BAMFORD, J. (1979). *Speech-hearing tests and the Spoken Language of Hearing-impaired Children.* London: Academic Press.

BERLINER, K.I., TONOKAWA, L.L., DYE, L.M. and HOUSE, W.F. (1989). Open-set speech recognition in children with a single-channel cochlear implant. *Ear Hear.* **10**, 237–242.

BLAMEY, P.J., SELIGMAN, P.S., DOWELL, R.C. and CLARK, G.M. (1987a). Acoustic parameters measured by a formant-based speech processor for a multi-channel cochlear implant. *J. Acoust. Soc. Am.* **81**, 38–47.

BLAMEY, P.J., DOWELL, R.C., BROWN, A.M., CLARK, G.M. and SELIGMAN, P.M. (1987b). Vowel and consonant recognition of cochlear implant patients using formant-estimation speech processors. *J. Acoust. Soc. Am.* **81**, 48–57.

BOOTHROYD, A. (1986). *SPAC Test Version II: A test of the perception of speech pattern contrasts.* New York: City University.

BREEUWER, M. and PLOMP, R. (1985). Speechreading supplemented with auditorily presented speech parameters. *J. Acoust. Soc. Am.* **79**, 481–499.

CLARK, G.M., BLAMEY, P.J., BROWN, A.M. et al. (1987). *The University of Melbourne – Nucleus Multi-Electrode Cochlear Implant.* Basel: Karger.

COOPER, H.R., READ, T.E., ALEKSY, W. and BOOTH, C.L. (1990). *The HIPPS Profile of Perceptual Skills.* University College Hospital, London.

DeFILIPPO, C.L. and SCOTT, B.L. (1978). A method for training and evaluation of the reception of on-going speech. *J. Acoust. Soc. Am.* **63**, 1186–1192.

DORMAN, M.F., HANNLEY, M., McCANDLESS, G. and SMITH, L. (1988). Auditory/phonetic categorization with the Symbion multichannel cochlear prosthesis. *J. Acoust. Soc. Am.* **84**, 510.

DORMAN, M.F., DANKOWSKI, K., McCANDLESS, G., PARKIN, J.L. and SMITH, L. (1991). Vowel and consonant recognition with the aid of a multichannel cochlear implant. *Q. J. Exp. Psychol.* in press.

FANT, G.M. (1956). On the predictability of formant levels and spectrum envelopes from formant frequencies. In: Halle, M., Lunt, H. and Maclean, H. (eds), *For Roman Jakonson.* The Hague: Mouton.

FAULKNER, A., BALL, V. and FOURCIN, A.J. (1990a). Compound speech pattern information as an aid to lipreading. *Speech, Hearing and Language: Work in Progress,* Vol. 4, pp. 63–80. University College London, Department of Phonetics and Linguistics.

FAULKNER, A., FOURCIN, A.J. and MOORE, B.C.J. (1990b). Psychoacoustic aspects of speech coding for the deaf. *Acta Oto-Laryngol. Suppl.* **469**, 172–180.

FAULKNER, A., POTTER, C., BALL, G. and ROSEN, S. (1989). Audiovisual speech perception of intervocalic consonants with auditory voicing and voiced/voiceless speech pattern presentation. In: *Speech, Hearing and Language: Work in Progress,* vol. 3, pp. 85–106. University College London, Department of Phonetics and Linguistics.

FOURCIN, A.J. (1981). Laryngographic assessment of phonatory function. *Proceedings of the Conference on the Assessment of Vocal Pathology*, ASHA Reports 11, ASHA, Rockville, Maryland.

FOURCIN, A.J. and ABBERTON, E. (1971). First applications of a new laryngograph. *Med. Biol. Illus.* 21, 172–182.

FOURCIN, A.J., ROSEN, S.M., MOORE, B.C.J., DOUEK, E.E., CLARKE, G.P., DODSON, H. and BANNISTER, L.H. (1979). External electrical stimulation of the cochlea: Clinical, psychophysical, speech-perceptual and histological findings. *Br. J. Audiol.* 13, 85–107.

FOURCIN, A., DOUEK, E., MOORE, B., ABBERTON, E., ROSEN, S. and WALLIKER, J. (1984). Speech pattern element stimulation in electrical hearing. *Arch. Otolaryngol.* 110, 145–153.

FULLER, H. (1987). Equipment for speech audiometry and its calibration. In: Martin, M. (ed.), *Speech Audiometry*, pp. 75–88. London: Whurr.

GANTZ, B.J., TYLER, R.S., KNUTSON, J.F., WOODWORTH, G., ABBAS, P., McCABE, B.F. et al. (1988). Evaluation of five difference cochlear implant designs: Audiologic assessment and predictors of performance. *Laryngoscope* 98, 1100–1106.

GIMSON, A.C. (1962). *An Introduction to the Pronunciation of English*. London: Edward Arnold.

HOCHMAIR-DESOYER, I.J., HOCHMAIR, E.S. and STIGLBRUNNER, H.K. (1985). Psychoacoustic temporal processing and speech understanding in cochlear implant patients. In: Schindler, R.A. and Merzenich, M.M. (eds), *Cochlear Implants*, pp. 291–304. New York: Raven Press.

KING, A.B. (1987). Speech perception tests for the profoundly deaf. In: Martin, M. (ed.), *Speech Audiometry*, pp. 171–177. London: Taylor & Francis.

LUDWIGSON, C. (1974). Construction and evaluation of an audio-visual test (the Helen test). *Scand. Audiol.* Suppl. 4, 67–75.

LYREGAARD, P. (1987). Towards a theory of speech audiometry tests. In: Martin, M. (ed.), *Speech Audiometry*, pp. 33–62. London: Taylor & Francis.

MILLER, G.A. and NICELY, P.E. (1955). An analysis of perceptual confusions among some English consonants. *J. Acoust. Soc. Am.* 27, 338–352.

OWENS, E., KESSLER, D.K., TELLEEN, C.C. and SCHUBERT, E. (1981). The Minimal Auditory Capabilities battery. *Hear. Aid J.* 34, 9–34.

PLANT, G. and MACRAE, J. (1987). Testing visual and auditory visual speech perception. In: Martin, M. (ed.), *Speech Audiometry*, pp. 179–206. London: Taylor & Francis.

PICKETT, J.M. (1980). *The Sounds of Speech Communication: A primer of acoustic phonetics and speech perception*. Baltimore: University Park Press.

RISBERG, A. and AGELFORS, E. (1986). Levels of measurement in pre- and postoperative testing of cochlear implant subjects. Speech Transmission Laboratory, Quarterly Progress and Status Report, pp. 45–59. Royal Institute of Technology, Stockholm.

ROSEN, S. (1989). Temporal information in speech and its relevance for cochlear implants. In: Fraysse, B. and Cochard, N. (eds), *Cochlear Implant: Acquisitions and Controversies*, pp. 3–26. Basel: Cochlear AG.

ROSEN, S. and BALL, V. (1986). Speech perception with the Vienna extra-cochlear single-channel implant: a comparison of two approaches to speech coding. *Br. J. Audiol.* 20, 61–84.

ROSEN, S. and FOURCIN, A.J. (1986). Frequency selectivity and the perception of speech. In: Moore, B.C.J. (ed.), *Frequency Selectivity in Hearing*, pp. 373–487. London: Academic Press.

ROSEN, S., MOORE, B.C.J. and FOURCIN, A.J. (1979). Lipreading with fundamental frequency information. *Proceedings of the Institute of Acoustics Autumn Conference*, Windermere 1979, paper 1A2:5-8. Institute of Acoustics.

ROSEN, S., WALLIKER, J., BRIMACOMBE, J.A. and EDGERTON, B.J. (1988). Prosodic and segmental aspects of speech perception with the House/3M single channel implant. *J. Speech Hear. Res.* **32**, 93–111.

SHANNON, R.V. and MULLER, C. (1990). Temporal modulation transfer functions in patients with cochlear implants. *J. Acoust. Soc. Am.* in press.

SUMMERFIELD, Q. (1985). Speech-processing alternatives for electrical auditory stimulation. In: Schindler, R.A. and Merzenich, M.M. (eds), *Cochlear Implants*, pp. 195–222. New York: Raven Press.

TONG, Y.C., CLARK, G.M., BLAMEY, P.J., BUSBY, P.A. and DOWELL, R.C. (1982). Psychophysical studies for two multiple-channel cochlear implant patients. *J. Acoust. Soc. Am.* **71**, 153–160.

TROUGHEAR, R. and DAVIS, P. (1979). Real-time, micro-computer based voice feature extraction in a speech pathology clinic. *Austr. J. Commun. Dis.* **7**, 4–21.

WALLEY, A.C. and CARRELL, T.D. (1983). Onset spectra and formant transitions in the adult's and child's perception of articulation in stop consonants. *J. Acoust. Soc. Am.* **51**, 1309–1317.

WALLIKER, J.R., ROSEN, S. and FOURCIN, A.J. (1986). Speech pattern prostheses for the profoundly and totally deaf. In: *IEEE Conference Publication No. 258*. International Conference on Speech Input/Output: Techniques and Applications, London, England, pp. 194–199.

WARREN, R.M. (1970). Perceptual restoration of missing speech sounds. *Science* **167**, 392–393.

Chapter 17
Children and Multichannel Cochlear Implants

STEVEN J. STALLER, ANNE L. BEITER and JUDITH A.
BRIMACOMBE

Introduction

In the last few years, the application of cochlear implants in children has
moved from limited investigational to widespread clinical application.
During the last decade, over 500 children have received either single-
channel (3M/House) or multichannel (Nucleus/Cochlear, Chouard)
implants world wide. Although initially the application of implants in
children was somewhat controversial because of the unknown implications of long-term electrical stimulation and placement of an intracochlear
electrode in children, the accumulation of data demonstrating performance improvements (Berliner et al., 1985; Mecklenburg, 1987; Hasenstab,
1988; Luxford et al., 1988; Busby et al., 1989; Miyamoto et al., 1989; Staller
et al., 1989, 1990), along with a reasonable complication rate (Staller et
al., 1989a; Cohen, 1990), have allayed many concerns. In addition, the
profound negative effect that early-onset deafness has on the development
of speech perception, speech production and language competence, as
well as on the development of the central auditory nervous system, has
highlighted the need for effective early intervention (Needleman, 1977;
Webster and Webster, 1977; Neville, 1984).

Clinical considerations surrounding the implantation of children dictate
a much broader and longer-term perspective than is typically taken when
working with adult implant patients. When dealing with children, the
clinical team must consider many developmental issues that are not
relevant to adults and the many individuals who have an impact on a child's
life, including family members, teachers of the deaf, rehabilitation
professionals and peers. In addition, the decision to implant a child creates
a life-long relationship between the implant team and the patient.

Patient Selection

Purpose of the preoperative evaluation

The preoperative evaluation period is typically more extensive for children and has multiple purposes. In addition to determining candidacy for implantation, the preoperative evaluation should establish whether the child's current amplification is appropriate or if an alternative sensory aid (hearing or vibrotactile) should be considered on a trial basis. The trial may vary in length depending on the child, but should include training in auditory skill development to determine whether benefit is derived from more conventional sensory devices. If the child does not understand the concepts necessary to program the speech processor after surgery, these must be taught preoperatively.

Selection criteria

The selection criteria which we recommend, listed in Table 17.1, reflect factors which are relevant to success with an implant that have been learned from experience with implanted children over the last few years. They are by necessity quite general, because each child must be considered in the light of his or her own particular circumstances. The exclusion medical criteria (e.g. cochlear agenesis and active middle-ear infection) represent potential adverse conditions postoperatively and are discussed in more detail below.

Table 17.1 Paediatric patient selection criteria

Selection criteria
* Bilateral profound deafness
* Ages 2–17 years
* No radiological contraindications

Candidates should:
* Demonstrate little or no benefit from amplification
* Be enrolled in an educational programme with a strong auditory/oral component
* Be psychologically and motivationally suitable
* Have appropriate family and educational expectations and support

---

The support network (social, family and educational/rehabilitative) available to children is even more critical to success with an implant than for adults. The child's family must develop appropriate expectations regarding the impact that the implant will have on their child. This can only occur if they have accepted the child's deafness and have a reasonable understanding of the implant process and the device itself. In spite of repeated counselling it is not uncommon for parents to expect their child to 'hear normally' postoperatively. Older adolescents and teenagers participate more directly in the decision-making process, and often the family assists in helping these youngsters understand the process more fully.

The recommendation for a strong auditory/oral component in the child's educational programme stems from the assumption that maximising listening skills is a prerequisite to effective use of any auditory prosthesis. This is not to imply that only purely oral programmes are appropriate, but that stress should be placed on auditory/oral training in whatever programme the child is enrolled in.

The audiological criteria include bilateral profound deafness and a lack of significant benefit from conventional amplification. The latter criterion is rather difficult to define precisely because benefit must be considered in light of each child's particular circumstances and environment, as well as the level of performance that might reasonably be expected from the implant. As might be anticipated, performance with a cochlear implant varies greatly from subject to subject. Therefore, predicting the level of postoperative performance a given child will achieve is extremely tenuous. However, based on performance data gathered to date (discussed in detail below), aided benefit is defined as access to spectral information at a segmental level. This generally can be determined clinically by administering a variety of open- and closed-set speech materials. If a child demonstrates significant open-set speech recognition or significant above-chance performance on closed-set word identification tests using monosyllabic or spondaic word materials, then he or she is not considered to be an implant candidate.

The team concept

The range of considerations necessary to evaluate, implant, programme and rehabilitate a deaf child requires a team of professionals with a broad spectrum of clinical expertise. Under optimal circumstances, the clinical team should include an audiologist, surgeon, speech pathologist, psychologist, teacher of the deaf and team coordinator. The coordinator is often one of the other professionals playing a dual role. Most often it is the audiologist's responsibility to coordinate the efforts of team members to ensure an efficient evaluation process. The teacher of the deaf is a critical member of the cochlear implant team. This is the person who will implement the rehabilitation programme and provide the intensive training recommended eventually to optimise the information the child receives through the implant. Team members should have experience in dealing with deaf children, as well as knowledge of the particular cochlear implant system, including the fitting system and associated software. The interaction of team members is particularly critical during the preoperative evaluation period. This is often a time of stress for the child and the family. Free and open communication between the family and the implant team can help reduce unnecessary concern.

Although the team may interact most closely during the evaluation and initial postoperative period, the long-term success of a child depends on periodic reappraisal. Questions should be asked at least annually to ensure the child's continued progress. Appropriate questions might include:

1. Is the equipment working properly?
2. Have the child's electrical thresholds and/or dynamic ranges changed, requiring a modification of the speech processor program?
3. Is the educational programme serving his or her needs, and is it taking advantage of the auditory input provided by the implant?
4. Should additional support services be requested?
5. Are social/peer interactions supporting the child's continued use of the implant, or is he or she a potential non-user?

Preoperative candidacy flow

The preoperative assessment sequence that is recommended is outlined in Figure 17.1. The various steps in the evaluation process proceed from general to specific and may take several months to complete, particularly if an extended hearing aid (or vibrotactile) trial is recommended. The candidate may withdraw or be discharged at each phase of the evaluation. Although not explicitly stated, counselling is often provided both formally and informally at various stages.

The initial intake, medical and audiological evaluations are designed to make a preliminary determination regarding general candidacy and to inform the child and his or her family about the implant and the process associated with receiving it. If after the preliminary evaluations the child is considered to be generally suitable, the sensory aids are evaluated for appropriateness. This may require fitting of new aids or the recommendation of a vibrotactile device if no benefit is demonstrated from hearing aids. Whenever sensory devices are modified, a trial period of at least 8 weeks is recommended during which time auditory training should continue. This allows for determination of whatever potential benefit the child may derive from the new aids and provides the best possible conditions to establish an optimal preoperative baseline. If changing aids results in sufficient improvement, the child ceases to be a candidate for implantation. The preoperative trial period can also provide the opportunity to teach young children the concepts necessary to program the speech processor. The child's understanding of concepts such as 'on/off', 'loud/soft', and 'same/different' assists the audiologist in fitting cochlear implants as well as hearing aids.

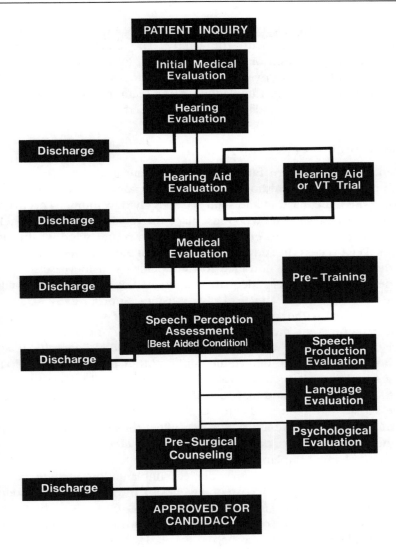

Figure 17.1. Recommended sequence of preoperative evaluation procedures. This process is extensive and may take place over a number of weeks. Note that discharge may occur at several points within the process. (Reprinted with permission from Mecklenburg (1988).)

If a child continues to be a candidate after the initial evaluations and hearing aid trial, a series of in-depth evaluations is scheduled to determine precisely his or her speech perception and production skills along with his or her language competence. These evaluations are conducted under the best-aided condition to provide a realistic baseline for comparison with postoperative results and to allow determination of the best possible aided benefit to determine candidacy. Once these evaluations are completed the entire implant team typically meets to discuss their recommendations among themselves and with the family. The team may or may not recommend implantation or suggest additional evaluation, counselling or a trial period to improve the child's chances for success. If the recommendation is against implantation, the team may suggest changes in sensory aids or in the child's rehabilitation or educational setting.

Medical/surgical evaluation

Implantation in children raises medical and surgical considerations not encountered in adults. Although the cochlea is adult size at birth (Eby and Nadol, 1986), the mastoid and skull are actively developing. This presents a challenge to the surgeon who must place the receiver/stimulator package in a thinner mastoid and create access to the round window through a smaller facial recess. In addition, since the distance between the mastoid and the round window entrance to the cochlea will increase for over a decade in young children, adequate redundancy or slack must be available in the electrode lead. The lead also must be appropriately secured to prevent gradual withdrawal from the intracochlear space.

The preoperative medical evaluation typically includes a thorough history, physical examination, laboratory testing and radiographic imaging. The history attempts to determine, among other things, the aetiology of deafness and when it occurred. Laboratory tests and a physical examination can assist in diagnosis and may identify the presence of any active disease process that may contraindicate surgery. High-resolution CT scans can determine cochlear patency, which may affect the choice of ear to implant and the ability to insert the long intracochlear electrode associated with most multichannel implants.

Aetiological implications for cochlear implantation include cochlear anatomy, new bone growth (osteoneogenesis), the viability of the auditory nerve and the distribution of spiral ganglion cells. Obviously, the failure of the cochlea to develop (cochlear agenesis) contraindicates placement of the electrode array. However, partial dysplasias of the cochlear duct may not always contraindicate surgery. Cochlear dysplasias can range from a bulbous basal turn to the complete elimination of cochlear turns and the presence of a single 'common cavity'. Although an intracochlear electrode can typically be inserted into these anomalous cochleae, the unknown characteristics of frequency representation may make appropriate programming difficult or perhaps impossible in some children.

New intracochlear bone formation is a common sequela of postmeningitic hearing loss. Although originally thought to be a contraindication of long intracochlear electrode insertion, this philosophy is changing. Even the few children with completely ossified cochleae have received partially inserted electrode arrays. Only the electrodes physically within the cochlea are programmed and, although less than optimal, all of these children detect sound and some are able to perform more complex perceptual tasks (Staller et al., 1988).

Although the absence of a viable acoustic nerve is extremely rare, such a condition would clearly contraindicate implantation. More frequently, disease processes may severely reduce the number and distribution of viable spiral ganglion cells and afferent dendrites. Aetiologies, such as Waardenburg's syndrome and in some cases meningitis, may severely reduce the population of ganglion cells (Hinojosa and Lindsay, 1980; Hinojosa and Marion, 1983). This has implications for optimal use of multielectrode devices that are predicated on the ability to stimulate subpopulations of neurons discretely.

Audiological evaluation

The audiological evaluation is designed to determine the child's perceptual skills, to assist in the determination of candidacy and to provide a baseline for postoperative comparison. The areas of assessment include aided and unaided sound detection, speech perception and lipreading enhancement. With the exception of unaided detection thresholds, audiological tests are conducted in the best-aided condition. Although evaluations are usually conducted at conversational loudness levels (e.g. 70 dB SPL), higher intensity stimuli are presented if the child is unable to detect sound at 70 dB. However, the inability to detect conversational level signals is a significant clinical and social detriment, irrespective of how well a child performs speech-perception tasks at very high intensities.

The selection of evaluation measures is complicated by the lack of standardised speech perception tests for hearing-impaired children. Most tests utilised with implanted children have been derived from batteries designed for profoundly deaf adults (e.g. Minimal Auditory Capabilities (MAC); Owens et al., 1981) or from instruments designed for less profoundly hearing-impaired children (e.g. Word Intelligibility by Picture Identification (WIPI) – Lerman, Ross and McLauchlin (1965); Kindergarten Phonetically Balanced Word Lists (PBK) – Haskins (1949)). Many young profoundly deaf children do not have adequate language or cognitive competence to perform these tests reliably.

The audiological battery developed by the authors is listed in Table 17.2. The core tests in this battery comprise the Early Speech Perception Battery (ESP) that was developed by Moog and Geers (1990) at the Central Institute for the Deaf (CID) (Figure 17.2). The ESP has several major strengths: (1) it incorporates a hierarchy of skill levels; (2) the vocabulary is appropriate for young deaf children; (3) pictures and objects depict the auditory stimuli allowing meaningful reinforcement for even very young children; (4) stimuli may be presented live voice or recorded. Two levels

Table 17.2   Speech perception evaluation*

Early Speech Perception (ESP) Battery (standard or low verbal version)
   Pattern perception
   Spondee identification
   Monosyllable identification
Northwestern University Children's Perception of Speech (NU-CHIPS)
Glendonald Auditory Screening Procedure (GASP) Words
Minimal Auditory Capabilities (MAC) Battery Spondee Recognition
Central Institute for the Deaf (CID) Sentences of Everyday Speech
Phonetically Balanced Kindergarten (PBK) word lists
Measure of speechreading
   Craig Lipreading Inventory: Word subtest
   CID Sentences of Everyday Speech

---

*Recorded versions of these tests should be administered whenever possible.

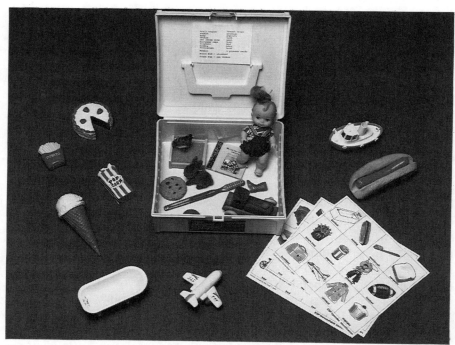

Figure 17.2.   Items of the CID Early Speech Perception Battery.

of complexity are available within the battery, both of which allow
assessment of suprasegmental (pattern) and segmental (spectral) skills.
The standard battery uses pictured stimuli that range in difficulty up to 12-
item spondaic and monosyllabic word identification tasks. A low-verbal

battery is also available for very young children. A limited number of objects are selected based on the child's vocabulary and presented live voice. Again, both pattern perception and closed-set word identification are assessed.

In addition to the ESP battery, the Northwestern University Children's Speech Perception (NU-CHIPS) (Elliott and Katz, 1980) is used to assess closed-set word identification in children who achieve ceiling scores on the ESP, and who have more sophisticated vocabulary. NU-CHIPS is a four-item, forced-choice word identification test which uses recorded monosyllabic stimuli. Four open-set word recognition measures are also included in the audiological battery. Three of the tests use word stimuli (Glendonald Auditory Screening Procedure (GASP) – Erber and Alencewicz (1982); MAC Spondee Recognition – Owens, Kessler and Telleen (1981); and PBK) and one uses sentence materials (MAC: CID Sentences of Everyday Speech – Owens, Kessler and Telleen, 1981). The open-set word tests range in complexity from the GASP, which uses common words of differing length, to PBK which uses monosyllabic words. Although the GASP was originally designed as a closed-set screening procedure, it is useful when modified in this application as an open-set procedure, because the vocabulary is appropriate for even very young children.

Assessment of lipreading enhancement is also incorporated into the audiological test battery. CID sentences are used for older children and the word subtest of the Craig Lipreading Inventory (Jeffers and Barley, 1977) is appropriate for children with less complex vocabularies. The Craig is a four-alternative forced-choice test which uses pictured materials. Visual enhancement is measured by comparing the difference in performance in the lipreading-alone condition with the lipreading-plus-sound condition.

Speech/language assessment

Although speech production and language competence are not generally major factors in determining candidacy for implantation, they are certainly a major component in determining long-term success. Auditory deprivation adversely affects the normal development of speech and oral language and, conversely, with appropriate training, sensory input from an auditory prosthesis can potentially improve delayed or deviant production and language. Changes in the quantity and quality of speech production are some of the most rapid consequences of implantation in young children.

The areas of speech/language assessment include: (1) imitative and spontaneous articulation, (2) non-segmental voice characteristics (i.e. pitch, intensity etc.), and (3) receptive and expressive language (Tobey et al., 1990). A variety of instruments, both formal and informal, is available to assess the speech production and language competence of paediatric candidates. Older children with more complex linguistic abilities allow greater flexibility in selecting language and speech measurement tools. Younger children may require less formal assessment through elicited or spontaneous language samples. The specific test battery to be employed must necessarily be tailored to each child depending on such factors as age at onset of deafness, duration of deafness, communication mode, educational setting and cognitive abilities.

Speech production and non-segmental voice characteristics can be assessed at both an analytical and a synthetic level. The Ling Phonetic Level Evaluation (PLE) determines the extent to which particular sound patterns exist and the rate at which sound patterns can be repeated and alternated. It was originally designed as a diagnostic teaching technique to determine the level at which to begin intervention; when used in assessment, the PLE provides a logical sequence to identify and evaluate phonemes in a child's repertoire. It also provides insight into the child's stimulability for each phoneme. The Ling Phonologic Level Evaluation provides a means to assess how sound patterns observed in the PLE are used for meaningful communication. This is achieved through analysis of spontaneous speech/language samples. Changes in the imitative production of individual phonemes (analytical) generally precede spontaneous changes or changes at the overall level of speech intelligibility (synthetic) (Ling, 1976).

Reliable assessment of speech intelligibility is difficult, especially with more deviant production. Linguistic context of the material, listener familiarity with the subject and the material all serve to bias intelligibility ratings. One method of assessing speech intelligibility is to have children read or imitate short sentences or phrases and have a panel of raters listen to recordings of the child's utterances. The judges write down what they hear, and the percentage of words correctly identified is calculated. A list of 36 sentences was developed specifically for hearing-impaired children by McGarr (1983). The sentences may be used for older children or keywords may be extracted and presented in one- or two-word phrases for younger children.

Whenever possible, receptive and expressive language assessments should be made using standardised instruments. The use of standardised tests provides an appropriate metric for determining the relevance of change across time for a given child, as well as facilitating performance comparisons across subjects. Unfortunately, there is a paucity of tests with normative data on hearing-impaired children. Appendix I provides a list of speech and language tests that have been used with paediatric cochlear implant candidates.

Two tests which do provide normative data are the Grammatical Analysis of Elicited Language (GAEL) and the Rhode Island Test of Language Structures (RITLS). The GAEL is designed for use with deaf children using oral or total communication whilst the RITLS is primarily designed for children using total communication. The GAEL comprises three levels: presentence, simple sentence and complex sentence. A nice feature of this test is the continuity provided across a broad range of ages and linguistic complexity.

Psychosocial evaluation

The psychosocial milieu of a deaf child is one of the most critical factors in assessing candidacy for implantation. It also contributes substantially to the long-term 'success' or 'failure' of the implant process. The interaction of the family constellation, peers and rehabilitative/educational professionals is important for effective use of the implant. Assessment of psychosocial parameters during the evaluation process typically includes a psychologist in consultation with a teacher of the deaf. Optimally the psychologist should have experience in dealing with hearing-impaired children and be familiar with sign language.

Determining the level of expectations on the part of the family and the child, the motivation for seeking a cochlear implant and the support system available to the child are three critical goals of the psychosocial evaluation. The acceptance of the child's deafness by the family may contribute to more realistic estimates of the benefits provided by a cochlear implant. Expectations that the implant will provide 'normal hearing' are not uncommon and may require extended counselling. In addition, many families feel that the implant will 'fix' the problem of hearing loss, rather than considering it as a tool in the long-term process of rehabilitation and education within which they must play an active role. Defining that role is an important part of the evaluation process.

Implant teams use a variety of tools and techniques (e.g. standardised non-verbal performance intelligence measures, interviews, questionnaires etc.) in an attempt to quantify the psychosocial variables. When dealing with older children it is important to separate the expectations and motivations of the family from those of the child. It is critical that adolescents have their own reasons for wanting an implant and that they realise the extent of the implantation process, including the need to wear external hardware that is similar in size to a body hearing aid. Many adolescents may echo the interests of their family rather than conveying their true feelings.

The influence of peer interactions and the educational environment cannot be underestimated. A child may be an excellent implant candidate and yet quickly become a non-user, if his or her peers do not use spoken language to communicate or if he or she is ostracised because of the use of an implant. The teacher on the team can provide valuable input in determining the appropriateness of the educational setting and the availability of ancillary support services.

Paediatric Considerations in Speech-processor Programming

Pre-programming training

Approximately 4–6 weeks are required for postoperative healing of the implant site. Especially with the younger children, training should continue during the recovery period to teach the basic perceptual skills necessary to program the speech processor. At the most basic level, the clinician teaches the child to make a clear behavioural response to a visual, tactile or auditory stimulus. Additionally, the initial programming sessions will be easier for all involved when the child is familiar with the tasks expected of him or her and if he or she is already comfortable with the external equipment. Children should be encouraged to try on the speech processor and headset and, ideally, to meet and observe another child or adult with a cochlear implant during a programming session. Such practice sessions tend to reduce the stress often associated with the initial fitting of the device.

The basic perceptual skills recommended to program the speech processor effectively include: presence/absence, soft/loud, same/different and loudness scaling. The concept of presence/absence is established by teaching the child to make time-locked behavioural responses to discrete stimulation. Such responses are trained using visual and/or tactile stimulation in conjunction with operant conditioning techniques, such as those typically applied in standard paediatric audiometric testing. Once the child is conditioned to respond to a stimulus, this response pattern can be transferred successfully to the auditory modality using electrical stimulation through the cochlear implant.

The concept of soft/loud is more difficult to teach, especially with children who have had little or no auditory experience. However, when programming the processor, it is important to establish, for each electrode pair, the end points of the loudness growth function (i.e. threshold and maximum comfortable loudness). This should ensure that the ongoing loudness variations occurring in speech will fit comfortably into the child's electrical dynamic range. For children who understand the concept of little/big, this similar comparison can be used when training soft/loud. When using the visual or tactile modality, the presentation of a less-intense stimulus is paired with a small object, whilst a more intense stimulus is paired with a large one. To facilitate understanding, the difference between the two visual or tactile stimuli should be as large as possible. Any functional low-frequency hearing in the contralateral ear can be used effectively in training the soft/loud distinction. Although this concept is initially more difficult to teach and then to transfer to the auditory modality, even very young children demonstrate a rudimentary understanding of 'loud' after brief exposure to changes in loudness resulting from electrical stimulation.

Depending upon the child's age and previous exposure to sound, the more advanced concepts of loudness scaling and same/different can also be introduced. Whilst these concepts are not necessary to create a wearable program or MAP* for the child, they are used to refine the MAP by equalising loudness levels across electrode pairs. Usually, the more difficult concepts of loudness scaling and same/different are taught over time, as the child gains experience with listening through the cochlear implant. In teaching the idea of a progression from soft to loud, the clinician may use props, such as objects of graduated size. At first, the loudness scaling exercise should be modified into a two-alternative forced-choice task, in which the child chooses between two adjacent points on the loudness growth scale. Once the louder level has been chosen, the clinician adds the next progressive step and removes the softer choice. As the child becomes more experienced with scaling, the audiologist increases the number of steps available. Figure 17.3 depicts paediatric materials that have been developed and provided to clinicians to teach the concept of loudness scaling. Pictures of faces and glasses of water simplify the concept for younger children. A more abstract representation of increasing loudness is used for teaching the concept to older children.

Training for same/different can take the form of presenting the child with many concrete examples of the distinction coupled with two auditory, visual or tactile signals. For example, pairing the same or different objects with stimulus trials representing soft/soft, loud/loud, soft/loud and loud/soft permits the clinician to train the concept and obtain information about loudness balance without requiring specific information from the child about which of two sounds is louder.

Programming the speech processor

An IBM PC-based Diagnostic and Programming System (Figure 17.4) with customised software provides maximal flexibility in fitting the cochlear implant to the child's individual electrical current requirements. The team of clinicians uses basic play audiometry to program the device. During the test sessions, it is critical that the audiologists have many age-appropriate reinforcing activities available, in order to keep the child's interest. Depending on the child's attention span, test sessions will need to be broken up into short segments, with frequent small breaks away from the test room. One audiologist is responsible for presenting the computer-controlled test stimuli. A second clinician is responsible for keeping the

---

*Acoustic parameters that are extracted and digitally encoded by the speech processor determine the stimulus parameters for each stimulus pulse delivered to the selected electrode pair. The information used to define these stimuli is stored within the speech processor and is referred to as the MAP.

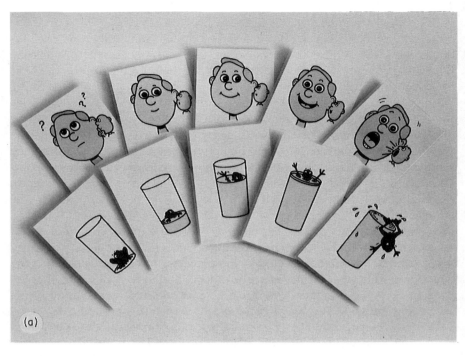

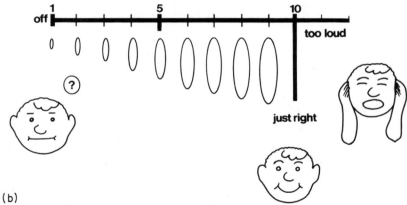

Figure 17.3. Materials used to teach the concept of loudness scaling. (a) Literal pictures of faces and glasses of water make the concept more concrete for younger children. (b) A more abstract representation of increasing loudness is used for teaching the concept to older children.

child on task, making behavioural observations and reinforcing responses (Figure 17.5). Using the concepts of presence/absence and soft/loud, as discussed above, in conjunction with traditional play audiometric techniques, threshold and comfortable loudness judgements for electrical stimulation are determined for each electrode pair. These values set the

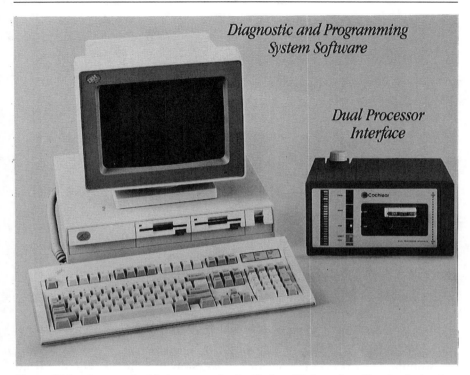

Figure 17.4. Computerised fitting system for the Nucleus 22-channel cochlear implant system. The Dual Processor Interface (DPI) accommodates both the original Wearable Speech Processor and the newer Mini-Speech Processor.

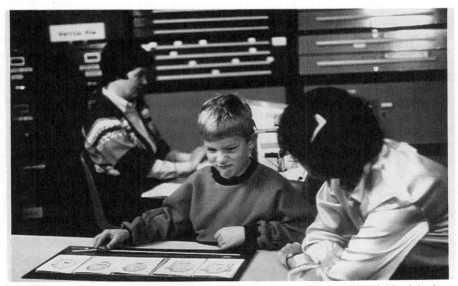

Figure 17.5. The use of two clinicians allows one to focus attention on the child, while the other presents computer-controlled stimuli.

child's electrical dynamic range and define how the loudness variations that occur in speech and environmental sounds will fit into this dynamic range and be perceived by the child after the processor is programmed.

As mentioned earlier, a full appreciation of soft/loud (the concept needed to set the upper limits of electrical stimulation for the child) seems to require that the child have some direct experience in the auditory modality. Thus, it is important to provide experience as soon as possible with everyday sounds as processed through the implant system. Ideally, enough information is obtained during the first day of initial stimulation that a MAP can be made for the child to wear home. This may mean that initial programs use only a few of the available electrodes. After experiencing sound even for a short period of time, small children begin to use words such as 'stop' or non-verbal signs during psychophysical testing to signal that the stimulus has become loud.

With the Nucleus multichannel cochlear implant, the standard psychophysical stimulus used to obtain threshold and maximum comfortable loudness level judgements is a 250-Hz constant current pulse train with a 50% duty cycle (500 ms on/off). Very young children may quickly find this stimulus uninteresting and adapt to it. The clinical impression is that, because there is no apparent response to the stimulus, the child is not hearing. This situation may result in clinicians progressively increasing the stimulation level until a startle or aversion response is elicited from the child. In an attempt to avoid this, recent versions of the programming software allow the audiologist to use a live-voice speech stimulus when determining thresholds and comfort levels. Because the stimulus is 'speech-like', it may be more interesting to the child, making it easier for the audiologists to obtain overt conditioned responses or to observe subtle changes in behaviour that are time-locked to stimulus presentation.

The initial goal in programming the processor is to create a comfortable MAP that allows the child to detect sound across the speech frequency range. This is normally accomplished, even with the youngest children, during the first few days of electrical stimulation. This task also is made easier when clinicians use play materials that are age appropriate, do not require an elaborate behavioural response and maximise the number of responses that can be obtained during the activity. To keep the child's interest during the session, a variety of materials should be available that are reinforcing to the child. After a MAP is made, the audiologists check to ensure that sounds are not too loud and that the child can reliably detect ongoing speech as well as specific speech sounds at conversational listening levels. It is not unusual to find threshold and comfortable listening levels changing during the first few days of device use as the child gains some experience with hearing. It is recommended that initial comfort level settings be conservative, so that there is little likelihood that the child will have a negative reaction, especially to loud environmental sounds.

Table 17.3 Number of electrodes programmed

Time	2–5 years		2–17 years	
	Mean	s.d.	Mean	s.d.
Day 1	7.3	5.1	10.5	5.6
Day 3	11.3	3.3	14.1	3.7
Day 30	16.8	4.2	17.6	3.61
6 months	17.0	3.2	18.3	3.15
12 months	17.5	3.5	18.2	3.5

All available electrode pairs may not be used during the initial programming, especially in the youngest children. However, as these children gain experience with the programming tasks and the auditory sensations provided by the cochlear implant, the number of electrode pairs that are programmed can be increased. Table 17.3 presents the mean number of electrode pairs programmed after 1 day and at 1 month and 6 months post-initial stimulation. Even with the youngest children, experienced clinicians are often able to program the majority of electrodes within 1 month of initial tune-up.

For those few very young children who initially have not been trained successfully to make reliable conditioned responses, standard audiological behavioural observation techniques can be used to estimate threshold and comfortable loudness levels. Responses that have been noted to electrical stimulation are the following:

1. No apparent responses.
2. Aversion responses.
3. Quieting.
4. Searching.
5. Questioning.
6. Facial expression change.
7. Threshold level responses only.
8. Comfort level responses only.
9. Conditioned responses.

Children with less auditory experience may show more subtle responses initially than other children. In cases where reliable conditioned responses cannot be obtained, estimations of dynamic range are made for individual electrode pairs and are used to generate a MAP. After programming the speech processor, the clinicians observe the child for any changes in behaviour when sound occurs in the environment, as well as for behaviours which suggest that sounds are uncomfortably loud. After observing the child, the program is modified until the audiologists are confident that sound is being adequately perceived and is not uncomfort-able. Once these young children gain some experience with the auditory sensations provided through the implant, they can be conditioned successfully so that more accurate measurements of threshold and comfortable loudness levels can be obtained for use in reprogramming.

Generally for all children, a reprogramming session is scheduled approximately 1 month following the initial 2- to 3-day session. Threshold and comfortable loudness levels are re-evaluated, and additional channels may be added to the program. In addition, modifications to the child's MAP can be made over time, as the child becomes more sophisticated in loudness scaling and equalising comfortable loudness levels across the electrode array. The Nucleus multichannel implant is designed specifically to extract and transmit certain speech features known to be critical to accurate speech perception. Spectral information is delivered to specific electrode pairs following the tonotopic organisation of the cochlea. Thus, high-frequency information in the speech signal is sent to more basal electrodes and low-frequency information to electrodes placed more apically within the cochlea. A MAP contains frequency boundaries for each active electrode, as well as the threshold and comfort levels necessary for translating sound pressure level information into stimulation parameters. Since the overriding goal in the implantation of profoundly deaf children is to provide access to the acoustic signal, most importantly for the development of speech and spoken language, paediatric training and assessment materials should consist of meaningful linguistic information. As a child's abilities to use electrical stimulation for speech discrimination, identification and/or recognition increase, the adequacy of new MAPs can be evaluated using informal speech tests, such as closed-set identification of words or short sentences of varying length and spectral composition.

Programming mode

The cochlear implant can produce two types of stimulation: bipolar and common ground. With bipolar stimulation, current flows between the active electrode and a specific return electrode that is within close proximity. As depicted in Figure 17.6a, when using bipolar stimulation, the current flow within the cochlea can be widened by progressively increasing the distance between the active and return electrodes. In contrast, common ground stimulation occurs between an active electrode and a ground or return made up of all of the other electrodes connected together. Typically, the lowest thresholds are obtained in this mode because of the wider current spread. Figure 17.6b illustrates the current distribution in common ground for an electrode array placed in saline. It should be noted that, although the majority of current is localised at the active electrode, there is a small amount of current flowing to each

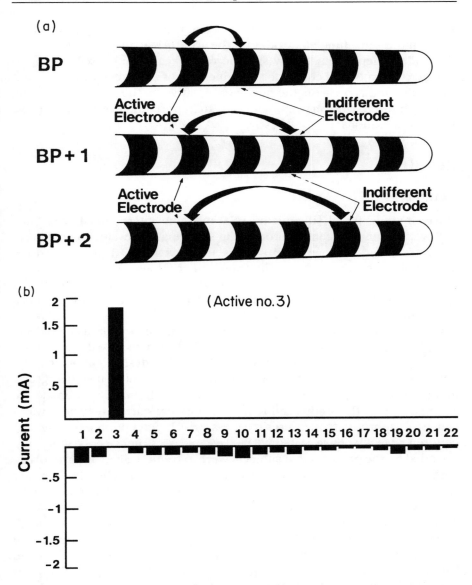

Figure 17.6. Illustration of current distribution with different modes of programming. Note that, although common ground links all indifferent electrodes together, the majority of current is restricted to a narrow region in the vicinity of the active electrode.

electrode on the array. However, because the majority of current is located at the active electrode, normal tonotopic pitch perception can be achieved when using this mode of stimulation.

It is recommended that all children initially be tested and programmed in common ground. Common ground represents a pseudo-monopolar mode where the designated active electrode uses a common return made up of all the remaining electrodes on the array. Thus, the integrity of each electrode, independent of any specific return, can be assessed. Common ground is the mode of choice for identification of any damaged or aberrant electrodes and represents the most conservative method of programming young children who may not be able to report unpleasant or unusual auditory sensations.

Results

Methods

Thirty investigational sites in the USA and nine international sites have followed a common clinical protocol in selecting and evaluating children. Subjects under the age of 10 years underwent an 8-week intensive preoperative training period. The training period allowed children to be evaluated longitudinally prior to surgery to ensure that amplification was optimised and that the concepts necessary for programming the Nucleus device could be learned.

In view of the heterogeneous nature of the population of deaf children, a single-subject, repeated-measures research design was used where each subject served as his or her own control. This design eliminated the unavoidable influence of inadequate matching inherent in matched group designs, because the salient variables related to performance are unknown. At the outset of the study (and to a certain extent currently), there was a paucity of appropriate measures to assess speech perception in young deaf children (Mecklenburg, 1986). The lack of assessment tools was compounded by the problem that subjects were extremely diverse, particularly with respect to age and language competence, thereby limiting the applicability of any given measure to a subset of the experimental sample. Because of these two problems, an extensive battery of evaluation measures was compiled from which specific age-appropriate tests were chosen for each subject. In order to evaluate changes in performance before and after implantation, attempts were made to administer the same battery of tests pre- and postoperatively to a given subject. For each subject, change in performance on a test after implantation was analysed for statistical significance ($P<0.05$) using the Thornton and Raffin (1978) derivation of the binomial model. In order to summarise performance across subjects, tests were organised within the following categories: (1) sound detection, (2) environmental sound identification, (3) prosodic speech perception (timing and rhythm), (4) closed-set word identification, (5) open-set word recognition, (6) lipreading and (7) speech production. Ideally, at least one test was attempted within each category for all subjects. Overall improvement within each category required subjects to demonstrate statistically significant improvement on at least one-third of the measures administered.

Recorded measures were used predominantly and were administered in sound field at 70 dB SPL. The few tests that were not recorded were administered monitored live voice, also at 70 dB SPL. Preoperatively, subjects were assessed in their best-aided condition. A subject may have used one or two hearing aids, a vibrotactile device or, in some cases, both hearing aids and a vibrotactile device. Preoperatively, subjects who could not detect sound at 70 dB SPL, even with high-gain hearing aids, were fitted with a vibrotactile device or were tested at higher stimulus intensities that corresponded with their most comfortable listening levels. Postoperative evaluations were conducted in the implant-alone condition, even in the few cases where contralateral hearing aids were worn by the children in their day-to-day environment. Therefore, in order to achieve postoperative improvement, a child's performance in the implanted ear must have exceeded his or her preoperative performance in the better-hearing ear at a statistically significant level. Evaluations were conducted preoperatively and at 6-month intervals postoperatively.

Subjects

As of April 15, 1990, 309 children were implanted with the Nucleus 22-channel cochlear implant world wide. Performance data have been gathered from 80 English-speaking subjects who have been wearing their devices for at least 12 months.

Selection criteria included bilateral profound deafness, no significant benefit from amplification, an absence of medical contraindications, appropriate expectations on the part of the child and family, and educational settings that included an auditory/oral component. Children in manual communication settings were not considered candidates and neither were adolescents who did not use spontaneous differentiated vocalisations during communication.

Demographic information on the 80 subjects from whom performance data were acquired is reported here. Most subjects were deafened at an early age. The mean age at onset of deafness was 2.8 years (s.d. = 3.6 years), whilst the mean age at implantation was 9.8 years (s.d. = 4.7 years). The youngest child implanted was 2 years, 1 month (2;1 years) of age. Fifty-five per cent of the subjects were prelinguistically deafened (at or before 2 years of age). Thirty-four per cent of all subjects were deaf at birth (congenitally deaf).

The distribution of the aetiologies of deafness is presented in Table 17.4. Half of the subjects were deafened as a result of meningitis whilst the aetiology of deafness was unknown for 38%. Although meningitis was the most frequently occurring aetiology, the presence of osteoneogenesis has

Table 17.4 Aetiologies of deafness

Cause of deafness	Percentage of subjects
Meningitis	50
Unknown	38
CMV	3
Mondini	2
Waardenburg	1
Other	6

not precluded insertion of a long intracochlear electrode in most cases. Although some drilling was required in 26% of subjects for whom data were reported, partial insertion of the electrode array (<16 electrodes) only occurred in 6% of subjects. An analysis of the number of electrodes inserted as a function of the aetiology of deafness was also performed. Due to the small numbers of subjects in some aetiological groups, categories were collapsed into meningitis, unknown and other. Mean insertion depth for the meningitis group was 18.0 mm (s.d. = 4.78) compared with 19.9 mm (s.d. = 3.98 and 2.36) for the unknown and other groups, respectively. The mean insertion depth was sufficient to allow intracochlear placement of all 22 active electrodes for all three groups.

Complications

There have been 21 (6.8%) medical/surgical complications in the 309 children implanted to date. Eight (2.6%) complications required surgical intervention and the remainder resolved medically, expectantly, or through programming or external hardware changes. Eight (2.6%) subjects developed postoperative flap infection or necrosis. Four of these required surgical intervention, three were treated with antibiotics and one minor irritation was resolved with moleskin. One subject developed delayed-onset unilateral facial paresis and was explanted. This subject has recovered 70% function of the lower face and 30% function in the orbital area. She has been reimplanted in the contralateral ear and currently wears her device daily.

Migration of the internal receiver/stimulator package occurred in three (1.0%) subjects. Two occurred subsequent to flap infections and subsequent surgical intervention, whilst the third occurred shortly after initial surgery. Two of these cases required surgical revision and the third was resolved by inactivating the basal electrodes that were not intracochlear. One electrode was inappropriately placed in a hypotympanic air cell. The device was replaced and the child is currently wearing her new implant during all waking hours.

There have been eight (2.6%) cases of internal device failure. Six of these had unknown causes whilst two were thought to be due to external agents (e.g. blow to the head). Seven subjects have been explanted and reimplanted and are currently wearing their devices daily. One subject has yet to be reimplanted.

The remaining complications were considered minor and included transient mild dizziness, local skin irritation, transient loud sounds, facial nerve stimulation and electrode faults. All of these complications resolved spontaneously or were eliminated through replacement of external equipment or through reprogramming.

Speech perception

With the exception of one subject with an inappropriately placed electrode array, all subjects detected sound at conversational levels with their cochlear implants. Detection thresholds with the Nucleus device are typically a function of microphone and preamplifier characteristics rather than a function of patient variables. Therefore, the variability in detection thresholds across frequency and across subjects is quite small (Figure 17.7) (Staller, 1990). Although an isolated electrode may not elicit an auditory percept in a few patients, the inherent flexibility in programming the Nucleus device universally has provided moderate-intensity sound detection to all paediatric subjects.

Only four subjects (1.6%) use their devices for less than 3 hours per day and are considered to be minimal users or non-users. All of these

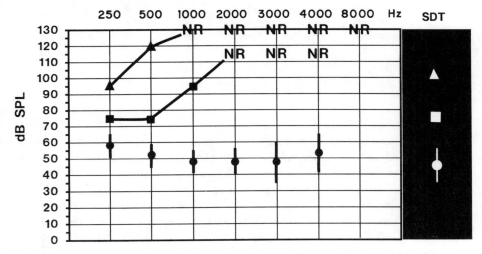

Figure 17.7. Preoperative median unaided (filled triangles) for the implant ear and best-aided (filled boxes) detection thresholds in dB SPL. Postoperative (filled circles) mean and standard deviation sound field detection thresholds with the cochlear implant (dB SPL).

subjects are adolescents who were deafened at an early age. Although a number of adolescents with long-term deafness use their implants successfully, they are subject to numerous psychosocial pressures that may constrain success, particularly if benefit from the implant is somewhat limited.

Assessment of auditory-alone speech perception was divided into three categories: (1) prosodics, i.e. the perception of the timing, duration and intonation of speech, (2) closed-set, i.e. the ability to identify a word from a small set of alternatives, and (3) open-set, i.e. the ability to recognise unrehearsed words and sentences without cues or contextual information. For the subjects tested within each category, significant postoperative improvement ($P<0.05$) was demonstrated by 66% for prosodics, 63% for closed-set, and 46% for open-set words (Figure 17.8).

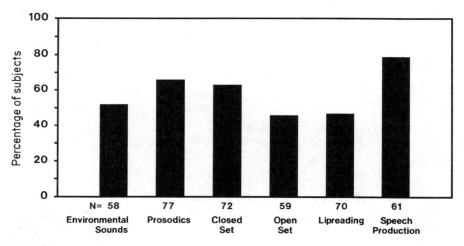

Figure 17.8. Percentage of subjects achieving significant improvement ($P<0.05$) within each perceptual category. (Reprinted with permission from Staller et al. (1990b).)

In order to evaluate performance on a test-by-test basis, paired comparisons are shown in Tables 17.5 and 17.6. These tables present preoperative and postoperative group means on the prosodic, closed-set and open-set tests. On the nine prosodic tests, postoperative performance was significantly better than preoperative performance on all of the measures. However, the magnitude of difference tended to be larger for those measures designed to be used with children (e.g. Discrimination After Training (DAT) – Thielemeir (1984) and Monosyllable/Trochee/Spondee (MTS) – Erber and Alencewicz (1976)).

A similar analysis on five closed-set word identification measures is presented in Table 17.5. With the exception of the Word Intelligibility by

Table 17.5 Prosodic and closed-set tests

Test	n	Best-aided preoperative (%)		12-month postoperative cochlear implant (%)	
Prosodic tests					
MTS: stress	37	45.3	(17.6)	68.0	(22.4)[c]
MTS(P): stress	5	39.8	(20.0)	90.0	(6.2)[c]
MAC: spondee same/different	39	62.1	(17.0)	72.2	(18.3)[b]
ANT: stress	4	45.0	(37.9)	100.0	(0)
MAC: noise/voice	38	59.5	(19.0)	73.2	(19.4)[b]
Iowa: male/female	16	51.0	(16.2)	65.9	(17.6)[b]
Iowa: no. of syllables	16	36.5	(17.5)	53.9	(19.5)[c]
DAT[d]	62	6.0	(3.0)	9.9	(2.5)[e]
TAC[d]	42	0.9	(1.3)	2.0	(2.0)[b]
Closed-set tests					
MTS: Word	40	14.8	(13.3)	45.3	(31.3)[c]
MTS(P): Word	5	14.7	(10.7)	61.7	(22.8)[a]
ANT: Word	25	18.7	(11.7)	54.3	(34.6)[c]
NU-CHIPS	14	31.3	(8.8)	40.9	(11.8)[a]
WIPI	16	18.0	(8.5)	22.8	(10.1)[b]
MAC: four-choice spondee	31	34.7	(17.6)	47.7	(26.9)[b]

[a]$P<0.05$.
[b]$P<0.01$.
[c]$P<0.001$.
[d]Assessed both prosodic and closed-set skills with a maximum score of: DAT 12 levels, TAC 10 levels.
[e]DAT was not statistically analysed because of the non-linear increase in complexity across levels. Clinical significance was considered to be an increase of 2 levels or 1 CID category. The mean postoperative improvement was clinically significant.
Values in parentheses are the standard deviations.

Table 17.6 Open-set tests

Test	n	Best-aided preoperative (%)		n	12-month postoperative cochlear implant (%)	
NU No. 6: word score	21	0.4	(1.0)	26	4.2	(9.4)
GASP: words	21	DNT		22	27.3	(33.3)
PBK: word score	7	1.1	(2.0)	19	9.4	(23.1)
Spondee recognition	23	2.3	(5.1)	34	11.3	(18.3)[a]
CID sentences	16	0.6	(2.0)	32	13.1	(25.4)[a]
BKB sentences	1	0		4	63.0	(27.6)
GASP: sentences	21	DNT		21	29.5	(38.0)

[a]$P<0.01$
Values in parentheses are the standard deviations.
DNT = did not test.

Picture Identification (WIPI) test, the postoperative means were all significantly improved over preoperative performance.

Pre- and postoperative scores on seven open-set measures are shown in Table 17.6. The open-set tests used recorded materials, except when given to a few younger subjects who attended more appropriately to live-voice administration. Paired comparisons are not presented because very few subjects were able to take open-set tests preoperatively with hearing or vibrotactile aids. Significant open-set performance was defined as recognition of at least two words. Under the clinical protocol, two tests (GASP words and sentences), originally designed to be administered closed-set, were presented open-set. These two measures were the only open-set tests which used vocabulary that was appropriate for younger children.

Twenty-seven (46%) of the 59 subjects tested with open-set measures achieved statistically above-chance results postoperatively. The range of performance across subjects varied widely. In general, tests using single-word stimuli (GASP words, PBK, NU no. 6 (Tillman, Carhart and Wilbur, 1966) and Spondee Recognition), particularly monosyllabic words, were more difficult than sentence materials (GASP, CID and BKB (Bench and Bamford, 1979) sentences). Six subjects were able to score 80% or greater on one or more of the open-set measures.

Improvements in auditory-alone speech perception suggest that many children are able to perceive pattern and stress cues and to make fine segmental contrasts with their multichannel cochlear implants. This ability aids in the perception of vowel transitions and formant frequency distinctions fundamental to word recognition.

Speech production

Improvement in speech production is an important, although less direct, benefit of implantation. A hierarchy of production skills was evaluated to determine the elemental (segmental) changes in the children's speech, the changes in suprasegmental speech patterns (i.e. melody, rhythm and intonation) and the effect of these changes on overall intelligibility. Accurate production of a particular speech element typically can be elicited after modelling by a clinician (imitatively) before it occurs in the child's spontaneous speech. Therefore, elicited measures document emerging skills that subsequently may be incorporated into the child's spontaneous repertoire.

To evaluate both elicited and spontaneous production, phonemes were acquired imitatively and extracted from a taped spontaneous language sample. The phonemes were analysed using the Ling Phonetic Level Evaluation (PLE) (imitative) and the Ling Phonologic Level Evaluation (spontaneous) (Ling, 1976). The segmental portion of the PLE evaluates simple sounds (e.g. /ba/) to more complex sounds involving multiple consonants (e.g. /stra/). Performance on the PLE was analysed using a numerical rating scale that was developed by Iler-Kirk and Hill-Brown (1985) and modified by Tobey et al. (1989). Accurate production of individual phonemes was assigned a score according to both the consistency of production and the complexity of the environment in which the sounds were produced. The hierarchy of production environments ranged from a single production of the phoneme in isolation to repeated production of the phoneme while varying its pitch. Higher scores on these measures therefore may reflect the acquisition of greater numbers of phonemes or more consistent production of existing phonemes. Imitative production of non-segmental speech features and spontaneous production of both segmental and non-segmental features was assessed using a similar rating scale. However, only the consistency of production was rated.

Speech intelligibility was evaluated using sentence materials developed by McGarr (1983). Each child was asked to read or repeat 36 sentences. The child's utterances were recorded and unfamiliar listeners were asked to write down what the child had said without knowledge of the materials used. The percentage of keywords correctly identified by the listeners was reported as an intelligibility score. In addition, spectral analyses of recorded utterances were performed to determine the immediate impact of sound from the implant on speech, compared to the children's speech with the processor turned off. Details of the acoustic analyses are the subject of a separate report (Tobey et al., 1990).

The PLE was performed on 45 subjects both pre- and postoperatively. Group mean preoperative and 12-month postoperative performance by these subjects on the segmental and non-segmental subtests are presented in Figure 17.9. Two non-segmental and seven segmental categories were

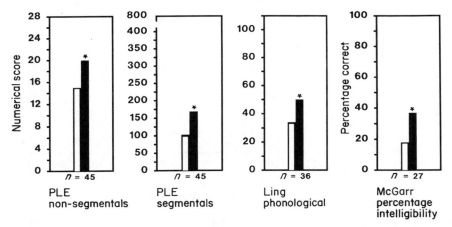

Figure 17.9. Group mean pre- and 12-month postoperative performance on four tests of speech production. * Indicates significant postoperative improvement in group mean scores. (Reprinted with permission from Staller et al. (1990b).)

defined by Tobey et al. (1989) to represent clinically relevant levels of performance. Fourteen (31%) and 30 (67%) of the 45 subjects, tested both pre- and postoperatively with the PLE, improved at least one clinical category on the non-segmental and segmental subtests, respectively. Group mean performance improved pre- to postoperatively from 14.9 to 20.1 (on a 28-point scale) on non-segmentals and from 102.9 to 179.1 (on an 832-point scale) on segmentals. Spontaneous production for 36 subjects on the Ling Phonologic increased from 34.3 to 51.2 (on a 110-point scale) after 12 months of experience with the cochlear implant. This difference was statistically significant ($P<0.001$). In addition, 27 subjects were evaluated both pre- and postoperatively for intelligibility with the McGarr materials. Seventeen (63%) of these subjects were significantly more intelligible after 12 months of implant experience. As a group, intelligibility increased from 18% to 36.5% pre- to postoperatively on this measure. When the data on all subjects for all measures of speech production are collapsed, 79% of the 61 subjects tested demonstrated significant ($P<0.05$) postoperative improvement in speech production.

Lipreading

Lipreading enhancement was assessed using a variety of test materials. Lipreading of words and sentences was evaluated by comparing lipreading alone with lipreading plus sound from the speech processor on the same test. The assessment of lipreading enhancement in younger children is

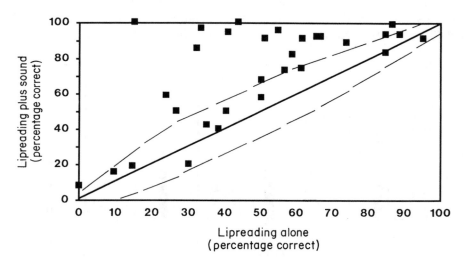

Figure 17.10. Postoperative scores on lipreading-alone vs lipreading-plus-sound conditions obtained from 30 subjects administered CID sentences. Significant improvement was demonstrated by 63% (19 of 30) of the subjects in the lipreading-plus-sound condition, over the lipreading-alone condition. (Reprinted with permission from Staller et al. (1990a).)

difficult. Few appropriate materials are available for younger subjects and many of these subjects are unwilling to perform the same task twice (under different sensory conditions). However, 70 of the 80 subjects completed at least one lipreading measure. The most frequently used test was the CID sentences subtest of the MAC Battery, which was administered live voice and scored as the number of key words correctly repeated. Performance of individual subjects on this measure is displayed in Figure 17.10. Eighteen of the 30 subjects (60%) improved significantly in the lipreading-plus-sound condition over the lipreading-alone condition. The mean percentage correct score was 72.1% with sound compared to 49.9% for lipreading alone. Considering performance across all test measures, 47% of the 70 subjects tested with at least one lipreading measure demonstrated statistically significant improvement in the lipreading-plus-sound condition compared to lipreading alone.

Language

Perhaps one of the most difficult decisions facing the parents of a profoundly deaf child relates to the establishment of a communication mode for their child. Should the child learn oral language, manual language or some combination of the two? We know that deaf children demonstrate normal language acquisition, as evidenced by those children who are exposed from a very early age to sign language and acquire it as their primary language (Curtiss, 1989). A critical issue in the application of cochlear implants in young children is whether the auditory signal provided by the implant can enhance the potential for the development of spoken language. This should not be construed to mean that children who use sign language cannot be considered as cochlear implant candidates. However, to gain maximum benefit from an auditory prosthesis, significant emphasis must be placed on auditory skill development in young children. Children who are congenitally deaf or deafened early in life, during the formative language learning years, are more likely to be enrolled in total communication programmes than children deafened later. For these children to develop functional speech and language, a strong auditory/oral component must be incorporated into their educational programme. Certainly, there will be many variables that influence a child's potential to develop spoken language when using a cochlear implant — some quite obvious, such as age at onset of deafness, age at implantation, duration of deafness and access to appropriate training.

Although the development of linguistic skills in children with cochlear implants cannot be attributed directly to the implant, it is important to assess any changes in the language abilities of these children over time. Measures of expressive and receptive language abilities, as well as an assessment of the child's functional use of language, should be obtained.

Assessment tools will vary, depending upon the child's age, communication mode, linguistic competence and cognitive development. Following the evaluation, individualised management programmes can be designed to build upon existing language and auditory abilities.

Due to the heterogeneity of the subjects in this study, it was inappropriate to choose a single language instrument for evaluation purposes. In fact, more than a dozen different language measures were used. Clinicians chose tests that were the most appropriate for the child who was in evaluation. Of the 80 subjects, 68 received a language evaluation. Of these, 36 children were given the Peabody Picture Vocabulary Test (PPVT-R) (Dunn and Dunn, 1965) both preoperatively and at 12 months postoperatively. This test measures single-word receptive vocabulary and is appropriate for children of various ages and linguistic competence. Results are presented in Table 17.7. As a group,

Table 17.7   Peabody Picture Vocabulary Test ($n = 36$)*

	Preoperative	12-month postoperative (years)	Change (years)
Mean chronological age	9.8	10.7	0.9
Mean age equivalency	5.2	7.6	2.4
Mean difference	4.6	3.1	1.5

*Receptive vocabulary for these children increased at a rate that exceeded their chronological age.

these children demonstrated delayed receptive vocabulary skills, both pre- and postoperatively. However, it is extremely encouraging to note that single-word receptive vocabulary increased at a much faster rate than would be expected based solely on maturation. This suggests that children can use the auditory information provided by the cochlear implant for language learning.

The following case report illustrates how this information can contribute to the increase in general language abilities: this boy had normal hearing and speech and language development until the age of 3 years when he was deafened due to meningitis. A profound bilateral sensorineural hearing loss was confirmed and the child was fitted with binaural amplification. He failed to demonstrate any benefit from amplification or tactile input during the 2 years prior to implantation. He received a multichannel cochlear implant at 5;5 years. Preoperatively and 12 months postoperatively, the clinician administered the receptive and expressive portions of the PPVT-R and the Preschool Language Scale (PLS) (Zimmerman, Steiner and Pond,

1974). Preoperatively, receptive and expressive performance was approximately 3 years below age level. Postoperative results with both instruments were consistent with significant gains in both expressive and receptive language abilities. Over the 12-month period, single-word receptive vocabulary, as measured by the PPVT-R, increased from an age equivalency of 2 years to 4;7 years. On the PLS, a measure that assesses the early stages of auditory comprehension and verbal ability, this boy's age equivalency increased from 2 years to 5;6 years, and from 2;3 years to 4;10 years on the receptive and expressive portions respectively. This child's primary mode of communication is oral/aural, supplemented with cued speech.

Long-term follow-up

The results presented above reflect evaluations performed after 12 months of experience with the Nucleus implant. Unlike postlinguistically deafened adults, children assimilate the novel code provided by the device over a longer period of time in conjunction with consistent training. Although the data above demonstrate broad-based improvement, they do not provide insight into the rate of change in skill level or whether improvements in performance will continue with longer-term use of the device.

Figure 17.11 presents group mean performance on closed-set and open-set measures preoperatively and at 6-month intervals postoperatively up to 24 months. Because of the small number of subjects who have worn the device for longer periods of time, the sample sizes are different at each interval and, consequently, are not a direct comparison of the same subjects. In spite of this limitation, a clear trend of continued improvement across time is evident for all measures. Furthermore, there does not appear to be any evidence of a performance plateau across subjects even though there is variability in the test/retest performance of individual subjects. Based on these data and on single-channel implant data in children (Berliner et al., 1985), it is reasonable to assume that progressive improvements in performance will continue with additional implant experience.

Educational considerations

The cochlear implant team needs to provide support services to the educational setting in terms of in-service training on how the cochlear implant system works, how to troubleshoot the system and what auditory behaviours the teacher should expect from the implanted child. The in-service training should enable the teacher to feel more confident when working with the child and help to integrate additional auditory training into the regular classroom routine. Individual needs will vary from child

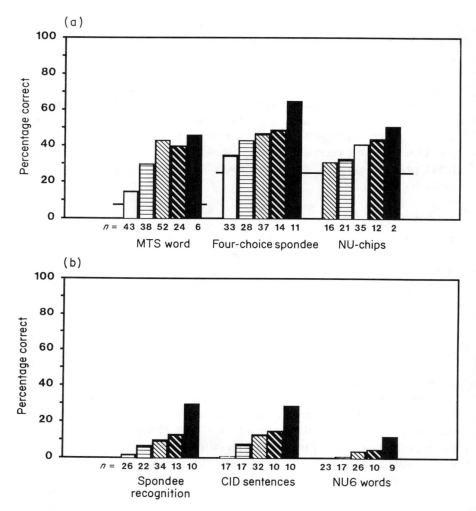

Figure 17.11. Group mean performance at 6-month postoperative intervals for selected (a) closed-set and (b) open-set tests of speech perception. (Reprinted with permission from Staller et al. (1990a).)

to child and also over time for a given child. The implant centre should discuss the concepts the child needs in order to refine the MAP and discuss with teachers of the deaf how these concepts can be taught to the child. A flow of information in both directions is to be encouraged: from the implant centre to the educational setting and vice versa. It is critical to remember that the teacher is responsible for the child's overall academic progress. Auditory skill development is only one area of concern.

In many educational settings for the hearing impaired, FM radio aids have gained widespread acceptance as assistive devices used to improve the signal-to-noise ratio. These can be particularly useful in classrooms with poor acoustics or larger numbers of students, or in situations where hearing-impaired students are mainstreamed with regular students. Most auditory trainers and personal FM systems can be directly interfaced with cochlear implant speech processors through an auxiliary input jack. Care should be taken to determine that appropriate voltage and impedance matching occurs between the FM output and speech processor input. In most cases this can be determined by contacting the manufacturer. Cross-talk between the FM signal of transcutaneous implant systems and the FM signal from the auditory trainer will sometimes occur. An attenuating cable can easily be constructed to minimise the interaction between these two signals. Again, the manufacturers can usually assist in determining the need for such a cable and in its fabrication.

Cochlear Corporation manufactures an optional 'Audio Input Selector (AIS)' which acts as an impedance and voltage matching device for various direct inputs to their speech processor. These inputs may include television, radio or auditory trainers. The AIS also provides a separate environmental microphone, allowing the child to monitor his or her own voice along with that of the teacher.

Discussion

The experience to date of children with multichannel cochlear implants has been positive. The children as a group have performed well; however, there still remains a complex interaction of factors that contribute to the 'success' demonstrated by any given child. The ongoing interaction of all team members with the child and his or her family is crucial to maximising the benefit derived by implanted children. For example, quantitative changes in auditory behaviour may not be demonstrated by young children until they have had over 6 months' experience with the device. During this time, parents and/or teachers may become concerned that the child is not progressing as rapidly as anticipated. All members of the team should be sensitive to the fact that auditory skill development in both normally hearing and hearing-impaired children is a long-term process. During this time, parents may need reassurance. As the child grows, the team will continue to play an important role in helping him or her meet the progressively more difficult challenges he or she will face educationally and socially.

The decision of *when* to undergo cochlear implantation is one of the more difficult questions facing the parent of a profoundly deaf child. On the one hand, there is the prospect of the development of future 'better' devices. Therefore, the parent faces the logical question of 'How long should I wait?'. Certainly, the prospect of the development of better devices influences this decision. However, parents also must weigh the consequences of sensory deprivation during the critical language learning period and the empirical evidence that postoperative performance is related to the duration of deafness. Based on the ability to place the cochlear implant package successfully, the acceptably low medical/surgical risks, and on the evidence of substantial benefit associated with cochlear implantation even in children as young as 2 years, it seems appropriate to recommend performing surgery as soon as possible. Of course, this presumes: (1) the ability to reliably diagnose profound deafness; (2) a demonstration of no significant benefit from an appropriately fitted sensory device(s) after intensive habilitation; and (3) consensus among team members with respect to candidacy. With adolescents, the decision of when to implant needs to take into consideration the child's motivation and feelings about receiving the device. Does the adolescent really want the implant or are their external pressures influencing his or her decision?

Although much has been learned, the long-term impact of multichannel cochlear implants remains to be determined. Effective auditory stimulation in early childhood is necessary for the development of oral language skills. Multichannel cochlear implants may provide this input and potentially minimise the impact of sensory deprivation on these children.

Appendix I: Tests of Speech and Language

1. Assessment of Children's Language Comprehension (ACLC)
2. Expressive One-word Picture Vocabulary Scale (EOWPT)
3. Fisher–Logemann Test of Articulation Competence
4. Grammatical Analysis of Elicited Language (GAEL)
5. Mean Length of Utterance (MLU)
6. Peabody Picture Vocabulary Test – Revised (PPVT-R)
7. Phonetic Level Speech Evaluation (PLE)
8. Phonologic Level Speech Evaluation
9. Preschool Language Scale (PLS)
10. Pre-speech Infant Transcription
11. Rhode Island Test of Language Structures (RITLS)
12. Test for Auditory Comprehension of Language (TACL, TA)

Name of test.................	Assessment of Children's Language Comprehension (ACLC)
Author(s)......................	R. Foster, J. Giddan and J. Stark
Source	Consulting Psychologists Press, Inc. 577 College Ave, Palo Alto, CA 94306
Purpose of test.............	To assess the comprehension of different word classes in different combinations of length and complexity
Name of test.................	Expressive One-word Picture Vocabulary Test (EOWPT)
Author(s)......................	Morris F. Gardner

Source	Academic Therapy Publications 20 Commercial Boulevard, Novato, CA 94947
Purpose of test	To measure expressive single-word vocabulary and to provide an estimate of a child's verbal intelligence

Name of test	Fisher–Logemann Test of Articulation Competence
Author(s)	H.B. Fisher and J.A. Logemann
Source	Test of Articulation Competence, Houghton and Mifflin, New York (1971)
Purpose of test	To assess production of vowels, consonants and consonant clusters

Name of test	Grammatical Analysis of Elicited Language (GAEL)
Author(s)	J. Moog, V. Kozak and A. Geers
Source	Central Institute for the Deaf 818 South Euclid Street, St Louis, MO 63110
Purpose of test	To evaluate receptive and expressive grammatical aspects of spoken and/or signed English under standardised testing conditions

Name of test	Mean Length of Utterance (MLU)
Author(s)	R. Brown
Source	A First Language: The Early Stages, Harvard University Press, Cambridge, MA, pp. 51–59 (1973)
Purpose of test	To provide a measure of language development based on the average length of utterances in an appropriate language sample

Name of test	Peabody Picture Vocabulary Test – revised: Form M (PPVT-R)
Author(s)	L. Dunn and L. Dunn
Source	American Guidance Service Circle Pines, MN 55014
Purpose of test	To measure receptive vocabulary for Standard American English and to provide an estimate of a child's receptive verbal intelligence

Name of test	Phonetic Level Speech Evaluation (PLE)
Author(s)	Daniel Ling
Source	Ling, D. (1976). Speech and the Hearing Impaired Child: Theory and Practice, pp. 147–169. Washington DC: A.G. Bell Assn. Clinical performance categories defined by E. Tobey (1989)

Purpose of test............	To provide clear teaching goals for speech production. The PLE determines the presence of specific sound patterns, assesses the stage at which the child differentiates between motor speech patterns and evaluates the rate at which speech sounds can be alternated and repeated
Name of test................	Phonologic Level Speech Evaluation (Ling Phonological Analysis)
Author(s)......................	Daniel Ling
Source	Ling, D. (1976). *Speech and the Hearing Impaired Child: Theory and Practice*, pp. 144–162. Washington DC: A.G. Bell Assn. Clinical performance categories defined by E. Tobey (1989)
Purpose of test............	To sample a child's phonological development before and during training
Name of test................	Preschool Language Scale (PLS)
Author(s)......................	I. Zimmerman, V. Steiner and R. Evatt Pond
Source	The Psychological Corp. Harcourt Brace Jovanovich, Minneapolis
Purpose of test............	To assess the early stages of receptive and expressive language development and to evaluate maturational lags in language
Name of test................	Pre-speech Infant Transcription
Author(s)......................	K. Oller
Source	Oller, K. (1978). Infant vocalization and the development of speech. *Allied Health and Behavioral Sciences* 1:523–549. Oller, K., Eilers, R., Bull, D. and Carney, A. (1985). Pre-speech vocalizations of a deaf infant: a comparison with normal metaphonological development. *Journal of Speech and Hearing Research* **28**, 47–63
Purpose of test............	To evaluate the speech production of pre-speech children receiving cochlear implants and other deaf children whose vocalisations cannot be reliably identified as meaningful speech sounds (phonemes), using a normal infant vocalisation transcription system (Oller, 1978)
Name of test................	Rhode Island Test of Language Structure (RITLS)
Author(s)......................	E. Engen and T. Engen
Source	University Park Press Baltimore, MD
Purpose of test............	To measure a child's comprehension of the basic grammatical structures and relationships of English

Name of test	Test for Auditory Comprehension of Language (TACL and TACL-R)
Author(s)	Elizabeth Carrow-Woolfolk
Source	DLM and Teaching Resources Allen, TX
Purpose of test	To measure receptive auditory comprehension of specific grammatical forms

Acknowledgements

The authors gratefully acknowledge Carol Liebermann and Karyen Harris for editorial assistance, Destyn Hood, Patti Arndt and Tamara Betz for database management, and Dianne Mecklenburg and Marilyn Demorest for study design.

References

BENCH, R.J. and BAMFORD, J. (1979). *Speech–Hearing Tests and Spoken Language of Hearing-impaired Children*. London: Academic Press.

BERLINER, K.I., COURTNEY, B., EISENBERG, L.S., FRAVEL, R.P., FRETZ, R.J., HILL-BROWN, C., HOUSE, W.F., ILLER-KIRK, K. and LUXFORD, W.M. (1985). The cochlear implant: an auditory prosthesis for the profoundly deaf child. *Ear Hear.* 6(suppl. 3), 1s–69s.

BUSBY, P.A., TONG, Y.C., ROBERTS, S.A., ALTIDIS, P.M., DETTMAN, S.J., BLAMEY, P.J., CLARK, G.M., WATSON, R.K., DOWELL, R.C., RICKARDS, F.W. and NICHOLLS, G.H. (1989). Results for two children using a multiple-electrode intracochlear implant. *J. Acoust. Soc. Am.* 86, 2088–2102.

COHEN, N. (1990). Complications of cochlear implants in children. Paper presented at Colorado Otology/Audiology Conference, Breckenridge, Colorado, March 4–9.

CURTISS, S. (1989). Issues in language acquisition relevant to cochlear implants in young children. In: Owens, E. and Kessler, D.K. (eds), *Cochlear Implants in Young Deaf Children*, pp. 293–305. Boston, MA: College-Hill Press.

DUNN, L. and DUNN, L. (1965). *Peabody Picture Vocabulary Test-Revised (PPVT-R)*. Circle Pines, MN: American Guidance Service.

EBY, T.L. and NADOL, J.B. (1986). Postnatal growth of the human temporal bone. Implications for cochlear implants in children. *Ann. Otol. Rhinol. Laryngol.* 95, 356–364.

ELLIOTT, L.L. and KATZ, D.R. (1980). *Northwestern University Children's Perception of Speech (NU-CHIPS)*. St Louis: Auditec.

ERBER, N.P. (1982). *Auditory Training*. Washington DC: Alexander Graham Bell Association for the Deaf.

ERBER, N.P. and ALENCEWICZ, C.M. (1976). Audiologic evaluation of deaf children. *J. Speech Hear. Dis.* 41, 256–267.

HASENSTAB, S.M. (1988). Developing spoken communication in a cochlear implant child. *Hear. Ins.* 39(11), 18–20, 76.

HASKINS, J. (1949). *Kindergarten Phonetically Balanced Word Lists (PBK)*. St Louis: Auditec.

HINOJOSA, R. and LINDSAY, J.R. (1980). Profound deafness; associated sensory and neural degeneration. *Arch. Otolaryngol.* 106, 193–201.

HINOJOSA, R. and MARION, M. (1983). Histopathology of profound sensorineural deafness. In: Parkins, C.W. and Anderson, S.W. (eds), *Cochlear Prostheses: An International Symposium*, pp. 459–484. New York: New York Academy of Sciences.

ILER-KIRK, K. and HILL-BROWN, C. (1985). Speech and language results in children with a cochlear implant. *Ear Hear.* **6**, 36s–47s.

JEFFERS, J. and BARLEY, M. (1977). *Speech Reading 'Lipreading'*. Springfield, IL: Charles C. Thomas.

LERMAN, J., ROSS, M. and McLAUCHLIN, R. (1965). A picture-identification test for hearing-impaired children. *J. Audiol. Res.* **5**, 273–278.

LING, D.L. (1976). *Speech and the Hearing Impaired Child: Theory and Practice*. Washington DC: Alexander Graham Bell Association for the Deaf.

LUXFORD, W.M., HOUSE, W.F., HOUGH, J.V.D., TONOKAWA, L.L., BERLINER, K.E. and MARTIN, E. (1988). Experiences with the nucleus multichannel cochlear implant in three young children. *Ann. Otol. Rhinol. Laryngol.* **97**, 14–16.

McGARR, N.S. (1983). The intelligibility of deaf speech to experienced and inexperienced listeners. *J. Speech Hear. Res.* **26**, 451–458.

MECKLENBURG, D.J. (1986). Cochlear implants in children. *Semin. Hear.* **7**, 341–446.

MECKLENBURG, D.J. (1987). The Nucleus children's program. *Am. J. Otol.* **8**, 436–442.

MECKLENBURG, D.J. (1988). Device fitting in children. Second Symposium on Cochlear Implants in Children, Denver, CO.

MIYAMOTO, R.T., OSBERGER, M.J., ROBBINS, A.J., RENSHAW, J.J., MYRES, W.A., KESSLER, K. and POPE, M.L. (1989). Comparison of sensory aids in deaf children. *Ann. Otol. Rhinol. Laryngol.* **98**, 2–7.

MOOG, J.S. and GEERS, A.E. (1990). *Early Speech Perception Battery*. St Louis, MO: Central Institute for the Deaf.

NEEDLEMAN, H. (1977). Effects of hearing loss from recurrent otitis media on speech and language development. In: Jaffe, B. (ed.), *Hearing Loss in Children*, pp. 640–649. Baltimore: University Park Press.

NEVILLE, H. (1984). Effects of early sensory and language experience on the development of the human brain. In: Mahler, J. and Fox, R. (eds), *Neonate Cognition: Beyond the Blooming Buzzing Confusion*. Hillsdale, NJ: Erlbaum.

OWENS, E., KESSLER, D., TELLEEN, C. and SCHUBERT, E.D. (1981). *The Minimal Auditory Capabilities Battery*. St Louis: Auditec.

STALLER, S.J. (1990). Perceptual and production abilities in profoundly deaf children with multichannel cochlear implants. *J. Am. Acad. Audiol.* **1**, 1–3.

STALLER, S.J., BEITER, A.L., ARKIS, P.N., DOMICO, E. and SPIVAK, L.G. (1988). Paediatric performance with partial insertion of multichannel cochlear implants. Presented at the Annual Meeting of the American Speech, Language and Hearing Association, Boston, November 19.

STALLER, S.J., BEITER, A.L., BRIMACOMBE, J.A. and MECKLENBURG, D.J. (1989a). Clinical trials of the Nucleus 22 channel cochlear implant in profoundly deaf children. In: Fraysse, B. and Cochard, N. (eds), *Cochlear Implant: Acquisitions and Controversies*, pp. 183–195. Toulouse: Paragraphic.

STALLER, S.J., BEITER, A.L., TOBEY, E.A., BRIMACOMBE, J.A., MECKLENBURG, D.J. and KOCH, D.B. (1989b). Speech perception and production abilities of children with multichannel cochlear implants. Presented at the Annual Convention of the American Academy of Otolaryngology, New Orleans, September 26.

STALLER, S.J., BEITER, A.L., BRIMACOMBE, J.A., MECKLENBURG, D.J. and ARNDT, P.L. (1990a). Paediatric performance with the nucleus 22 channel cochlear implant system. *Am. J. Otol.* in press.

STALLER, S.J., BEITER, A.L., TOBEY, E.A., BRIMACOMBE, J.A., MECKLENBURG, D.J. and KOCH, D.B. (1990b). Speech perception and production abilities of children with multichannel cochlear implants. *J. Am. Acad. Otolaryngol. Head Neck Surg.* in press.

THIELEMEIR, M.A. (1984). *The Discrimination After Training Test.* Los Angeles: House Ear Institute.

THORNTON, A.R. and RAFFIN, M.J. (1978). Speech discrimination modeled as a binomial variable. *J. Speech Hear. Res.* **21**, 507–518.

TILLMAN, T., CARHART, R. and WILBUR, L. (1966). A test for speech discrimination composed of CNC monosyllabic words (NU auditory test No. 6). *USAF School of Aerospace Medicine*, Report 55–66.

TOBEY, E.A., STALLER, S.J., BEITER, A.L., MECKLENBURG, D.J. and BRIMACOMBE, J.A. (1989). Speech production results of children with the Nucleus 22 channel cochlear implant system. Presented at the 34th meeting of the Ear, Nose and Throat devices panel, Washington DC, November 13–14.

TOBEY, E.A., ANGELETTE, S., MURCHISON, C., NICOSIA, J., SPRAGUE, S., STALLER, S.J., BRIMACOMBE, J.A. and BEITER, A.L. (1990). Speech production abilities of children with a multichannel implant. *Am. J. Otol.* in press.

WEBSTER, D.B. and WEBSTER, M. (1977). Neonatal sound deprivation affects brain stem auditory nuclei. *Arch. Otol. Laryngol.* **103**, 392–396.

ZIMMERMAN, I., STEINER, V. and POND, R. (1974). *Preschool Language Scale (PLS).* Minneapolis, MN: Harcourt Brace Jovanovich.

Chapter 18
Effects of Cochlear Implants in Children: Implications for Rehabilitation

MARGERY N. SOMERS

Introduction

The pervasive effects of deafness on the development of communicative and linguistic skills in children are well known. An auditory prosthesis that can improve speech perception offers the potential for improved speech and language. Until the advent of the cochlear implant, the hearing aid was the only prosthesis that improved speech perception abilities of hearing-impaired children. Deaf children with no residual hearing to amplify to a meaningful range had a poor prognosis (Erber and Hirsch, 1978); now, they are children who can benefit from a cochlear implant. When such children began to use the 3M/House cochlear implant in 1981, there was hope that the implant could improve speech perception abilities and thus result in improved speech and language. Such improvement is especially important for children so deaf that they traditionally have been unable to benefit from hearing aids (Thielemeir, Tonokawa and Peterson, 1985).

The more severe the hearing loss, the more difficult communication becomes (Boothroyd, 1978). For a child, this communication handicap is even more devastating. A deafened adult has previously established a language and speech base; a child, however, robbed of normal hearing during the crucial developmental years, is left not only with problems of understanding others but also with severely delayed language and defective speech.

This chapter will discuss which children with the 3M/House cochlear implant benefit most from the device and which children appear to gain only minimal benefit. Similarities and differences will be examined in speech perception abilities provided by the 3M/House single-electrode and Nucleus multichannel cochlear implants. These are the two cochlear implants currently used in children (although the 3M/House cochlear implant is no longer being manufactured). Educational implications for rehabilitation and training will be discussed for all implant children. Follow-up programmes, intervention strategies and sequences of instruction for the cochlear implant child will be outlined.

Performance Differences with the 3M/House Cochlear Implant

In the last 8 years, 296 children have received the 3M/House single-channel cochlear implant. The authors are now studying this population retrospectively and are examining the performance levels of various groups of children; from this they can describe factors that appear to effect beneficial use of the device.

Subject characteristics include a mean age at time of surgery of 7.8 years, with a range from 2;2 years to nearly 18 years. The majority (59%) of the children were deafened by meningitis. Other causes include Mondini deformity, trauma, maternal toxaemia, maternal infection, maternal rubella, ototoxicity, hereditary and unknown congenital cause. Thirty-four per cent of the subjects are congenitally deaf (Johnson, 1987).

The mean age at onset of deafness was 1.6 years, with a median of 1 year. Only 13% of the children were deafened after the age of 3. Thus, the vast majority were prelingually deaf. Consistent with this fact, the majority of children (67%) used total communication. They used sign language as the focus for communication development. The average duration of deafness before implantation was 6.1 years and ranged from 6 months to nearly 18 years (Johnson, 1987).

Pre-implant, there was no detection of speech within the speech range with powerful hearing aids (Figure 18.1) (Thielemeir, Tonokawa and Peterson, 1985). Thresholds post-implant average 53 dB HL across the speech frequencies. The children can detect, but not necessarily discriminate, medium- and high-intensity speech and environmental sounds (Thielemeir, Tonokawa and Peterson, 1985). Once sounds are detected, however, the child has the potential to learn to attach meaning to acoustic events.

Although these clinical data show that the cochlear implant raises thresholds to the speech range (Thielemeir, Tonokawa and Peterson, 1985), improves discrimination scores on individual words over time (Johnson, 1987) and, for a small number of children, provides spectral information (Geers and Moog, 1988), the effect of training on auditory development with the cochlear implant is a crucial consideration.

To evaluate the effects of the 3M/House cochlear implant in conjunction with different types of educational training, the speech perception abilities provided by the implant were first examined. Then a comparison was made

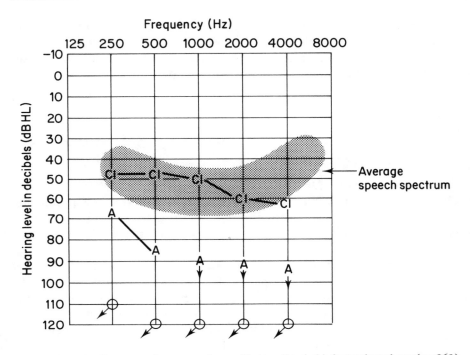

Figure 18.1. Median pre- and postoperative warble-tone thresholds for implanted ears ($n=260$) in children with 3M/House cochlear implants. (A = aided thresholds; O = unaided thresholds; CI = thresholds with cochlear implant.)

between the different categories of speech perception abilities and an established indicator of deaf children's potential for oral skill development.

Moog and Geers developed speech perception categories with corresponding speech intelligibility categories for profoundly deaf children (Geers and Moog, 1987). The graph shown in Figure 18.2 shows that category 1 (minimal detection) is equivalent to the first speech perception category. Children have no pattern perception, minimal detection of sound and unintelligible speech.

Category 2 represents pattern perception. Children in this category can perceive suprasegmental aspects of speech. They can hear the rhythm of speech but cannot hear individual speech sounds as different from one another. Children in this category have the capacity to develop somewhat intelligible speech and basic, but not fluent, oral language skills. Category 3 represents the ability to recognise words. In this category children are discriminating words on the basis of phonemes, not just stress differences. They can actually hear differences in speech sounds. Children in category 3 can develop intelligible speech and good oral communication skills.

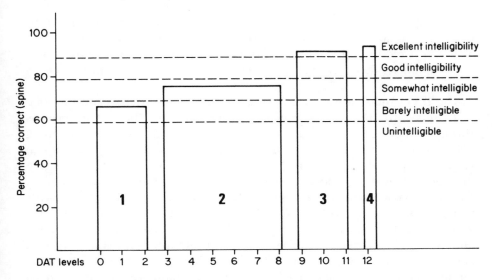

Figure 18.2. Speech Perception Index (Geers and Moog, 1987). Categories of speech perception abilities are defined as follows. Category 1: detection only. Category 2: pattern perception. Category 3: some word identification. Category 4: consistent word identification.

Category 4 represents consistent word recognition with the prognosis for very intelligible speech and fluent communication. Children in categories 3 and 4 have a good prognosis for developing oral skills. Fluent verbal communication and intelligible speech are all possible for children with word recognition skills.

The author divided 171 implant children with data on educational placement into six groups according to onset of deafness and educational communication training. The groups are: congenitally deaf children educated in total communication programmes ($n=49$); congenitally deaf children in oral programmes ($n=8$); prelingually deaf children who became deaf after birth but before 3 years of age in total communication programmes ($n=62$); prelinguals in oral programmes ($n=29$); postlingually deaf children, deafened after 3 years of age, in total communication ($n=11$) and in oral ($n=12$) programmes. The index developed by Moog and Geers was used to compare the mean performance level on the Discrimination After Training (DAT) test for these different groups of implant children to the speech perception and speech intelligibility levels of profoundly deaf children with hearing aids.

The DAT test (Thielemeir, Tonokawa and Peterson, 1985) is a speech discrimination test which was developed at the House Ear Institute (HEI) specifically for prelingually, profoundly deaf adults and children. The DAT test determines if the subjects have auditory capability to learn to discriminate speech, or some of the non-segmental aspects of speech. Training is incorporated as part of the test in an attempt to control, or at least minimise, the effect that previous auditory experience may have on test results.

The DAT stimuli are drawn from a monosyllable, trochee and spondee test used with HEI adult cochlear implant patients. The test progresses through a hierarchy of difficulty (Table 18.1). It begins with speechreading discrimination to determine that the child understands the task and can respond appropriately (level 1), and proceeds to auditory-only detection of speech (level 2), and auditory-only discriminations of non-linguistic (levels 3–5) or linguistic (levels 6–12) speech stimuli. Table 18.1 presents test stimuli and descriptions of each test level. Of the speech items, level 2 is a detection task and levels 3–5 are discriminations of gross durational and timing differences (long vs short, fast vs slow, one sound vs two sounds). Levels 6–8 are discriminations of different word stress patterns (monosyllable vs spondee, trochee vs spondee, monosyllable vs trochee) in an order of increasing difficulty. This order was based on the performance of prelingually deafened adult cochlear implant users (M. Thielemeir, unpublished data, 1981): levels 9 and 10 each contain two spondees; level 9 contains the easier discrimination as determined from adult implant user performance; level 11 contains three spondees; and level 12 contrasts four spondees.

The DAT test is administered live voice with the tester 1–2 ft (half a metre) behind the patient. The approximate voice level of the tester at the child's microphone is 75–80 dB SPL. The child responds by pointing to a picture, or by saying or signing the correct response. Each test item is

Table 18.1   DAT test items

Level	Description	Stimuli
1	Visual discrimination	'popcorn' vs 'cat'
2	Detection of voice	'ba' 'ba' 'ba'
3	Long vs short sound	'baaaaaaaa' vs 'ba ba'
4	Fast vs slow sound	'babababababa' vs 'ba ba'
5	One vs two syllables	'ba' vs 'ba ba'
6	Monosyllable vs spondee	'cat' vs 'popcorn'
7	Trochee vs spondee	'chicken' vs 'popcorn'
8	Monosyllable vs trochee	'cat' vs 'chicken'
9	Spondee vs spondee	'popcorn' vs 'toothpaste'
10	Spondee vs spondee	'popcorn' vs 'baseball'
11	Three spondees	'popcorn' vs 'baseball' vs 'toothpaste'
12	Four spondees	'popcorn' vs 'baseball' vs 'toothpaste' vs 'birdhouse'

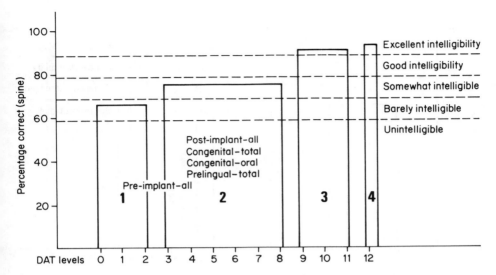

Figure 18.3. The group mean Discrimination After Training (DAT) scores were used to categorise groups of children with the 3M/House cochlear implant on the Speech Perception Index.

presented five times in random order. A level is passed if the child gets 90% correct responses. If the child scores below 90% for a given level, 5–10 min of intensive training are provided for those two, three or four items. Upon retest, if 90% correct competency is not achieved, an additional training session is given, then a final retest. The test is complete when two consecutive subtests in levels 3–9 are failed or one subtest in levels 10–12 is failed. The test score is the highest level passed.

Figure 18.3 shows the means of the DAT scores for groups of the following children placed in Category 2 after implantation. They are congenitally and prelingually deaf children educated in total communication settings, congenitally deaf children who had oral communication settings and the most recent follow-up mean DAT score for all post-implant children. Category 2 indicates enough speech perception to aid proper stress and rhythm in speech production. This ability is the foundation of usable, somewhat intelligible speech, but not of fluent oral communication skills.

It is not surprising that children in total communication programmes do not have the auditory basis for fluent oral communication. Specific auditory training in developing the use of audition is required to optimise benefits of the implant. Total communication programmes that do not focus on audition would not promote maximal benefit from the implant. Also, congenitally deaf children who have no auditory memory or previous verbal language will find it difficult to attach sound cues meaningfully.

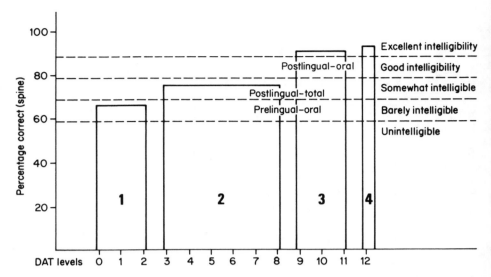

Figure 18.4. The group mean DAT scores were used to categorise children with the 3M/House cochlear implant. Postlingual children in oral settings demonstrate the best performance.

Figure 18.4 shows results of children who gain enough speech perception through the cochlear implant to facilitate speech and language. These are prelingually deaf children educated in oral settings, postlingually deaf children educated in total communication environments, and postlingually deaf children from oral education. Two groups are between categories 2 and 3. A small number of children had fully developed speech and language before they became totally deaf. Many of the young children had rapidly deteriorating speech before they received a cochlear implant. The implant effectively offers enough speech perception for these children to maintain and, in many cases reinstate, a very intelligible level of speech.

Consequently, all children benefit to some degree from the 3M/House cochlear implant. Children who benefit most either learned to speak before they lost their hearing or, if they experienced a prelingual onset of deafness, had intensive oral training.

Comparing the 3M/House and Nucleus Multichannel Implants

In October 1986, clinical trials for the multichannel implant began for children aged 2–10 years. In 1987 the first young child was implanted with the Nucleus multichannel cochlear implant at the House Ear Institute. Since that time, over 200 children (ages 2–18) have been implanted with the Nucleus device. The multichannel implant is designed to process speech by providing both first and second formant information. Its electrode array spans one and a half turns of the cochlea, thereby providing spectral information. The auditory information that is potentially provided by the Nucleus implant opens new possibilities for profoundly deaf children. The possibility that profoundly deaf children, especially those of preschool age, can hear and utilise the spoken communication code of the Nucleus device giving improved auditory performance compared to the 3M/House device is exciting. The importance of the potential benefits of a cochlear implant for a preschool child centres on the availability of increased auditory stimulation at a time when the child is focused in auditory learning and communication acquisition. If a young child has enhanced auditory input afforded by the cochlear implant during the period of communication acquisition, an improved mastery of the spoken communication code is likely to occur.

Now that a multichannel cochlear implant is being used for children, it is important not only to compare their processing capabilities, but also to examine performance differences between children with the Nucleus multichannel device and those with the 3M/House single-electrode cochlear implant. Direct comparison of Nucleus and 3M/House implantees will enable us to specify differences in capabilities that the devices provide. Additionally, cochlear implants, regardless of type of device, need to be compared to the traditional hearing prosthesis used with children – hearing aids.

Hence, the author's group conducted a 3-year comparative study (Somers, 1991) to determine differences between the two cochlear implant devices available for children and compare those devices to hearing aid use. Since communication mode had been found to be an important variable, children were investigated with different hearing devices in total communication and oral settings. The results of the first year are summarised below.

The option of the cochlear implant for children has brought about numerous questions relating to the development of speech perception skills. Physicians, speech and hearing professionals, and parents want to know if the cochlear implant affects auditory capabilities enough to facilitate oral language development and intelligible speech. If so, is oral programming necessary to maximise the benefits of the cochlear implant or can a child in a total communication programme develop speech perception skills to the same level? This question of educational intervention (total communication or oral) is pertinent to hearing aid children as well; it has still to be ascertained whether speech perception development differs between children using different educational communication methods.

Otologists and other professionals are also concerned with auditory ability comparisons between hearing aid users who have measurable residual hearing and cochlear implant users who, with the implant, have speech detection thresholds similar to aided thresholds of hearing aid users. Few control group studies with hearing aid users have been implemented. Aided speech perception information has been hypothesised as being more important for developing spoken language than pure-tone threshold (Boothroyd, 1978; Luterman and Chasin, 1981; Geers and Moog, 1987). Initial investigations have reported similar (though not equal) speech perception performance on some measures between implant users and profoundly deaf hearing aid users who have aidable, usable, residual hearing (Boothroyd, 1989; Osberger, 1990; Staller, 1990).

Studies have indicated an inverse relationship between speech intelligibility and hearing acuity: speech intelligibility decreases as the degree of hearing loss increases (Hudgins and Numbers, 1942; Boothroyd, 1976; Jensema and Trybus, 1978; Osberger and McGarr, 1978). Hearing prostheses which improve hearing in deaf children offer the possibility for improved speech and language development. The more speech a child can perceive, the easier the child can learn to understand and produce it. If the primary goal of a cochlear implant is to facilitate the hearing-impaired child's acquisition of spoken language, then the effectiveness of that device must be judged in terms of the extent to which it improves the ability to perceive speech (Geers and Moog, 1988). Additionally, training children to listen and utilise their residual hearing improves auditory abilities as well. The better a child listens, the better he or she will process speech auditorily (Hirsch, 1978; Erber, 1982; Erber and Boothroyd, 1987).

Approximately 70% of hearing-impaired children are educated in total communication programmes that use sign language in addition to oral communication (Office of Demographic Studies, 1984). This report did not categorise by hearing loss. However, it is assumed that the majority of children who are candidates for cochlear implants are in total communication programmes due to their poor prognosis for auditory-based instruction. In fact, 61% of all children with cochlear implants are educated in total communication settings. The remainder are in auditory-based instruction (27% in auditory–oral programmes for the hearing impaired, 9% mainstreamed) (Somers, 1987; Staller, 1990). These figures represent a large population of children in total communication programmes whose potential benefit from the cochlear implant needs to be assessed.

Speech perception performance was compared between prelingually deaf children who use cochlear implants and children who use hearing aids and have usable aidable residual hearing ($n=68$). The children were either in total communication or in oral programmes. Thus, there were four groups of children: hearing aid children in total communication programmes ($n=16$), hearing aid children in oral programmes ($n=14$), cochlear implant children in total communication programmes ($n=13$) and cochlear implant children in oral programmes ($n=13$). Additionally, a fifth control group of hearing aid children without usable hearing was tested and this group comprised children considered to be cochlear implant candidates ($n=12$). There were an equal number of Nucleus and 3M/House users in each implant group. This study involved seven research sites (schools for the deaf and implant centres throughout the country) and was implemented in the Spring of 1989.

Subject Selection

Subjects in all groups were aged between 4 and 8;11 years. The mean age for the implant users was 81 months (6;9 years) and was 75 months (6;3 years) for the children with hearing aids. Age of onset of deafness was 7 months for the hearing aid subjects and 11 months of age for the cochlear implant subjects. Subject demographics for the four study groups appear in Table 18.2. In order to control for differences in language abilities, only subjects who became deaf before the age of 3 years were chosen for investigation. The greatest interest was in assessing prelingual children because these children had not developed full language competence prior to losing their hearing. Children had to have been in their school setting for at least 1 year and all children were judged to be of at least average intelligence.

Table 18.2 Demographic information for four study groups

	Oral		TC	
	HA	CI	HA	CI
No. of subjects	14	13	16	13
Onset (months)				
Mean	2.7	9.6	11.3	12.2
Range	0–27	0–32	0–35	0–36
Age at test (months)				
Mean	69.7	87.6	80.3	74.5
Range	54–86	55–99	57–104	54–106
Sensory aid				
One HA	2	–	1	–
Binaural HAs	12	–	15	–
CI/3M	–	6	–	6
CI/Nucleus 22	–	7	–	7
Aetiology				
Congenital	13	4	11	4
Adventitious				
Meningitis	–	5	1	6
Other	1	4	4	3

HA = hearing aid.
CI = cochlear implant.
TC = total communication.

Strict hearing selection criteria were applied to all children who were potential participants in the study. Essentially, hearing aid subjects were required to demonstrate some degree of residual hearing. Hearing aid children had unaided, better-ear, three-frequency (500, 1000 and 2000 Hz), pure-tone average thresholds between 100 and 110 dB. All cochlear implant children had three-frequency, better-ear, pure-tone averages greater than 110 dB. The control group also had no aidable residual hearing (pure-tone averages greater than 110 dB), but they wore hearing aids. Hearing aid subjects speech reception thresholds (SRT) were required to be better than 67 dB SPL; the control group had SRTs greater than 67 dB SPL.

Test Materials

Five speech perception subtests were administered to all subjects to evaluate pattern perception through to open-set comprehension. The Early Speech Perception (ESP) Test (Moog and Geers, 1988b), Subtest A was used to assess pattern perception by having the children discriminate among one-syllable, trochee, spondee and three-syllable words. Subtests B and C of the ESP were used to assess spondee and monosyllable identification, respectively. A closed-set sentence subtest from the Pediatric Speech Intelligibility Test (PSI) (Jerger and Jerger, 1984), in which the child discriminates between five simple sentences comprising two or three critical elements, was used as a measure of connected language processing. Stimuli from the Glendonald Auditory Screening Procedure (GASP) which consists of 10 sentences presented open-set were used to assess connected language comprehension. Test stimuli were recorded and presented at an average level of 76 dB SPL at 3 feet (1 m) from the child.

Results

The mean percentage correct for all five study groups on the five speech perception measures, including the implant control group, is shown in Figure 18.5. Performance differences can be seen as a function of speech-perception task for these children; pattern perception emerges the least difficult whilst open-set comprehension is the most difficult task. Table 18.3 displays the means and standard deviations for all study groups.

Children educated in oral settings performed higher on all speech-perception tasks compared to those educated in total communication settings. There were significant differences between the two combined groups of oral subjects and the two combined groups of total communication subjects on pattern perception and spondee subtests. The mean score

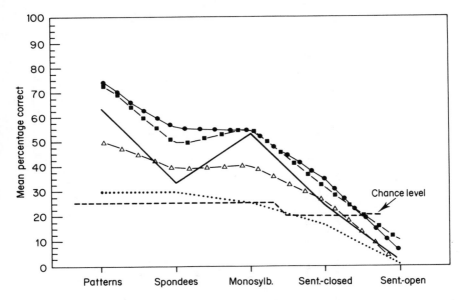

Figure 18.5. Performance for the four study groups and the control group on the five speech perception measures tested. — = Total communication cochlear implant ($n=13$); ∎ — ∎ = oral communication cochlear implant ($n=13$); △ — △ = total communication hearing aid ($n=16$); ● — ● = oral communication hearing aid ($n=14$); ···· = cochlear implant control hearing aid ($n=12$).

for the oral communication subjects was 73%, and the mean score for the total communication subjects was 56% on the ESP-A. The analysis of variance indicated a significant main effect of educational method for ESP-A ($P<0.05$). The mean score for the oral communication subjects was 51% and the mean score for the total communication subjects was 37% on ESP-B. The analysis of variance indicated a significant main effect of educational method ($P<0.05$). This can be seen in Table 18.4.

In order to determine whether an interaction effect existed between education method and prosthesis, t-tests were applied to determine significant differences between the oral and total communication hearing aid users (Figure 18.6) and oral and total communication cochlear implant users (Figure 18.7). Significant differences were found on pattern perception and spondee identification between oral communication and total communication hearing aid users ($P<0.05$). No significant differences were found between the oral and total communication cochlear implant groups on any of the speech perception measures.

The author applied t-tests to performance data comparisons on the five speech perception measures for cochlear implant and hearing aid users in both oral and total communication settings. No significant differences ($P<0.05$) existed between cochlear implant and hearing aid users with the

Table 18.3 Mean values and standard deviations for the five speech-perception measures for the four study groups and the control group

| | Hearing aid (% correct) | | | | Cochlear implant (% correct) | | | | Cochlear implant control group (% correct) | |
| | Oral communication (n=14) | | Total communication (n=16) | | Oral communication (n=13) | | Total communication (n=13) | | (n=12) | |
	Mean	s.d.	Mean	s.d.	Mean	s.d.	Mean	s.d.	Mean	s.d.
Sent.-open set	6.2	14.5	0.0	0.0	10.0	18.4	1.5	3.8	0.0	0.0
Sent.-closed set	35.0	15.1	26.3	12.2	31.7	24.2	24.4	11.3	16.7	9.1
Monosyllable	54.5	24.9	40.6	12.1	55.1	12.0	53.2	33.5	25.7	12.0
Spondees	55.8	25.3	39.1	17.4	49.2	28.2	33.5	28.9	29.9	9.0
Patterns	73.2	33.3	50.5	28.1	74.4	24.9	63.7	23.1	29.9	16.5

Table 18.4 Analysis of variance (ANOVA)*

Source	Mean square	F
ESP-A		
Group (HA or CI)	0.056	0.713
Communication mode	0.362	4.553†
Group × communication mode	0.068	0.855
Explained	0.164	
Residual (error)	0.080	
ESP-B		
Group (HA or CI)	0.079	1.337
Communication mode	0.266	4.514†
Group × communication mode	0.009	0.148
Explained	0.119	
Residual (error)	0.059	

*Significant main effect for communication mode shown when the two oral groups are compared to the two total communication groups.
†$P<0.05$.
HA = hearing aid; CI = cochlear implant.

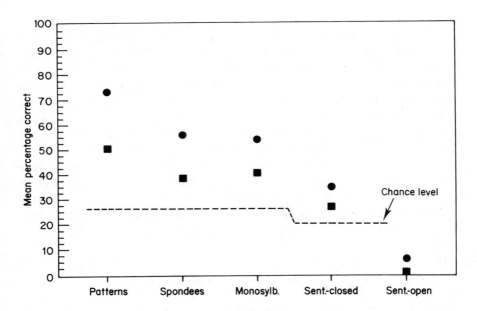

Figure 18.6. Hearing aid users in oral education programmes perform significantly higher than children in total communication programmes on pattern perception and monosyllable identification. ($P <0.05$) ■ = total communication hearing aid ($n = 16$); ● = oral communication hearing aid ($n = 14$).

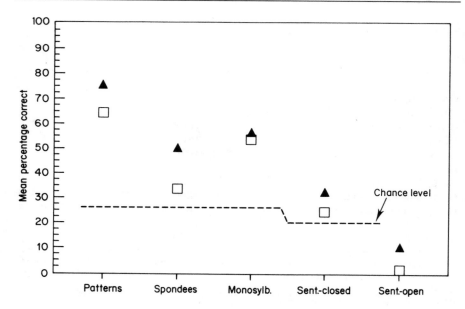

Figure 18.7.   Data are displayed for the two groups of cochlear implant users on the five speech perception measures. □ = Total communication cochlear implant ($n = 13$); ▲ = oral communication cochlear implant ($n = 13$).

same educational method on any of the speech perception measures. The two groups performed comparably. Hence, the cochlear implant appears to provide the almost-totally deaf child with the same auditory capacity as a profoundly deaf child in the mid-profound range (100–110 dB). Conversely, the control group performed lower than all groups on all speech perception measures except one (spondee identification); t-tests were applied comparing performance data between the cochlear implant control group and the implant groups (both total and oral combined) to determine if significant differences existed. Significant differences were found for all speech perception measures except spondee identification ($P<0.05$). If the children in the implant groups had not been implanted, they would have been expected to perform just as poorly, because their unassisted hearing acuity was essentially the same as that of the control group.

As indicated, although oral implant users performed higher than implantees in total communication settings, there were no significant differences between the two groups. In an attempt to determine which implantees were performing highest, the Nucleus implant children were separated in oral settings ($n=7$) from the entire oral implant group. These children performed higher on all measures than all other groups – both implant and hearing aid. Thus, these Nucleus users performed better than

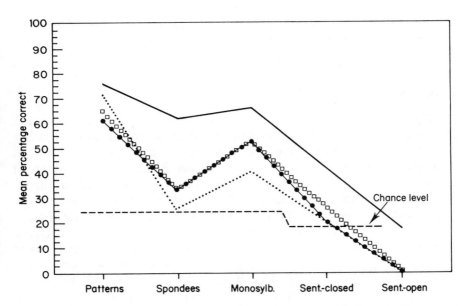

Figure 18.8. Subjects grouped by device and communication mode show that Nucleus implantees educated in oral communication settings perform significantly higher ($P < 0.05$) on spondee and monosyllable identification than any of the other implant groups. ···· = oral communication, 3M ($n = 6$); — = oral communication, Nucleus 22-channel ($n = 7$); □–□ = total communication, 3M ($n = 6$); ●–● = total communication, Nucleus 22-channel ($n = 7$).

hearing aid children in the mid-profound range. Children with residual hearing at higher levels (i.e. 90–100 dB and severely hearing-impaired children) need to be tested to ascertain comparable levels between cochlear implant users and hearing aid users who (unaided) are profoundly and severely deaf.

Grouping of the implant subjects by device and communication mode is shown in Figure 18.8. The small numbers (six and seven per group) were not sufficient to apply t-tests, hence a non-parametric test was applied. A Mann–Whitney U test shows that the oral Nucleus children ($n=7$) performed significantly higher ($P<0.05$) than the three other implant groups on spondee and monosyllable identification. These two subtests are particularly important for determining oral language potential (Moog and Geers, 1988b). These Nucleus subjects scored at this level and, hence, the Nucleus cochlear implant appears effective for the development of oral communication abilities for children trained in oral education settings.

Although controls could not be placed on onset of deafness at the beginning of the study, a multiple regression analysis was run with all of the 68 subjects to determine whether age at onset of deafness (up to 3 years of age) was predictive of performance. Low positive correlations were found ranging from 0.11 to 0.38 for all measures, i.e. onset of deafness did not predict performance in these subjects to any meaningful degree.

Discussion

Comparative performance on five tape-recorded speech perception measures were obtained from prelingually deaf children who wore either cochlear implants or hearing aids. Although caution must be taken in generalising from first year, initial data, trends indicate that, regardless of hearing device, children in oral communication settings perform higher on speech perception tasks than children in total communication settings. Those with hearing aids and the Nucleus cochlear implant in oral settings show the highest performance potential. According to Moog and Geers' Speech Perception Index (Moog and Geers, 1988b), these children would be expected to develop intelligible speech and oral language given continued training. Thus the acceleration of speech perception development to enhance oral communication development appears to be possible for prelingual, profoundly deaf children.

The cochlear implant appears to provide the almost-totally deaf child with the same auditory capacity as a hearing aid child who has hearing in the mid-profound range (100–110 dB). According to the Speech Perception Index these children would otherwise have a very minimal chance of developing intelligible speech. With the cochlear implant, however, these children's hearing, now raised to the mid-profound level, gives them a basis from which (with training) oral communication is possible. All children benefit from cochlear implants as is seen from comparison of both oral and total communication implants to the control group, but it does appear that orally educated implantees benefit to a greater extent.

The Nucleus cochlear implant combined with oral training appears to give the almost-totally deaf child an auditory capacity better than hearing aid children in the mid-profound range. Since the average length of cochlear implant use was only 1 year for Nucleus users, it can be speculated that with further device use and training, scores of this group on speech perception tasks may eventually compare with scores of severely deaf children. This has far-reaching implications. Most severely deaf children develop intelligible speech and fluent oral communication. Although special education may still be needed, the prognosis for severely deaf children is generally excellent.

Performance on connected language tests, both closed- and open-set, was low for all groups; there were no significant differences between any of the groups on either of the connected language measures. This indicates that, regardless of device or educational method, most children with such minimal acuity cannot use hearing alone to process connected language.

Since connected language more closely represents 'real-life' communication (as opposed to single words), this is an important indicator of functional abilities. It will be important to continue to follow these children to ascertain the continued effect of hearing device and educational method on their perception of connected language over time.

There does not appear to be a meaningful relationship between onset of deafness (up to 3 years of age) and speech perception performance in the cases studied. Although the multiple regression analysis did not yield any high correlation coefficients between onset of deafness and performance, a meaningful correlation may be seen in future years. However, with the prelingually deaf population, differences in performance between congenital and adventitiously deafened children may not become apparent (auditory performance differences between prelingual and postlingual profoundly deaf children are apparent in both hearing aid and implant paediatric populations). It may be that congenital children take longer to reach the same maximum auditory skill levels as those deafened adventitiously.

First year data from the author's 3-year study indicate trends that reveal important implications for developing speech perception skills in prelingually deaf children with cochlear implants and hearing aids. Data obtained in future years will allow a comparison of rates of auditory skill acquisition for study groups as well as performance differences over time. Studying educational method in combination with different hearing devices gives us important information for maximising the auditory potential of profoundly deaf children.

Educational Follow-up: Rehabilitation Programmes

The option of the cochlear implant has continued to bring about numerous questions. Parents and professionals want to know if the cochlear implant effects auditory capabilities sufficiently to facilitate communication. If so, what rehabilitation strategies would best maximise the benefits of the cochlear implant? How should these postoperative rehabilitation programmes be managed?

With appropriate auditory intervention and directed attention to auditory input, the cochlear implant can provide the opportunity for improved speech intelligibility and accelerate language acquisition. Along with these opportunities, however, come many difficulties and challenges for both the families and the professionals involved with these children.

Many implant centres across the USA have developed postoperative management programmes in conjunction with the children's educational facilities. Often the implant centre invites the child's teacher to be a part of the implant decision. Personnel from the implant centre then coordinate the implantation process (evaluation, surgery and training) with the child's school. Additionally, some of the required post-implant evaluations may be carried out at the school.

The child's school will also typically be responsible for the bulk of the postoperative rehabilitation programme. It is clear that the teacher of the deaf must be brought into the programme in a more active role than is currently practised by many implant centres in the USA.

Enhancing Auditory Information: Objectives and Strategies

Attempts to utilise residual hearing of children through cochlear implants have been an integral part of both educational and habilitative endeavours. Primarily two approaches to optimising auditory input received through the cochlear implant have been utilised. These two approaches (the synthetic and analytical approaches) have been used for decades to maximise the use of residual hearing for children with hearing aids. Although specific target objectives may be different for children with cochlear implants, general strategies and intervention techniques are similar to those used with hearing aid children.

Synthetic approach

The synthetic or 'top down' (Ling, 1978) approach facilitates auditory skill acquisition throughout the child's daily routine in a natural, holistic environment. Although the environment may be structured to maximise auditory interactions, auditory skills develop primarily through language experience. Teachers and peers concentrate on auditory input by integrating and emphasising audition in classroom and play situations. Educators have developed conversational strategies (Stone, 1991), cognitive sequences (Grammatico, 1980) and specific curricula (Trammel, 1976) to support the synthetic approach to auditory skill acquisition. Children with cochlear implants educated with the synthetic approach develop much the same as hearing aid children (Stone, 1991) and appear to follow the same auditory skill acquisition sequences.

When using the synthetic approach, it may be difficult to see improvements when children are first implanted as auditory skills begin to emerge. At this stage the teacher may find it helpful to identify emerging auditory skills (Somers, 1990) and track changes in such skills over time (Table 18.5).

Table 18.5 Listening skill development sequence

Objective	Strategy
1. The child will accept the cochlear implant during all waking hours	The adult will introduce and encourage the child's acceptance of the cochlear implant
2. The child will attend to a listening activity/talk	The adult will help the child focus attention on a particular person and/or object
3. The child will develop a 'listening set'	The adult will help the child develop anticipation of forthcoming sounds
4. The child will respond to the presence of environmental sounds	The adult will stimulate the child's response to sound by facial expression, by body movement (hands up to ears), and by verbal expressions, i.e. 'I heard that'
5. The child will respond to the presence and absence of environmental sounds	The adult will stimulate the child's response to the presence and absence of environmental sound by facial expression, movement, verbal expression
6. The child will respond to the presence of voice	The adult will encourage the child's response to voice, through facial expressions (smiling, laughing), vocalisation or body movements
7. The child will associate meaning to environmental sounds	The adult will take advantage of natural occurrences to point out sound sources
8. The child will associate meaning to vocal inflection	The adult will react to situations with appropriate vocal inflections
9. The child will respond and associate meaning to sounds at increasingly greater distances	The adult will introduce familiar sounds at increasingly greater distances: (a) up to 2 feet (0.6 m) (b) 2–5 feet (0.6–1.5 m) (c) 5–10 feet (1.5–3.0 m) (d) from across the room (e) from outside the room or out-of-doors
10. The child will discriminate among different environmental sounds	The adult will provide opportunities for the child to focus in on the differences between and among sounds
11. The child will discriminate among different speech sounds using pitch, intensity, duration and number of syllables as variables	The adult will present speech sounds and encourage the child to focus in on the differences within each of the four variables
12. The child will discriminate among different voices	The adult will help the child focus in on different voices, e.g. female voice vs male voice
13. The child will turn to the source of sounds (localise)	The adult will direct the child's attention to sounds from various locations within the room and will encourage the child to locate the sources with increasing independence
14. The child will discriminate among large segments of spoken language, e.g. two different songs	The adult will provide the child with appropriate models of large segments of spoken language and encourage the child's discrimination
15. The child will discriminate among short segments of spoken language, e.g. phrases and expressions	The adult will present different phrases and expressions to the child and encourage the child's discrimination
16. The child will discriminate among different words	The adult will present known vocabulary to the child and encourage the child's discrimination

Analytical approach

The analytical approach focuses on development of specific skills designed to enhance auditory input being provided by the cochlear implant speech processor. Although there are children with the 3M/House device who receive spectral information, primarily temporal aspects of speech are provided by the implant. Discriminating long vs short sounds, short vs fast sounds and interrupted vs uninterrupted sounds are the first target objectives for these children. As these children gain auditory competence, the clinician or teacher can then advance to phonemic discriminations such as voicing, manner or place discriminations. Discrimination between words (spondees and monosyllables), short phrases and sentences is attempted simultaneously as the children begin to process words and connect language through their hearing. Although comprehension of open-set language is realistic for only a small number of implantees, the opportunity for the child to process and respond to language auditorily is important for maximising the potential of the hearing device.

If the analytical approach is used, it is important to determine which speech cues the child is perceiving through his or her speech processor. In another investigation, collaborating with Boothroyd, the author investigated the perception of speech pattern contrasts in almost-totally deaf (>110 dB) children with cochlear implants ($n=26$) and profoundly deaf children with hearing aids ($n=30$) with usable, residual hearing (100–110 dB). Speech pattern contrast testing identifies which acoustic speech features are being perceived by the listener.

Subjects were between 4 and 8 years of age and had prelingual (<3 years) onset of deafness. There were equal numbers of children in each group in total and oral communication settings and equal numbers of 3M/House and Nucleus users.

The Imitative Speech Pattern Contrast test (IMSPAC) is administered by having the child repeat stimulus nonsense syllables indicative of predetermined speech pattern contrasts: initial consonant continuance, final consonant voicing, initial consonant place, vowel height, initial consonant voice, vowel place, syllabification and intonation. The child's repetitions are recorded and then identified by listeners in a four-choice task. Final correct scores are adjusted for chance and then graphed to display contrast distinctions perceived.

Initial analyses of ten subjects suggest that the perception of acoustic speech patterns represents the signal input provided by the hearing device. For example, results for the children with the single-electrode implant suggest that they are perceiving primarily time and intensity information. Children with 3M/House and Nucleus cochlear implants make final consonant voicing, syllabification and vowel height discriminations. Nucleus users are additionally able to make vowel, intonation and, to a lesser degree, place distinctions. Nucleus users perceived those contrasts reflective of spectral speech cues similarly to the hearing aid users, but poorly relative to the contrasts representing suprasegmental feature information.

The investigation of speech pattern contrasts has important implications for the evaluation and understanding of speech-processing strategies of cochlear implant systems. Additionally, knowledge of children's perception of speech cues can be used for effecting children's rehabilitation and programming.

Despite the application of research knowledge and the combined efforts of parents and professionals, many children with cochlear implants do not benefit from their implant sufficiently to permit the acquisition of spoken communication. An intensive auditory programme integrated both into the educational and home setting will ensure that the cochlear implant child has the best possible chance of maximising the effect of the cochlear implant. Specific auditory objectives coupled with specific strategies can assure the optimisation of potential of the cochlear implant (as listed in Table 18.5).

These objectives are general guidelines for children beginning use with a cochlear implant. It is important to remember that these children have had a history of failure with listening. Consequently, trust in listening must be developed. Adults working with the child must be patient and reinforcing. Success with an implant can and will occur if first the adults trust the listening process and secondly the child is given repeated, guided opportunities to listen and respond.

Conclusions

Attempts to utilise residual hearing of hearing-impaired children through amplification devices have been an integral part of both educational and habilitative endeavours. There is a wealth of theoretical, clinical and practical literature, historically and currently, which addresses what, how and why amplification, coupled with aural habilitation, is important for hearing-impaired children. In addition, emphasis has increased over the years on the importance of the provision of sound and auditory training very early in the hearing-impaired child's life.

An intensive auditory programme integrated into both the educational and home settings will ensure that the cochlear implant child has the best possible chance of maximising the benefits of the cochlear implant.

References

BLAMEY, P., MARTIN, L. and CLARK, G. (1977). A comparison of three coding strategies using an acoustic representation of a cochlear implant. *J. Acoust. Soc. Am.* **17**, 82–97.

BOOTHROYD, A. (1976). Influence of residual hearing on speech perception and speech production by hearing-impaired children. Paper presented at the annual convention of the American Speech, Language and Hearing Association, Houston, Texas.

BOOTHROYD, A. (1978). Speech perception and sensorineural hearing loss. In: Ross, M. and Giolas, T.G. (eds), *Auditory Management of Hearing Impaired Children*. Baltimore, MD: Baltimore University Park Press.

BOOTHROYD, A. (1987). High performing cochlear implant users. Paper presented at American Speech, Language and Hearing Association, National Convention, New Orleans, USA.

BOOTHROYD, A. (1989). Hearing aid, cochlear implants, and profoundly deaf children. In: Owens, E. and Kessler, D.K. (eds), *Cochlear Implants in Young Children*, pp. 81–99. Boston, MA: Little, Brown & Co.

ERBER, N.P. (1982). Glendonald Auditory Screening procedure. In: *Auditory Training*, p. 104. Washington DC: Alexander Graham Bell Association for the Deaf.

ERBER, N.P. and HIRSCH, I. (1978). Auditory training. In: Davis, H. and Silverman, R. (eds), *Hearing and Deafness*, 4th edn. New York: Holt, Rinehart & Winston.

GEERS, A.E. and MOOG, J.S. (1987). Predicting spoken language acquisition in profoundly deaf children. *J. Speech Hear. Dis.* **28**, 67–91.

GEERS, A.E. and MOOG, J.S. (1988). Predicting long term benefits of the single channel cochlear implant in profoundly deaf children. *Am. J. Otolaryngol.* **37**, 224–250.

GRAMMATICO, L. (1980). Talk to your child. Presented at Alexander Graham Bell Convention, Portland, Oregon.

HUDGINS, C. and NUMBERS, F. (1942). An investigation of intelligibility of the speech of the deaf. *Genet. Psychol. Monogr.* **25**, 48–67.

JENSEMA, C. and TRYBUS, R. (1978). *Communication Patterns and Educational Achievement of Hearing Impaired Students*. Office of Demographic Studies, Washington DC, Ser. T, 2.

JERGER, S. and JERGER, J. (1984). *Pediatric Speech Intelligibility Test*. St Louis, MO: Auditec.

JOHNSON, J. (1987). Auditory and speech perception abilities of children with the 3M/House Cochlear implant. Presented at the National Convention of the American Speech, Language and Hearing Association, New Orleans.

LING, D. (1978). *Speech and the Hearing-impaired Child: Theory and Practice*. Washington DC: The Alexander Graham Bell Association for the Deaf.

LUTERMAN, D. and CHASIN, A. (1981). The deafness management quotient as an indicator of oral success. *Volta Rev.* **83**, 91–98.

MOOG, J.S. and GEERS, A.E. (1988a). Predicting spoken language acquisition of profoundly hearing-impaired children. *J. Speech Hear. Dis.* **52**, 84–94.

MOOG, J.S. and GEERS, A.E. (1988b). *Early Speech Perception Test for Profoundly Hearing-impaired Children*. St Louis, MO: Central Institute for the Deaf.

OFFICE OF DEMOGRAPHIC STUDIES (1984). *Trends in the Hearing Impaired Population*. Gallaudet University, Washington DC: Gallaudet College Press.

OSBERGER, M.J. (1990). Speech production abilities of children with implants and tactile aids. Presented at the Third Symposium on Cochlear Implants in Children, January. Indianapolis, IN.

OSBERGER, M.J. and McGARR, N. (1978). Pitch deviancy and intelligibility of deaf speech. *J. Commun. Dis.* **11**, 34–58.

SOMERS, M. (1987). Auditory development in a young multichannel cochlear implant child. Presented at the Annual Meeting of the American Auditory Society, September. New Orleans, LA.

SOMERS, M. (1990). Auditory Evaluation Instrument: Assessing emerging auditory skills. Paper presented at the Alexander Graham Bell Association National Convention, July, Washington DC, USA.

SOMERS, M. (1991). Comparing speech perception abilities in deaf children. Proceedings from the Third Annual Symposium on Children with Cochlear Implants, Indianapolis, IN. *Am. J. Otol.* in press.

STALLER, S. (1990). Pediatric performance with the Nucleus 22 channel cochlear implant. Presented at the Third Symposium on Cochlear Implants in Children, January. Indianapolis, IN.

STONE, P. (1991). Tucker–Maxon's experience with cochlear implant children. Proceedings from the Third Annual Symposium on Children with Cochlear Implants, Indianapolis, IN. *Am. J. Otol.* in press.

THIELEMEIR, M., TONOKAWA, L. and PETERSON, B. (1985). Audiological results in children with a cochlear implant. *Ear Hear. Monogr.* 6 (suppl. 3).

TRAMMEL, J.L. (1976). *Test of Auditory Comprehension.* North Hollywood, CA: Foreworks.

Chapter 19
Speech Production in Postlinguistically Deafened Adult Cochlear Implant Users

THEODORA READ

Introduction

The onset of a profound or total hearing loss after the acquisition of normal speech and language often results in problems with communication. The primary difficulty is usually in understanding the speech of other people. However, the loss of auditory feedback about the deafened person's own speech may result in deterioration of speech production skills. Much of the research carried out with adult cochlear implant users has been related to their perceptual abilities and, in particular, to speech–perception skills. In contrast, there has been relatively little research into changes in speech production as a result of using a cochlear implant although anecdotal evidence has been available for some time. Before discussing in detail the effects of a cochlear implant on speech production, it would be useful to describe the sorts of changes in speech production that may occur as a result of an acquired profound hearing loss. Whilst this chapter will concentrate on speech production, it is important to remember that speech production is not an isolated skill; it is interdependent with language skills and auditory and kinaesthetic perception.

Speech Changes following Hearing

There is a considerable amount of data in the literature describing the speech skills of congenitally deaf people. It is widely recognised that the expressive speech and language of people who are born deaf are likely to be more severely affected than people who developed normal speech and language before they became deaf. This may explain some comments in the literature which suggest that adults with an acquired loss have little or no speech deterioration. For example, Ling (1976, p. 78) suggests that, as adult speech production control mechanisms are well established, 'auditory feedback is therefore not essential'. Similarly, Espir and Rose (1976, p. 40) state: 'The onset of deafness in adults does not usually interfere with the ability to speak, except that some will tend to shout owing to difficulty gauging the loudness of their voice.' However, research which has investigated speech deterioration in postlinguistically deafened adults has found that this group do have speech problems and that they can be of a serious nature. It has also been demonstrated that there is a considerable amount of individual variation. Some adults retain excellent speech after being deaf for several years whilst others show marked deterioration after a short period of time.

There is broad agreement across the numerous studies of speech production that changes following an acquired loss tend to be in the prosodic and segmental aspects of speech production, and not in the language (syntax and lexicon) of the speaker. It is also noted that changes at the prosodic level (voice quality, rate of speech, intonation, pitch) tend to occur more frequently than at the segmental level (speech sounds).

In Penn's study (1955) 200 cases of acquired hearing loss were investigated (100 conductive losses, 100 sensorineural losses). Volume, pitch, voice quality and rate were shown to change and Penn identified relationships between the type of hearing loss and speech production patterns. Markides (1977) described problems with precision of articulation, rate of speech and intonation patterns, voice quality and loudness. Plant (1984) used a single subject design and found the following features: reduced rate of speaking, elongation of syllables, tendency to centring of vowels, deletion of final consonants, inability to use contrastive stress patterns and a tendency for fundamental frequency to rise in the articulation of high vowels. Binnie, Daniloff and Buckingham (1982) also investigated a single case and found similar changes in rate of speech and intonation patterns. In addition, syllabification of consonants, diphthongisation of vowels, reduction of consonant clusters and use of glottal stop were identified. Cowie and Douglas-Cowie (1983) also found that changes tended to occur in rate, voice quality, volume, pitch and intonation patterns. Parker (1983) gives an excellent review of these studies and also includes her own clinical observations to describe deterioration in adults with a profound acquired loss. Changes are summarised under suprasegmental (prosodic) features (breathing patterns, voice, intonation, timing and rhythm) and segmental features.

Parker (1983) introduces an important distinction between phonetic and phonological levels. If speech is described at the phonological level without narrow phonetic transcription, then initial phonetic changes may not be identified and 'speech may not be recognised as abnormal until deterioration approaches very marked and obvious levels'. Parker also calls attention to the fact that deaf adults may suffer from a voice problem caused by abnormal vocal fold function but that this may be overlooked and attributed to the hearing loss. Therefore it is important to involve the ENT consultant in voice assessment to exclude any laryngeal pathology prior to speech therapy intervention. In addition to describing speech deterioration, Cowie, Douglas-Cowie and Kerr (1982) investigated listener reactions to deaf speakers. They found that deaf speakers were not perceived as intelligent, organised, tidy, reliable or industrious. Listeners did not assume that the person was deaf. Not only do people with acquired profound hearing loss have problems with speech intelligibility, but they also have to cope with adverse reactions from listeners.

To summarise the findings of various studies, it was generally found that: postlinguistically deaf speakers are less intelligible than normally hearing speakers but more intelligible than congenitally profoundly deaf speakers; age of onset of deafness is a factor in intelligibility and speech takes time to degenerate; individuals vary considerably in the degree of speech deterioration that has occurred; and suprasegmental features of speech (voice quality, rate of speech, intonation patterns, pitch) are most likely to be affected.

Effects of Cochlear Implant Use on Speech Production

The speech of a postlinguistically, profoundly deafened person may show signs of deterioration, but will there be any improvement in speech production skills following the use of a cochlear implant?

It has been reported that cochlear implant users show improvements in voice quality, intonation patterns, volume control and intelligibility. However, the majority of investigations have used subjective or anecdotal evidence. There have been few objective studies so far, but those which have been carried out have found evidence of improvement in speech production skills. Several studies have investigated changes in habitual pitch mode. Iler-Kirk and Edgerton (1983) examined voice parameters in four cochlear implant users: two male and two female. They found that in the implant-on condition, the fundamental frequency of the two male subjects decreased and the variability in intensity also decreased. These movements were in the direction of normal voice production. The two female subjects also showed improvement but, in their case, fundamental frequency and variability in intensity increased in the direction of normal. Leder et al. (1987) also found that fundamental frequency decreased in male cochlear implant users and that this change was noted almost immediately. Four implant users were noted to have moved to more normal fundamental frequency values by Ball and Faulkner (1989). Low frequency irregularity (described as creaky voice) was also reduced with the implant. This reduction of creaky voice was observed by Waters (1986) in two out of three patients.

Use of contrastive stress patterns has also been examined. It has been observed that cochlear implant users show an improvement in the use of contrastive stress patterns (Leder et al., 1986; Waters, 1986; Medwetsky, Hanin and Boothroyd, 1989). However, it was noted that improvements in intonation patterns did not occur immediately but only following use of the implant for some months. Prolongation of sentences and pauses was identified as a problem for some deafened adults and was noted to have improved in some patients (Iler-Kirk and Edgerton, 1983; Waters, 1986; Leder, Spitzer and Kirchner, 1987).

There has also been some work using listener judgements to evaluate acceptability of speech. Frost and Carpenter (1987) devised a four-point scale which was not found to be sufficiently sensitive to pick up subtle changes in speech production, but was able to identify improvements in acceptability of speech and in intonation patterns for 12 cochlear implant users. Read (1989) evaluated 30 cochlear implant users and found that 57% were judged to have considerable improvement in speech production. Voice quality and voice volume were also noted to have improved in 53% and 60% of subjects respectively.

It is important that the previous subjective reports have been supported by objective research, but there is still a long way to go. The speech of larger numbers of implant users needs to be evaluated and objective measures need to be made of specific suprasegmental skills. Cochlear implant users are said to be able to control the volume of their voice but as yet there is no objective measure available. Leder et al. (1987) have demonstrated that prospective cochlear implant users have increased voice intensity. They recorded normally hearing and deaf subjects reading a set passage. Intensity values from the recordings were measured using an automatic intensity analyser (Kay Visi-Pitch 6087DS) at the beginning and end of each breath group. The breath group is defined as 'a section of utterance that is produced between two respiratory inspirations, and is marked by stress and intonation'. Subjects with normal hearing were recorded at a standard input level and intensity values were determined using a standard output level on the tape recorder. This procedure was not possible with the deaf speakers because of their highly variable speaking intensities and therefore calibration of the tape recorder was necessary. This process is described in detail in Leder et al. (1987). The results of this research indicated that voice intensity was significantly increased in the deaf speakers and that they produced wider intensity fluctuations. This is valuable information as it provides objective measurements where previously there was only anecdotal evidence. However, data from people who have received implants have not yet been presented. Contrastive use of stress has been investigated but so far only a small range of intonation patterns has been examined (place of nuclear stress and question/statement forms). Although the work which has been presented so far is valuable and interesting, there is still a considerable amount to investigate.

Speech Therapy with Cochlear Implant Users

The cochlear implant training programme at University College Hospital, London includes intervention on speech production skills by a specialist speech therapist where appropriate. A detailed speech production assessment is carried out with all prospective cochlear implant candidates. Those accepted onto the programme are reassessed at regular intervals post-implantation (after 'switch on', at 3 months, 6 months and 1 year post-implantation, then yearly thereafter). The same assessment procedure is used with adults with acquired hearing loss but not participating in the cochlear implant programme. The assessment procedure consists of a high-fidelity audio recording and a Visispeech histogram. Speech in a variety of different contexts is elicited for the audio-recording sample as intelligibility may vary depending on the familiarity and complexity of the language used. The sample consists of the following:

1. Sequential speech, i.e. counting up to ten, the days of the week.
2. A single word list (the list was developed to elicit a full range of contrasts, consonant clusters and polysyllabic words – narrow phonetic transcription is used).
3. A specially prepared passage. (The passage contains questions, answers, lists of words etc. in order to elicit different prosodic patterns.)
4. A voice loudness level task (the client has to repeat a sentence and alter the loudness of their voice with each repetition (Summers, Peake and Martin, 1981).)
5. A true conversation.

The recording procedure is based on the RNID Speech Assessment Procedure (Fisher, King and Wright, 1979) developed by Waters (1986) and further refined by Frost and Carpenter (1987). The second part of the assessment is a Visispeech histogram. Visispeech is a computer-based visual speech display developed at the Royal National Institute for the Deaf. The histogram mode shows the fundamental frequencies that have occurred in the sample and how often they have registered. The contour of the histogram will be highest over the frequencies that occur most and lowest over those that occur least. However, the histogram does not only indicate presence or absence of phonation. Characteristic histograms have been identified for normal and abnormal voice quality (Cook, Hooker and Webb, 1986). Statistics are also provided, especially pitch mode and range. The histogram therefore provides an objective assessment of voice quality. The author has noted that several of the implant patients prior to implantation have noticeably creaky voice. This quality is caused by irregular vocal fold vibration. Once they begin using the implant, vocal fold vibration becomes more regular and voice quality improves.

Figure 19.1 shows a characteristic histogram of normal voice. The pattern is similar to a normal distribution curve, indicating the habitual pitch mode at the height of the curve and a range of frequencies used either side of the mode. Figure 19.2 shows a histogram of a single-channel implant user with the implant off. This person has a markedly creaky voice quality, and this is represented on the histogram by several peaks either

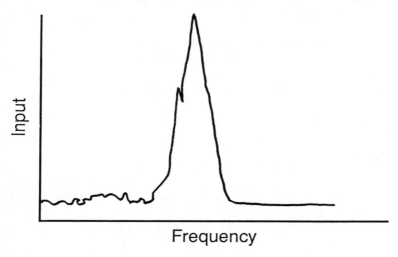

Figure 19.1.   Visispeech histogram: normal voice.

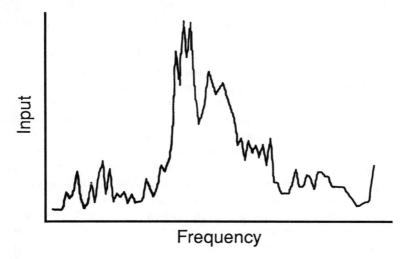

Figure 19.2.   Visispeech histogram: implanted patient, implant off.

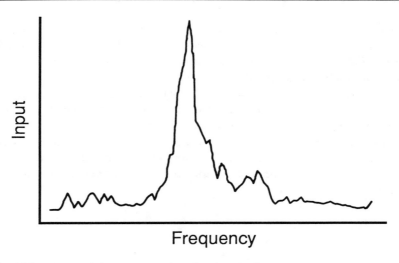

Figure 19.3.   Visispeech histogram: implanted patient, implant on.

side of the mode indicating irregular vocal fold function. Figure 19.3 shows the same patient with the implant on. The histogram has changed from one characteristic of a creaky voice to a pattern much more similar to normal voice quality. This demonstrates the benefit to this patient of the input from the implant. She is much more able to monitor her voice quality appropriately with the implant on. Changes in voice quality had previously been reported anecdotally. It is much more useful to have objective measures which can be compared over time with the same patient and across a group of patients. Accurate assessment is a vital prerequisite to speech therapy intervention.

As noted earlier in the chapter, speech deterioration is most likely to occur in suprasegmental speech features. Once the larynx has been examined, and any laryngeal pathology excluded, conventional approaches to achieving good breathing patterns and improving voice production can be used. With some deafened adults, it is necessary to include counselling as part of the speech production work as some people find it difficult to accept that their speech is abnormal. It would not usually be appropriate to work on expressive speech skills in isolation. A speech therapy session would typically include both perception and production work. Role reversal can be used, in production, to elicit skills achieved in perception. For example, the trainer presents a monosyllabic speech sample with either flat or falling pitch. Once the listener can discriminate between the two sounds consistently, the roles can be reversed. The listener then has to present the sound and the trainer has to identify flat or falling pitch.

Visual speech displays (for example Visispeech or Laryngograph) have proved to be extremely useful for both perception and production work, as they can demonstrate clearly pitch mode, intonation contrasts and voice quality. The use of visual feedback when the implant is new to the patient reinforces the sounds being heard: it facilitates perception and assists the patient in monitoring their production. It is essential to achieve carry-over of skills from the structured situation where a visual speech display is being used to a more natural communication situation. There is more to good communication skills than just speech production and so video recording is used to evaluate overall tension, eye contact and facial expression. Video can also be used within a therapy session for role-play and other social skill activities.

Conclusion

Adults with profound, acquired hearing loss may experience deterioration in speech production skills, especially in suprasegmental features of speech. Speech production skills have been shown to improve in cochlear implant users, particularly fundamental frequency, timing and use of contrastive stress. Therapeutic approaches to speech production skills with this group tend to be a combination of conventional methods and use of newer technology. For the future, there needs to be further research using objective measures to examine changes in speech as a result of using a cochlear implant and also more discussion of therapy techniques used with this group.

References

BALL, G. and FAULKNER, A. (1989). Speech production of postlingually deafened adults using electrical and acoustic speech pattern prostheses. In: *Speech, Hearing and Language: Work in Progress*, Vol. 3, pp. 11–32. University College London, Department of Phonetics.

BINNIE, C.A., DANILOFF, R.C. and BUCKINGHAM, H.W. (1982). Phonetic disintegration in a five-year-old following sudden hearing loss. *J. Speech Hear. Dis.* 47, 181–189.

COOK, J., HOOKER, D. and WEBB, J. (1986). The application of Visispeech to pathologies of voice. *Bulletin of the College of Speech Therapists* 411, 1–2.

COWIE, R. and DOUGLAS-COWIE, E. (1983). Speech production in profound post-lingual deafness. In: Lutman, M.E. and Haggard, M.P. (eds), *Hearing Science and Hearing Disorders*, pp. 183–200. London: Academic Press.

COWIE, R., DOUGLAS-COWIE, E. and KERR, A.G. (1982). A study of speech deterioration in post-lingually deafened adults. *J. Laryngol. Otol.* 96, 101–112.

ESPIR, M. and ROSE, C. (1976). *The Basic Neurology of Speech*. Oxford: Blackwell Scientific.

FISHER, J., KING, A. and WRIGHT, R. (1983). Assessment of speech production as a basis for speech therapy. In: Levitt, J., Hochberg, I. and Osberger, M.J. (eds), *Proceedings of the Conference on Speech for the Hearing Impaired*, City University, New York. Baltimore, MD: Baltimore University Park Press.

FROST, R. and CARPENTER, L. (1987). Design of a speech production assessment for use with deafened adults receiving single channel extracochlear implants. In: Banfai, P. (ed.), *Proceedings of the International Cochlear Implant Symposium*, pp. 297–305, Düren, W. Germany.

ILER-KIRK, K. and EDGERTON, B.J. (1983). The effects of cochlear implant use on voice parameters. *Otolaryngol. Clin. North Am.* **16**, 281–291.

LEDER, S.B., SPITZER, J.B. and KIRCHNER, J.C. (1987). Immediate effects of cochlear implantation on voice quality. *Arch. Oto-Rhino-Laryngol.* **244**, 93–95.

LEDER, S.B., SPITZER, J.B., MILNER, P., FLEVARIS-PHILIPS, C., RICHARDSON, F. and KIRCHNER, J.C. (1986). Reacquisition of contrastive stress in an adventitiously deaf speaker using a single channel cochlear implant. *J. Acoust. Soc. Am.* **79**, 1967–1974.

LEDER, S.B., SPITZER, J.B., MILNER, P., FLEVARIS-PHILIPS, C., RICHARDSON, F. and KIRCHNER, J.C. (1987). Voice intensity of prospective cochlear implant candidates and normal hearing adult males. *Laryngoscope* **97**, 224–227.

LING, D. (1976). *Speech and the Hearing-Impaired Child: Theory and Practice.* Washington DC: Alexander Graham Bell Association for the Deaf.

MARKIDES, A. (1977). Rehabilitation of people with acquired deafness in adulthood. *Br. J. Audiol.* Suppl. 1.

MEDWETSKY, L., HANIN, L. and BOOTHROYD, A. (1987). Objective changes in the speech of cochlear implantees. Paper presented at the Annual Convention of American Speech, Language and Hearing Association, New Orleans.

PARKER, A. (1983). Speech Conservation. In: Watts, W. (ed.), *Rehabilitation and Acquired Deafness*, pp. 234–250. London: Croom Helm.

PENN, J.P. (1955). Voice and speech patterns of the hard of hearing. *Acta Oto-Laryngol. Suppl.* 124.

PLANT, G. (1984). The effects of an acquired profound hearing loss on speech production; a case study. *Br. J. Audiol.* **18**, 39–48.

READ, T. (1989). Improvement in speech production following use of the UCH/RNID Cochlear Implant. *J. Laryngol. Otol.* Suppl. 18, 45–49.

SUMMERS, I., PEAKE, M. and MARTIN, M. (1981). Field trials of a tactile acoustic monitor for the profoundly deaf. *Br. J. Audiol.* **15**, 195–199.

WATERS, T. (1986). Speech therapy with cochlear implant wearers. *Br. J. Audiol.* **20**, 35–43.

Chapter 20
Electrical Tinnitus Suppression

JONATHAN W.P. HAZELL

Introduction

Tinnitus is an extremely common problem producing marked disability in an important minority of the population. Seven per cent of the whole population have consulted a doctor at some time or other about tinnitus, and from 0.5% to 1% find that their ability to lead a normal life is severely affected by the presence of tinnitus (Institute of Hearing Research, 1981).

The majority of patients adapt or habituate to the presence of a continuous noise in the ear or the head once they are reassured of a benign aetiology. In the UK, however, there are some 200 000 people who are severely affected by their tinnitus and many of them become depressed and even suicidal. Whilst the habituative process can be enhanced by specific counselling techniques and additional help can be gained from the fitting of appropriate tinnitus maskers, hearing aids or combination instruments, there are still many thousands of people who cannot be helped by these established techniques. It is possible that many of them could benefit from electrical tinnitus suppression (ETS), and that their numbers may well exceed those who are profoundly deafened and who could benefit from auditory rehabilitation by cochlear implantation. If this is so, then one of the future roles of cochlear implantation, particularly using single-channel extracochlear devices, may be as a means to control tinnitus. One-third of those with hearing losses have significant tinnitus as well, and this is often a most important problem in those who are profoundly or totally deaf. The effect of electrical stimulation on tinnitus needs to be assessed where this is (1) the prime object of such implantation, (2) where it is a desired subsidiary effect of implantation, and (3) where it is important that tinnitus should not be exacerbated.

In this chapter, the subject matter is the suppression of tinnitus by electric current. This begs the question as to what is actually happening when an electric current is applied to an ear with tinnitus. In some cases there is undoubtedly a masking effect. This is analogous to the effect of auditory masking when one sound becomes inaudible in the presence of another (total masking) or appears quieter (partial masking). These terms have come into common use as a result of the use of tinnitus maskers — 'white noise generators' — which are applied to an ear over a period of time as a therapeutic procedure (Hazell et al., 1985). Unfortunately, the so-called masking effect is indeed a very complex one that may be divided into the immediate effect of an external sound applied to the ear and the more long-term effect occasioned by the presence of external sound over time — in the latter there is a learning phenomenon whereby the tinnitus changes in its noticeability or detectability in the presence of external white noise (Berliner et al., 1987). Tinnitus suppression suggests a direct interference by the electric current with the neural patterns responsible for the sensation of tinnitus. It may be that this involves a process of hyper-polarisation, with the result of a refractory period during which it is impossible for the nerve to conduct this signal pattern (Aran and Cazals, 1981).

An Historical Perspective

Since 1800, when Volta constructed the first battery, numerous attempts have been made to suppress tinnitus and stimulate impaired hearing by electric currents. Volta's battery consisted of layers of 30 metal plates interspersed with brine-soaked board. He performed a number of physiological experiments examining the body's response to electricity, and these included the introduction of electrodes into each external ear canal. Attached to the voltaic cell, he perceived a noise which he described as tough material being torn and which he found altogether disagreeable. He did not repeat the experiment. Grappengiesser (1801) used five different electrode configurations to stimulate the ear in an attempt to cure deafness. However, he also noticed the effects of direct current on the tinnitus when it was present. He produced a classification of tinnitus depending on whether there was a response to electrical stimulation or not. Duchenne de Boulogne (1855) gave the first account of the use of the induction coil, which had just been introduced by Faraday, as a method of applying interrupted or alternating current to the ear. He placed one electrode in the external ear canal which was filled with water, the indifferent electrode being applied to the neck. Eight out of ten patients were said to have been cured of their tinnitus by this kind of electrical stimulation. MacNaughton Jones (1891) recorded his use of both galvanism and faradism in a book on tinnitus in 1891. He used a variety of electrodes involving both the eustachian tube and the external meatus. Often he was forced to admit that his treatment failed to achieve its objective. In this book (cited by Stephens, 1987) he says 'in cases of which it has done good, I have always been in doubt if the benefit was not as much derived from other treatment accompanying its use as from the Galvanism alone'. He was certainly able to identify the numerous interacting psychological and physiological components that determine whether tinnitus is a complaint or merely an experience.

Over the last 20 years there has been a revival of interest in treating tinnitus, and the number of publications on this subject has risen exponentially. This has resulted from the early work of Vernon (1977) and others, although an improved understanding of the auditory physiological mechanisms which may be responsible for tinnitus generation in the auditory system has been of paramount importance (Hazell and Jastreboff, 1989). It was natural that any renewed therapeutic attempts to deal with this extremely common and often debilitating condition should include renewed efforts to achieve ETS.

Transtympanic Electrical Stimulation

Aran and Le Bert (1968) devised a needle electrode placed through the tympanic membrane to measure the cochlear action potential and cochlear microphonic in humans, using an averaging computer. This transtympanic electrode was subsequently used by House and Brackmann (1974) to pass low-voltage, low-frequency electric current to the promontory. This was proposed as a test to differentiate between cochlear and retrocochlear deafness. Where the patient was deaf, and where an electrically induced sound could be heard, they proposed that the loss was principally one involving cochlear hair cells. Where there was no response to electrical stimulation they proposed that there was a neural and more central deficit. Although they did not record the effect of this stimulation on tinnitus where it was present, a beneficial and suppressive effect was obtained in about half the patients tested who had experienced tinnitus (Brackmann, D.E., personal communication). Graham and Hazell (1977) reported on nine patients in whom tinnitus was suppressed by an alternating current passed through a transtympanic needle electrode on the promontory. Aran and colleagues also reported the effects of tinnitus suppression using a transtympanic electrode (Portmann et al., 1979). They used a variety of different waveforms at different frequencies and intensities. They found five patients whose tinnitus was suppressed but only by positive pulses. Negative pulses elicited clear auditory sensations and they concluded that, when suppressing tinnitus, a pathological neural activity was inhibited. Von Wedel and colleagues (von Wedel, Strahlmann and Zorowka, 1989) used transtympanic electrodes for suppression of tinnitus in conjunction with a number of other therapeutic approaches: they describe the study of 462 patients where less than 10% were helped by ETS. From the author's own clinic, Rothera et al. (1986) used transtympanic stimulation with both alternating and direct currents to evaluate profoundly deaf patients for cochlear implantation. The protocol involved tinnitus suppression experiments, in cases where this symptom was experienced. Tinnitus was suppressed in some 50% of ears, and a.c. stimulation was found to be as effective as d.c.

Stimulation with a Round Window Electrode

Aran and colleagues (Cazals, Negrevergne and Aran, 1978) reported on the use of a Teflon-coated silver wire placed in the round window via an anterior tympanotomy. The bony part of the external meatus was drilled to make a small canal in which the electrode lead could be fixed with histoacrylic glue. The patient could then be tested over a number of days, at the end of which the electrode was removed by gently pulling on it. Tinnitus suppression occurred in five out of six patients but only in the ear under test and with the application of positive unbalanced rectangular pulses. Negative pulses were ineffective, but balanced, alternating current sources were not tried on this occasion. The patients all had profound hearing losses. Aran concluded that tinnitus inhibition was achieved by a reduction of pathological activity rather than a restitution of missing neuronal function. In 1981, they noted that round window electrical tinnitus suppression was effective in 60% of patients and always total. This was compared with promontory stimulation where the suppression was partial in 43% and complete in only 25%.

Transcutaneous Electrical Tinnitus Suppression

Hatton, Erulkar and Rosenberg (1960) found that positive d.c. currents were most effective at suppressing tinnitus using external electrode configurations. Fifteen patients reported electrical tinnitus suppression, against 80 who did not. ETS was least effective in the presbyacusis group (no effect in 10 out of 11 patients). Chouard, Meyer and Maridat (1981) were among other authors who noticed tinnitus suppression during round window stimulation, when totally deaf patients were assessed for cochlear implantation. A separate study was performed in which 71 patients with either unilateral or bilateral tinnitus were examined in their response to transcutaneous ETS. Different electrode configurations were used but the highest success rate was obtained with an asymmetrical pulse. Overall one-third of cases reported obtaining some relief from their tinnitus. It was recommended that the treatment should be repeated two or three times to achieve an effect. Chouard's experiments were repeated by Vernon and Fenwick (1985) who used large carbon-impregnated rubber pads placed in front of and behind the ear. The criterion for improvement in tinnitus was taken as a 40% change. This study included a placebo group where the subjects were informed that they would not feel the stimulus because of its high-frequency nature. In the placebo group, none of the 23 subjects reported any change of tinnitus. Five subjects (22%) reported a significant change in tinnitus during actual ETS. In only one case was this achieved with monophasic positive pulses. A second study was performed in which the electrodes were placed on each mastoid area to facilitate current flow across the cochlea. In this study one patient gave a positive response in the placebo trial and nine patients (33%) gave positive results to ETS. Vernon and Fenwick concluded that the results were disappointing and did not produce enough positive effects to warrant use of the technique as a relief procedure for tinnitus, although it may be that the responders represent an important subgroup.

Shulman, Tonndorf and Goldstein (1985) report on a transcutaneous electrical tinnitus suppressor called the Audimax. This device uses a 60-kHz sinewave which is modulated at different rates between 0.2 and 20 kHz. The concentric electrodes are applied to the skin and this produces a current flow through the skin of around 1 mA. Shulman (1987) reviewed the results of Audimax stimulation with the passage of time. Six out of 50 patients continued to use the device and there was an increase in the intensity of the original tinnitus reported in 21, with a rebound effect in 19. Lyttkens and colleagues (1986) also tested the Audimax in a double-blind, cross-over trial with a placebo unit. One of five patients reported a consistent positive effect from active stimulation and no effect at all from the placebo.

Cochlear Implants and ETS

The widespread application of the cochlear implant for the rehabilitation of total deafness has facilitated chronic electrical stimulation of the cochlea, at least with alternating current. Reports from Los Angeles in the early days of cochlear implants (House, 1976) indicated that tinnitus could be influenced, although it was interesting that in a few patients tinnitus suppression was only achieved after some months. The possibility also exists that, taking into account the very elementary electronics employed in the early devices, there may well have been some net current flow into the cochlea. Whether or not this was so, there was no real evidence in this group of deterioration of electrical thresholds for hearing and, in those patients where suppression or masking of their tinnitus was achieved, this proved to be a useful additional therapeutic benefit that a single-channel device might bestow in addition to its main purpose as an aid to lipreading.

More recently, Berliner et al. (1987) reported on a group of 65 subjects who were implanted for profound deafness in the Los Angeles Group and who had received pre- and postoperative tinnitus questionnaires. The tinnitus was improved in 53% of cases with the implant switched on but 11% found it was worse. It seemed that there was some predictive value in those who had worn hearing aids prior to becoming totally deaf and

Table 20.1 Perstimulus tinnitus (T) suppression (implant with sound processor): tinnitus severity vs response

	T significant problem	T slight problem	T no problem
Made tinnitus inaudible	1	0	2
Distracting background sound tinnitus still audible	0	0	4
Both of the above at different times	6	5	0
No effect	2	2	6

who had experienced a masking effect while using them. Hazell, Meerton and Conway (1989) have reported recently on the effects of tinnitus suppression in 29 out of a series of 50 patients fitted with the UCH/RNID single-channel cochlear implant for total deafness. The improvement in tinnitus, while using the sound processor, was not limited to the implanted ear in this case, and therefore it is suggested that some kind of central masking or learning effect occurs. The results indicated that there could either be a reduction in tinnitus awareness or it could become completely unnoticeable, and this may bear some relationship to the effects of acoustic masking of tinnitus.

In Table 20.1 the results of 28 patients from this study are shown, all of whom had tinnitus in the implanted ear (or bilaterally).

The first reports of a single-channel, round window electrode being used for tinnitus suppression alone were reported in France in 1983 by Fraysse and Lazorthes. They used a modified cardiac pacemaker with the electrode in the round window to continuously stimulate the ear with sinusoids. Two out of four patients obtained some long-term help with their tinnitus. Gersdorff and Robillard (1985) also reported on a patient who had permanent electrode placement for tinnitus suppression.

Electrical Tinnitus Suppression at UCH/RNID

A regular weekly tinnitus clinic has been held at University College Hospital since 1976. More than 7000 patients have been seen and managed, principally with counselling and prosthetic techniques (Hazell et al., 1985). The approach has been to develop a multidisciplinary team consisting of otologists, audiologists, therapists, psychologists and nurses working together to achieve an holistic and broadly based medical, surgical and psychological approach to tinnitus. In the initial stages of the work, where a single masking instrument was applied to the ear without any appropriate form of counselling, as the only form of treatment available, less than one-quarter of the patients gained any benefit (Hazell, Williams and Sheldrake, 1981). The author's group now finds that the proportion of patients who cannot be helped in any way amounts to less than 5% of the total of the referrals, even though many of these are tertiary referrals who have been seen and treated by other colleagues, often on many occasions.

In 1983, the UCH/RNID cochlear implant programme started with the aim of rehabilitating total deafness. This allowed the examination of the effects of electrical tinnitus suppression on those who had failed to respond to other therapies. The author's findings with transtympanic stimulation of the tinnitus ear suggested that it was possible to suppress tinnitus with a balanced alternating current in certain cases. However, the group was aware that Aran and his colleagues had cautioned against the chronic use of unbalanced current sources because of the possibility of damage to the cochlea (Cazals, Negrevergne and Aran, 1978).

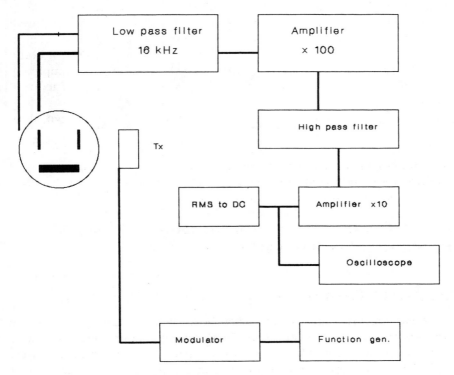

Figure 20.1. Apparatus for measuring waveforms at surface electrodes during electrical stimulation of implanted patients and temporary round window electrodes. Tx = 12-MHz transmitter, replaced by optical isolator and direct attachment with round window electrode. (Figures 20.1–20.3 were reproduced with permission from the *Journal of Laryngology and Otology.*)

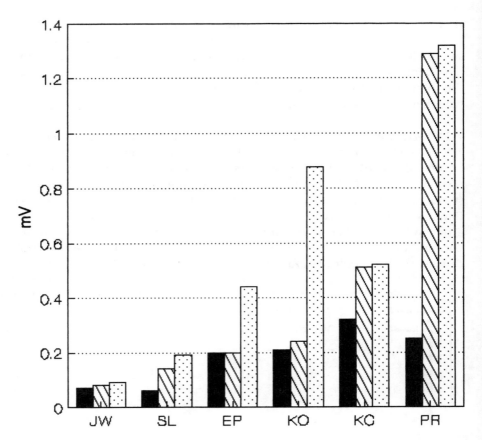

Figure 20.2. ETS using sinewaves on totally deaf patients with cochlear implants. ■ Threshold;
▨ tinnitus suppression; ⊞ loudness discomfort level.

ETS with Low-frequency Sinusoids in Patients implanted for Total Deafness

Six patients who had significant tinnitus had received a single-channel cochlear implant for their total deafness. They were tested to see how a sinusoidal current transmitted through their implant receiver would influence the tinnitus. In place of their wearable sound processor, an identical transmitter, connected to a function generator and modulator, was placed over the implant behind the patient's ear. Electrodes were attached to the scalp to record the surface potentials generated by the implanted round window electrode via an oscilloscope (Figure 20.1). The voltage required for the detection of a signal was recorded, together with its loudness discomfort level (LDL) and that required for tinnitus suppression. Figure 20.2 shows the responses obtained for 100 Hz sinewaves, indicating the wide intersubject variability that occurs in sensitivity and in tinnitus suppression. As a result of this experiment, one of the patients requested a device to produce continuous suppression.

ETS with Temporary Round Window Electrodes

Experience with both transtympanic and round window stimulation of the cochlea led to the conclusion that much better results could be obtained with a round window electrode, and that these resembled very much more closely the experience of a patient when finally fitted with a single-channel, round window, cochlear implant. Eight patients with severely disabling tinnitus in a dead ear were selected from the UCH tinnitus clinic. All patients had hearing in the contralateral ear, which was either normal or appropriately aided. In all cases, the tinnitus continued to be a severe problem despite the various approaches of the multidisciplinary team, and the use of pharmacological, psychological and contralateral masking techniques. Two patients had been obtaining minimal benefit as far as their tinnitus was concerned from the hearing improvement provided by a CROS hearing aid.

A platinum ball electrode was placed in the round window under local anaesthesia. This electrode is identical to the one attached to the cochlear implant; it has an inherent springiness which makes it easy to maintain in position, and it is insulated down to the platinum ball. Lignocaine is injected into the external meatus and an 'L'-shaped myringotomy incision is made in the tympanic membrane (see Gantz et al. (1988), Ryan (1989) for details of the technique). In the few cases where there was difficulty in positioning the electrode, a small anterior tympanotomy flap was raised, also under local anaesthetic. The test equipment used is described in Figure 20.1, and is similar to that used for sinusoidal stimulation of previously implanted patients, except that an optical isolator separates the function generator from the connection to the round window electrode.

The best results were obtained from electrical stimulation at low frequencies, and no suppression was achieved with sinusoids above 200 Hz, although earlier protocols had included frequencies up to 20 kHz. Three of our patients did not experience tinnitus suppression within the dynamic range of electrical stimulation in the dead ear, and their results are therefore not recorded. In Figure 20.3, the thresholds, LDLs and suppression levels are shown for five patients who experienced ETS. With the patient, HP, suppression only occurred very close to the loudness discomfort level. The patient, SA, who experienced total suppression of tinnitus, preferred the sound of her own tinnitus to the evoked sound from the suppressor current. Subsequent on the good results obtained with a temporary electrode, three patients have now been given single-channel

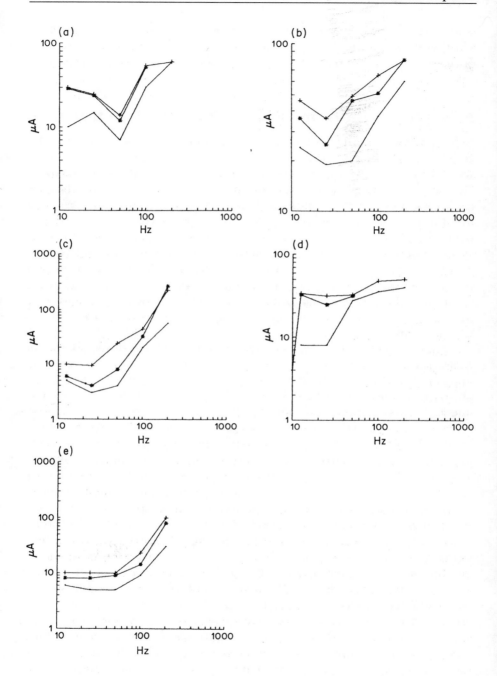

Figure 20.3. Results of ETS using a temporary round window electrode. (a) Patient HP – not suitable; (b) patient AF – awaiting implant; (c) patient SA – not suitable; (d) patient GP – received implant; (e) patient CD – received implant. ——— Threshold; +—+ suppression; —●— LDL.

(extracochlear) implants for electrical tinnitus suppression and use low-frequency sinusoids to suppress their tinnitus via their implants. A further patient awaits implantation in the near future. Favourable prognostic features in ETS would seem to be a low threshold, a wide dynamic range and suppression that occurs near the threshold of electrical hearing.

Case Results

GP is a 59-year-old male with a 16-year history of progressive unilateral otosclerosis. He had a right stapedectomy performed in 1981. This resulted in a dead ear, but he retains normal hearing on the left side. Tinnitus became more severe as time progressed, affecting his concentration at work, his ability to drive and sleep, and he had several periods of marked depression. Although hearing was helped by a CROS hearing aid system, his tinnitus continued to interfere with his life and in 1987 he received a UCH/RNID single-channel, round window implant and a 25-Hz suppressor.

On switching on the suppressor, his tinnitus is 'turned off' completely and, because of the very low thresholds at which suppression occurs, he is now barely aware of the sound created by the suppressor current. His life was immediately and dramatically changed, with a return to normal sleep patterns and other day-time activities. After a period of 3 months he began to get long periods of post-stimulus inhibition lasting up to 3 hours, particularly in the evening. He has been using his device continuously over a period of 18 months.

PR is a 39-year-old male who lost hearing in the right ear at the age of 6 and in the left ear at 32 as a result of meningococcal meningitis. He originally received a UCH/RNID cochlear implant in January 1983 for rehabilitation of his total deafness, but the tinnitus continued to be more troublesome than his deafness and was not helped by the masking effect of his sound processor. From March 1989 to January 1990 he was using a 100 Hz suppressor with his implant on a daily basis for a maximum of about 3 hours. He only uses the suppressor when his tinnitus is distressing, but reports great overall benefits from the device and describes the sound of the suppressor as much more pleasant than his tinnitus. He is a very skilled lipreader and (when the tinnitus is bad) uses the tinnitus suppressor in preference to his sound processor.

Cases where there is total deafness and severe tinnitus indicate the need for a suppressor that is analogous to the combination hearing aid and tinnitus masker used by those with partial hearing loss and tinnitus.

CD, a 51-year-old female with otosclerosis, had a right stapedectomy performed 10 years ago which was followed immediately by vertigo and hearing loss. Subsequent closure of a perilymph fistula did not improve matters. She continued to have a lot of problems with her balance until a membranous labyrinthectomy was performed 7 years later. This improved her balance but she continued to have a big problem with her tinnitus which consisted of a high-pitched whistle with associated low-frequency hum. There is currently a 50–60 dB mixed loss in the contralateral ear, for which she wears a BICROS hearing aid. Her tinnitus was affecting her concentration, ability to get off to sleep and also to get back to sleep if she woke in the night. It interfered with quiet recreational activities of all kinds. In 1989, a tympanotomy was performed and a round window electrode inserted. She was connected for 24 hours to a low-frequency sinusoid generator from which she obtained good tinnitus suppression. She received a cochlear implant in July 1989. She is now using her tinnitus suppression more or less constantly at a frequency of 48 Hz. The suppressor is used at about half volume and this changes what she describes as a fluctuating cocktail of noises into a single continuous tone which is easy to ignore. On switching off the device the tinnitus is quieter for some hours.

Discussion

Tinnitus is a symptom that needs very different management from hearing impairment, although they may exist jointly or separately. Although tinnitus is a widespread experience affecting 17% of the adult population (IHR, 1981), only 20% of those who experienced tinnitus ever consulted a physician (OPCS Monitor, 1983). Intrusiveness of tinnitus does not relate to any measurements of its loudness or pitch (Hazell et al., 1985), but to its learned or emotional significance (Hazell and Jastreboff, 1990). Loudness, unpleasantness and intrusiveness are part of a process of evaluation at a cortical level rather than depending directly on the tinnitus generator. With acoustic therapeutic maskers, 30% of those who are successfully fitted achieve a state of habituation following a period of symptom control, when the masker is no longer required (Hazell, Sheldrake and Meerton, 1987). In counselling a patient prior to implantation and ETS, it should be stressed that there may come a time when the device is no longer needed. It is best that patient selection and implantation take place within a multidisciplinary team skilled both in tinnitus management and in cochlear implantation.

There will inevitably be a temptation to recommend ETS as a surgical panacea for tinnitus, but at the present moment it plays a small, yet potentially very important, part in symptom control. It is obviously important to make sure that all patients are psychologically stable and, in particular, to determine that the tinnitus rather than some other problem is the cause of their distress. The author's group has identified a small group of tinnitus patients in whom the complaint of tinnitus is very definitely a cry for help, and not a problem in its own right. In such cases a large number of other psychosocial factors are involved.

In most cases, the small risk of damage to the cochlea from an unbalanced current source can usually be outweighed by the severity of the tinnitus. In approaching patients who have useful hearing in the affected ear, it would be important to have a much more guarded approach. The present experience is that tinnitus in a hearing ear can almost always be managed by other approaches, and symptom control can be achieved by masking and/or amplification.

In the past, the overall results of electrical tinnitus suppression have been disappointing. This may be because trials have often involved small numbers of patients in whom the exact pathology was not well identified. In many cases, it is not possible to identify the site of the tinnitus generator. The way in which the tinnitus is evaluated, or at least the distress which it causes, will vary enormously dependent on a wide variety of other factors. The trials of transdermal stimulation do show occasional responders, and more studies are needed to identify how good results may be predicted. Obviously, if electrical suppression of tinnitus can be achieved transdermally then this is preferable to an operative technique.

Great difficulties occur due to the response of tinnitus to any sort of professional intervention. Reassurance and counselling have a very powerful therapeutic effect and it is hard to initiate any trial of symptom control without counselling the patient. Tinnitus remains a sensation like pain; although it may be assessed by various techniques, it cannot yet be objectively measured in the same way as hearing impairment. In the past inappropriate criteria have been used for the evaluation of benefit. However, if we are able to establish electrical suppression of tinnitus, as a help not only to those patients who have tinnitus in a dead ear, but also to some of those with residual hearing, then it is possible that this might result in a much more potent and widespread application of cochlear implant technology than is currently in use for the rehabilitation of total deafness. For the time being, it would appear that, for a proportion of patients with distressing tinnitus in a dead ear, the application of low-frequency sinusoids through a single-channel cochlear implant has an important part to play in their management.

References

ARAN, J.M. and LE BERT, G. (1968). Les response nerveuse cochleaires chez l'homme, image fonctionnement de l'oreille et nouveau test d'Audiometrie objective. *Rev. Laryngol. (Bordeaux)* **89**, 361.

ARAN, J-M. and CAZALS, Y. (1981). Electrical suppression of tinnitus. In: *Tinnitus*, pp. 217–231. London: Pitman Books (Ciba Foundation Symposium 85).

BERLINER, K.I., CUNNINGHAM, J.K., HOUSE, W.F. and HOUSE, J.W. (1987). Effect of the cochlear implant on tinnitus in profoundly deaf patients. In: Feldmann, H. (ed.), *Proceedings of Third International Tinnitus Seminar,* Munster. Karlsruhe: Harsch.

CAZALS, Y., NEGREVERGNE, M. and ARAN, J-M. (1978). Electrical stimulation of the cochlea in man: hearing induction and tinnitus suppression. *J. Am. Soc. Audiol.* **3**, 209–213.

CHOUARD, C.H., MEYER, B. and MARIDAT, D. (1981). Transcutaneous electrotherapy for severe tinnitus. *Acta Oto-Laryngol.* **91**, 415–422.

DUCHENNE DE BOULOGNE (1855). *De l'éléctrisation localisée et de son application à la physiologie, à la pathologie et à la therapeutique.* Paris.

FRASER, J.G., COOPER, H.R., HAZELL, J.W.P., PHELPS, P.D. and LLOYD, G.A.S. (1986). The UCH/RNID Cochlear Implant Programme: Patient selection. *Br. J. Audiol.* **20**, 9–18.

FRAYSSE, B. and LAZORTHES, Y. (1983). Implantation chronique d'éléctrode au niveau de la fênetre ronde dans le traitement des bourdonnements. *J. Fr. d'Oto-Rhino-Laryngol.* **32**, 307–310.

GANTZ, B.J., TYLER, R.S., KNUTSON, J.F., WOODWORTH, G., ABBAS, P., McCABE, B.F., TYE-MURPHY, N., LANSING, C., KUK, F. and BROWN, C. (1988). Evaluation of five different cochlear implant designs: Audiological assessment and predictors of performance. *Laryngoscope* **98**, 1100–1106.

GERSDORFF, M. and ROBILLARD, T. (1985). Treatment of tinnitus by electrical stimulation of the ear. *Acta Oto-Rhino-Laryngol. (Belg.)* **39**, 583–612.

GRAHAM, J.M. and HAZELL, J.W.P. (1977). Electrical stimulation of the human cochlea using a transtympanic electrode. *Br. J. Audiol.* **11**, 59–62.

GRAPPENGIESSER, C.J.C. (1801). *Versuche den Galvanismus zur Heilung einiger Krankheiten anzuwenden.* Berlin.

HATTON, D.S., ERULKAR, S.D. and ROSENBERG, P.E. (1960). Some preliminary observations on the effect of galvanic current on tinnitus aurium. *Laryngoscope* **70**, 123–130.

HAZELL, J.W.P. and JASTREBOFF, P. (1990). Tinnitus mechanisms and management. *J. Otolaryngol.* **19**, 1–5.

HAZELL, J.W.P., MEERTON, L.J. and CONWAY, M.J. (1989). Electrical tinnitus suppression. *J. Laryngol. Otol.* Suppl. 18, 39–44.

HAZELL, J.W.P., SHELDRAKE, J.B. and MEERTON, L.J. (1987). Tinnitus masking – is it better than counselling alone? In: Feldmann, H. (ed.), *Proceedings of Third International Tinnitus Seminar,* Munster, pp. 239–250. Karlsruhe: Harsch.

HAZELL, J.W.P., WILLIAMS, G.R. and SHELDRAKE, J.B. (1981). Tinnitus maskers – successes and failures: A report on the state of the art. *J. Laryngol.* Suppl. 4, 80–87.

HAZELL, J.W.P., WOOD, S.M., COOPER, H.R., STEPHENS, S.D.G., CORCORAN, A.L., COLES, R.R.A. et al. (1985). A clinical study of tinnitus maskers. *Br. J. Audiol.* **19**, 65–146.

HOUSE, W.F. (1976). Cochlear implants. *Ann. Otol.* Suppl. 27, 34.

HOUSE, W.F. and BRACKMANN, D.E. (1974). Electrical promontory testing in differential diagnosis of sensori-neural hearing impairment. *Laryngoscope* **84**, 2163–2171.

INSTITUTE OF HEARING RESEARCH (1981). Epidemiology of tinnitus. In: *Tinnitus,* pp. 16–34. London: Pitman Books (Ciba Foundation Symposium 85).

LYTTKENS, L., LINDBERG, P., SCOTT, B. and MELIN, L. (1986). Treatment of tinnitus by external electrical stimulation. *Scand. Audiol.* **15**, 157–164.

MacNAUGHTON JONES, H. (1891). *Subjective Noises in the Head and Ears: Their Etiology, Diagnosis and Treatment.* London: Baillière, Tindall & Cox.

OPCS MONITOR (1983). Office of Population Censuses and Surveys. *General Household Survey: The Prevalence of Tinnitus 1981.* OPCS Monitor GHS 83/1, Dept M. OPCS, 10 Kingsway, London WC2.

PORTMANN, M., CAZALS, Y., NEGREVERGNE, M. and ARAN, J-M. (1979). Temporary tinnitus suppression in man through electrical stimulation of the cochlea. *Acta Oto-Laryngol.* **87**, 294–299.

ROTHERA, M., CONWAY, M., BRIGHTWELL, A. and GRAHAM, J.M. (1986). Evaluation of patients for cochlear implant by promontory stimulation. *Br. J. Audiol.* **20**, 25–28.

RYAN, R. (1989). Pre-operative cochlear implant assessment using a round window ball electrode. *J. Laryngol. Otol.* Suppl. 18, 11–13.

SHULMAN, A., TONNDORF, J. and GOLDSTEIN, B. (1985). Electrical tinnitus control. *Acta Oto-Laryngol.* **99**, 318–325.

SHULMAN, A. (1987). External electrical tinnitus suppression: a review. *Am. J. Otol.* **8**, 479–484.

STEPHENS, S.D.G. (1987). Historical aspects of tinnitus. In: Hazell, J.W.P. (ed.), *Tinnitus.* Edinburgh: Churchill Livingstone.

VERNON, J. (1977). Attempts to relieve tinnitus. *J. Am. Audiol. Soc.* **2**, 124–131.

VERNON, J.A. and FENWICK, J.A. (1985). Attempts to suppress tinnitus with transcutaneous electrical stimulation. *Otolaryngol. Head Neck Surg.* **93**(3), 385–389.

VOLTA, A. (1800). On the electricity excited by the mere contact of the conducting substances of different kinds. *Trans. R. Soc. Phil.* **90**, 403–419.

VON WEDEL, H., STRAHLMANN, U. and ZOROWKA, P. (1989). Effectiveness of various non-medicinal therapeutic measures in tinnitus. *Laryngo-rhino-otologie (FRG)* **68**, 259–266.

Chapter 21
The Experience of being Deafened

ALISON HEATH

Perhaps, indirectly, Hitler was to blame for my deafness. Until the age of 8 years, I was a very normal child and a member of quite a large family – I have three older sisters and a younger brother.

All my memories of being able to hear perfectly date from the war years and, surprisingly, I even have some recollection of hearing French spoken since I lived in Normandy for most of the first 3 years of my life and subsequently had a French governess.

The rest of my normal hearing years were in wartime Britain, at home in Hampshire where my parents ran a market garden and also used all available land to help with the war effort by keeping chickens, ducks, geese and Jersey cows.

When I reached school age my sister and I began to receive our education at home and this included piano lessons. Then the flying bombs began to fall and my mother, fearful for our safety, dispatched the three youngest members of her brood to Devonshire to stay with her eldest sister. It was while I was in the care of my aunt that I contracted an ear infection that remained untreated; the doctor whom we consulted apparently did not think it was a case for antibiotics.

We returned to Hampshire at the end of the war but the ear infection was still festering and may have been exacerbated by a heavy cold. Whatever happened, early in 1945 (just after my eighth birthday) I went down with bacterial meningitis and was admitted to Winchester hospital where, for a few days, I hovered between life and death. After treatment with streptomycin, I turned the corner and my recovery was slow and uneventful but, unfortunately, not complete. This I soon discovered for myself. I had a small bell with which to summon the nurse. One night I was playing with it lying on my left side. I shook the bell and no sound came so I went on shaking it. One of the nurses heard the din and duly expressed her annoyance at being called for no good reason. Not really concerned, I experimented further banging a ruler against the locker while

370

putting my hand over my good left ear and taking it away again. It was clear – one ear was deaf. Rather casually, I informed my mother when she next came to visit. Actually, she insisted that she had noticed herself as I had been asking her to repeat what she said. Whoever it was – I or my mother – who had first noticed the trouble, the medical staff were duly informed.

Just before I was discharged, a hearing test was performed. We were told that there was a complete loss in one ear and the other ear was slightly affected and that was it. My parents were not given any advice on how to cope with my hearing loss or even told about the effect it might have on my education in future.

At home I slowly recovered strength. At this stage my weakness and difficulty in walking, which was probably due to loss of balance rather than the inability of my 'matchstick' legs to hold me up, caused more concern than my hearing loss. When I was fit enough I was sent as a day pupil to a small private school. My progress was poor but I do not remember worrying too much about my deafness – unbeknown to myself my hearing impairment was already an educational handicap. As it was the custom in my family for us to attend boarding school as soon as we were old enough, at the age of 9 years I was sent to a preparatory school in Sussex.

In spite of a front seat in the classroom, I failed to keep up with the class though this must, in part, be blamed on the very sketchy and disrupted schooling that I had received in the foregoing years. The hearing in my one good ear deteriorated steadily and, to make matters worse, tinnitus set in. Both the hearing and tinnitus at this time were erratic. I can still remember sitting in class with my hand cupped over the good ear straining to hear the teacher and then, within minutes, the tinnitus – though I mentioned this to no one and could not even put a name to those strange noises – would start up and put an end to all possibility of following the lesson.

By now my parents were getting worried. My father, who was already a hearing aid user because he had been blown up in World War I and lost not only his hearing but also an arm, decided that I needed a hearing aid and bought me one of the cumbersome instruments of the day – it was American and bright pink. Needless to say, it was some time before I accepted and used it. My hearing got steadily worse and was very unpredictable. This caused me a lot of distress and, consequently, also worried my fellow pupils and the staff at the preparatory school. No one had any experience of hearing impairment in a child or how to cope with it and they did not really appreciate the effect it was having on my educational progress.

At last my parents sought professional advice through the RNID and I was moved to a very small private school run by a teacher of the deaf. Here I was introduced to the art of lipreading and also, following my father's example, began to make more use of my hearing aid. Two years later, when I was transferred to the Mary Hare Grammar School for the Deaf, I was inseparable from my aid, which was by now slightly smaller. I wore it from morn to night. Inexorably my hearing got worse – I gave up my piano lessons; they were not a pleasure any more. Nevertheless, I did sometimes have some 'good' days and was enjoying one such day when I went to see the ENT surgeon in Southampton for a medical report – he expressed some doubt as to whether I should be sent to a special school as my hearing appeared to be quite good. In a way, I think he was right. If only there had been units and peripatetic teachers of the deaf to support hearing-impaired children in mainstream education, I am sure that would have been the right provision for me. As it was, I was sent to the Mary Hare Grammar School for the Deaf – it was excellent as a special school for bright, deaf children but not, in my opinion, for deafened children.

My education was slowed down to the pace at which children with severe linguistic handicaps could proceed. I do not think I, nor any other deafened children in the school who could not sign, were ever fully 'accepted' by the deaf children there whose normal mode of communication was sign language, albeit surreptitiously, as we were supposed to use oral methods of communication at all times. My parents persuaded the headmaster to allow me to jump a form as I was bored by the slow pace of the lessons.

In spite of the fact that very few other children were ever seen outside the classroom with a hearing aid on, I continued to wear mine at all times. By now it was really essential to me, but there were days when I heard little and could not understand anyone well as I still used my hearing more than my lipreading. In fact my lipreading skills were so poor that one of the teachers tried to help by suggesting that I should leave my aid off sometimes and concentrate on improving my lipreading. Even then – I was about 16 at the time – there could still be occasions when my hearing briefly returned. I can remember listening to a lesson about 'laissez faire' while looking through the window – the teacher giving the lesson was so sure that I had not been paying attention that he made me write it down for him. He was most surprised when he got it almost word for word.

I managed to leave the Mary Hare 4 years later with a respectable number of 'O' levels to my credit. With the help of some private tutors, I prepared for the Oxford entrance examination and 'A' levels. They arranged for me to have individual sessions with them as I clearly could not manage in a group. It was also at this time that the full implication of my profound hearing loss became apparent to my family. In desperation my parents began to look around for a 'cure'. I had several appointments with a faith healer in Harley Street until we decided that he was a quack. My sister, who was then a medical student at St Thomas's and developing an interest in psychiatry, thought my hearing problem might stem from emotional problems and I duly found myself in the care of Dr Sargent for a short time. However, if my family found it difficult to accept my deafness it was not really so on my side. Although the idea of hearing again was pleasant to contemplate, deep down I really accepted my fate. My acquaintance with others in the same boat as myself at the Mary Hare helped me here.

My tutors at Somerville College always saw me alone instead of in a group of twos and threes as was the case with other undergraduates. They were also extremely patient for I was by now profoundly deaf and my lipreading still left much to be desired. Even the one-to-one sessions were difficult and quite a lot had to be written down. I did try to attend one or two lectures but soon decided that it was best to borrow notes from friends and spend the time more profitably reading in the library. Fortunately, I read history and, for this particular course, lectures did not feature too large and were not compulsory.

Despite my almost non-existent hearing and still rather indifferent lipreading, I was very happy at Oxford and made many friends, one of whom was to become my husband.

The transition from university to the world of work was not an easy one. I was not only deaf, but also had the disadvantage of being a woman. I can still remember my session with the Oxford Appointments Board; I did not understand the appointments officer well and, initially, all she could think of was that I should be a tutor for correspondence courses! However, later when I finally decided on a career in librarianship, she went out of her way to help. It was partly through her intervention that I finally got my first real job as a trainee librarian with the British National Bibliography.

It was shortly after I came down from Oxford, when I was job hunting, that I again paid a visit to an ENT surgeon to find out the reason for my still deteriorating hearing – there was hardly any left now. I still wore a hearing aid but there were times when even with the aid I heard nothing at all. This time the eminent consultant whom I saw pronounced that it was 'perceptive' deafness and that nothing could be done, but he did say I would not lose the scrap of hearing that I had then – I did and with it went all hope of a 'cure'. Like so many others in this situation, I resigned myself to being deaf and making my way in life with the help of my friends, family and many others who have gone out of their way to help me.

Now that I was totally deaf, my lipreading improved but I was still nervous, particularly with strangers, and often found it difficult to maintain the intense concentration that good lipreading needs.

I worked for 4 years, qualifying as a librarian through part-time study before I gave up my job to become a full-time housewife and mother. When the youngest of our three children reached school age I returned to work – life at home was rather lonely and we needed the money. Even a hearing mother with toddlers to care for finds it difficult and it was worse for me as I could not use the telephone, enjoy the television or the radio.

I was fortunate and secured a post in a small medical library and started to commute to London every day. As my husband is a teacher he was able to look after the children in the school holidays. Later, when the children were a bit older and more independent, I changed my job to become a curator in the British Library.

It was really due to my knowledge of medicine and the medical information services, acquired during the course of my work, that I became aware that there were some developments in the field of sensorineural deafness that might have some relevance to me. I read an article on cochlear implants and decided that it was time to find out if anything was going on in this country. Accordingly, I went to the RNID to enquire and was very excited when they told me that the first cochlear implant operation in this country was about to be performed at the Royal Ear Hospital (REH).

When it was ascertained that I was indeed totally deaf, I was given some literature about the UCH/RNID programme. I went to see my GP and asked to be referred for tests. Actually I got something of a rocket for wanting to be involved in what was clearly experimental surgery, but he did give me the letter of referral that I wanted. In spite of my spell in the fellows' library at the Royal College of Physicians, I did not have much experience of hospitals and it was with some trepidation that I went to keep my first appointment at the REH. I must have been a bit of a novice at making it clear to the receptionist that I was deaf and missed my turn because it was two solid hours before I saw anyone. I did better with the next couple of appointments, taking care to take my husband with me on the second occasion when Mr Hazell carefully explained all that was involved and answered the many questions that I had about the tests and the equipment.

The next time I went round for some 'tests of hearing' with Mr John Graham, I might not have been so unconcerned about them had I known what lay in store. I was laid flat out with my head tied up with wires for the electrical tests of hearing. It was still the early days of the programme and testing procedures and equipment were not quite as sophisticated as they are now. The wire with the electrode on the end for the promontory stimulation of the cochlea was pushed through the ear drum and wobbled around. After a time, being intent on listening to all the odd sounds which I heard and answering questions about their pitch, loudness and effects on my tinnitus, I finally managed to lie on the protruding wire – ouch! The next thing was the X-rays at the Royal National Throat, Nose and Ear Hospital, Grays Inn Road. They were very thorough and I spent an hour with the radiological technician, getting into various awkward positions and obediently maintaining them until the necessary pictures had been taken. Finally, there was the vestibular test and an interview with the clinical psychologist.

When I returned to the hospital to find out the results of all these tests it was a big let down to be told that I was not considered to be a suitable candidate for the multichannel implant they were then using. Only one ear responded well enough to the promontory stimulation tests and there was some residual labyrinthine function on that side which might be damaged by the insertion of a multichannel electrode.

As the tests had taken place over 6 months and I had been very excited at the prospect of being able to hear again – it had been difficult to think of anything else – I went back to the library and, much to the concern of one of my colleagues who happened to be there, broke down and wept in the cloakroom. However, there was a glimmer of light at the end of the tunnel. There was another device, an extracochlear implant, for which I might be a suitable candidate.

What seemed to be an interminable wait ensued. The device was a foreign one and difficult to obtain. In the meantime, the multichannel implant operation which was performed, failed and all implant work at the REH ceased. Finally, the long-awaited Austrian implants arrived and, although still very disappointed that I had not been accepted for the much vaunted multichannel device, I decided that the results they were getting from the Viennese single-channel device – some users were apparently able to recognise some speech without lipreading – were sufficiently good to make it worth while going ahead.

I saw the speech therapist, clinical psychologist and other members of the rehabilitation team. I had recordings made of my speech and did some tracking, repeating word-for-word stories that were read out to me, so that there would be good before and after results to compare.

I was booked to go into hospital early in March 1984 for a fortnight. I did not relish the idea of staying in hospital for so long, but decided that I would have to go through with it. I was not really concerned about the operation itself – Mr Graham Fraser and his team inspired me with a lot of confidence and I felt that I was in safe hands. Also, I looked forward, should the operation succeed, to hearing rather more than I had been told to expect, but it would not have been wise to have admitted to this as I might have been turned down for having unrealistic expectations. I worked with the REH cochlear implant team and with the research workers at University College, London right until the very last moment.

On the evening before the operation I went into Ward F in the Royal Ear Hospital to be prepared for an operation that was to last 4½ hours. The atmosphere was very relaxed and friendly and we all had our meals, when we were fit enough, at a communal table. I was awakened at 6 a.m. by the night duty nurse and took the ritual preoperation bath, had my injection and was told to stay in bed until they 'came for me'. I only felt one moment of real panic and that was just before the anaesthetist put me out – my stretcher was wheeled upstairs and I found myself lying flat on my back with a lot of strange faces looking down. Fortunately, I recognised the anaesthetist's assistant who had taken the precaution of visiting me the evening before. 'Do you remember me?' she said and that was all I knew until I came round late in the afternoon back in my cubicle in Ward F.

I did not feel any real discomfort though my head was wrapped up in a bandage that resembled a turban but one that was a bit more extensive and a good deal tighter. I was very sleepy and glad to take it easy. It was a comfort to have my husband with me at this point, although talking was difficult and I could not focus my eyes well enough to read. While I was still drowsy, I had my first experience of a ward round with Mr Fraser and his staff wanting to know how I felt – I just managed to reply to their questions.

I recovered rapidly and the huge bandage was removed. My hair was no pretty sight on one side so I went around with a head scarf for a couple of weeks until it grew again. The week after the operation while I was waiting for the wound to heal sufficiently well to be discharged, I did some work with the speech therapist. I am afraid I was not as appreciative of this as I should have been – speech therapy was something I had not bargained for. I did, however, learn some very useful things. In particular I learned to make a conscious effort to keep my voice low and quiet especially if I am a bit agitated about something. Like many deaf people, I tend to raise my voice and sound a great deal more annoyed and angry than I mean to be, which does not make for a calm relaxed atmosphere when there are problems to be sorted out.

Sadly, my mother who had been ill for several months with cancer died 2 days after the operation. I was most relieved that I was allowed out to attend her funeral in Devonshire with my family.

It was suddenly, on the fifth day after the operation, that the world started to go up and down whenever I moved. Fearing that what they had sought to avoid – damage to my residual balance function in the good ear by giving me an extracochlear implant – had happened, I mentioned it to Mr Hazell when he next visited me. I was given to understand that it was to be expected after major surgery but I found the moving horizons very disconcerting when I walked along the street or rode my horse – it was best to keep my eyes down.

After the metal clips, not stitches, had been rather painfully removed I was allowed home to recuperate before the most exciting part of all, the 'switch on'. However, the medical team were not too worried about this as they had already ascertained when I was still unconscious that the implant was working!

It was not actually as dramatic as it sounds because it was really a question of Mike Conway, the hospital physicist, getting the implant correctly adjusted for me and Huw Cooper, then a new member of the staff, ensuring that it was not adversely affecting my tinnitus. I had an appointment with Tracy Waters, the speech therapist, and we were delighted that I was immediately able to hear the rhythm of speech. I went home with the transmitter secured to my head with an elastic band and a scarf on the top. The sound of the traffic in the street was more than I could tolerate so I switched off for most of the journey home. I heard the voices of my family for the first time and listened to my daughter playing the viola. However, everything was very strange and did not really correspond to my memories of sound at this point.

When I went to church very shortly after the 'switch on', I could not even distinguish between the congregation singing and speaking but this changed rapidly. Before I had had the implant for 3 months, I could follow the service fairly well provided I did not lose my place in the service book. I also took great pleasure in listening to the lessons being read as I could track the speaker if I read from my own copy of the Bible at the same time – it was almost as though I could really hear. It was the same with the piano. The first time I tried I could not tell the difference between high and low notes but 3 weeks later I played some scales and my memories of learning the piano began to come back. It sounded a lot more natural. A little more experimentation established that I could hear the pitch changes for about one octave above middle C and two below.

I returned to work 5 weeks after the operation. Initially, there was not too much improvement in communication because our office is located in a busy part of central London and I not only had to contend with all the noise of a large open-plan office but also of traffic. I was, however, surprised to receive the first of many comments on the improvement in my speech from the head of my division. It had deteriorated considerably during the years of silence and, though still easily intelligible, the pitch had risen and, like so many other totally deaf people, it was not possible for me to modulate it to take into account the level of the background noise. Now it was the one thing I could hear well at all times; it became quieter and the pitch dropped. To some extent I can adjust the loudness to suit the situation but I still make some misjudgements. Some sounds, like those of electric fans, come across to me as unnaturally loud, so I tend to compensate by shouting when I don't need to. Since I have been corrected on numerous occasions, especially in restaurants when my husband finds it rather embarrassing if I speak too loudly when other people are only chatting quietly, experience has taught me to be more careful.

My inability, initially, to recognise the sounds I heard was sometimes amusing, frightening and even embarrassing. Every time someone coughed or sneezed I looked up and occasionally enquired what that strange noise was! Finally, a colleague who worked close to me came to work with a really bad cold, the sound effects of which I had to listen to for 3 days without respite. After that I became quite skilled in recognising coughs, sneezes, snuffles and so on. There was another time when, going down into the Oxford Circus underground station, I heard a strange wailing sound. Thinking it was some warning sound, I was not sure whether I ought to flee or dive for cover. A rapid glance round told me that there did not appear to be anything to worry about as my fellow passengers were going on their way unperturbed. A little further on all was explained – a music student, anxious to supplement his meagre grant money, was playing a saxophone!

At first I was unable to tolerate loud sound and switched off when I went out into the street but gradually I taught myself to face the din of the London traffic, until I was confronted with a police car on an emergency call. The noise quite literally almost knocked me flat. Now, like everybody else, although I do not like sirens, fire alarms and other loud noises, I have learned to take them in my stride and react to them appropriately. The world is certainly a safer place for me now.

Even in the early days there were improvements, not only for me, but also for my family as I learned to recognise a large number of environmental sounds. I could hear when someone was listening to the radio and no longer tried to start a conversation quite oblivious to the fact that their attention was elsewhere. When in a group situation it was a great relief to me to know, without continuously having to scan all the faces to see if someone was speaking, when I could safely proffer a comment without interrupting someone else. It seems strange how such a small thing can help to increase confidence in social situations.

There were other changes; I became more aware that my own activities could generate more noise than I realised. We have a cupboard in which saucepans, lids and other kitchen metal ware are piled none too tidily. The removal of one pan without due care can result in the entire contents spilling out on to the floor. The first time this happened and 'deafened' me, my family were not in the least bit sympathetic! I have always enjoyed singing when I hope no one is listening to my wildly untuneful voice and I now regained the art of whistling. I started to whistle while going about my household chores. Unfortunately, my family did not appreciate my 'music'. My mother-in-law came up with a saying that her own mother had used, many years ago, to silence her unladylike daughter, 'A whistling woman and a crowing hen is good for neither God nor men'.

After 6 months, although my speech had improved noticeably, there was still little perceptible improvement in my lipreading abilities as far as other people were concerned. I myself, however, did find conversations much easier partly because I felt a great deal more relaxed now that I could hear. And there was another gain – I was once again able to appreciate the richness and variety of human speech; that everyone has a voice as unique and distinctive as their features. It was at this stage that I met Dr Hochmair-Desoyer of Vienna when she came to attend a conference on cochlear implants. She also brought all her testing equipment so that she could adjust the processors of the people who had been fitted with her implant. Surrounded by interested onlookers in the small sound-proofed room at the RNID, she tested my new-found hearing and made some very fine adjustments to the sound processor. Immediately voices sounded a little bit less throaty and higher. Shortly after this, I found that I could recognise a few words without lipreading for the first time – initially it was numbers spoken slowly and distinctly in a quiet room. Some of the numbers which I confused, and still do, gave me an insight into the limitations of the implant – I could not tell the difference between thirty and forty easily because the fricatives 'f' and 'th' eluded me. I could now hear some fricatives such as 'sh', 't' and, faintly 's', which I had not initially been able to hear.

There were also some sounds which had, uncannily, been shut out such as the fire alarm at work. I felt a great deal more independent now that I could identify it and respond as necessary – to stop talking until the din died down if I was in conversation with someone and it was just a test or to leave the building if it was a real fire drill. It was great not to have to rely on other people to tell me this. There was another sound which I had not been able to hear: the chiming of our grandmother clock which had originally belonged to my parents. I could still remember watching fascinated while my father wound it up and made it chime if he had to reset it. It sounded exactly as I remembered it when I had last heard it more than 30 years ago.

After the first few weeks, I really became dependent on the implant and hated to be caught without a charged-up battery – it uses two to three batteries per day – and would prefer to buy one rather than endure the silence. Before I had the implant, no one could have convinced me that to acquire the ability to hear environmental sounds was going to be important but now, even if I am not talking to someone, I feel out of touch if I cannot hear the traffic, the sounds of people moving round the house, my son's pop music, the din made by the dishwasher, washing machine or coffee-maker in the kitchen. After Dr Hochmair-Desoyer's visit, the improvement in my ability to understand speech, which had been my main reason for wanting the implant, really began to become evident, not only to myself, but also to my family, friends and colleagues at work. After years of speaking at the rate I could lipread, my husband must, unconsciously, have begun to speak faster as I began to understand him more easily. When I was caught with a flat battery or was temporarily without my implant, he began to notice the difference and to comment on the fact that it was much more of an effort to communicate with me. On such occasions I also tended to speak too loudly – and still do. It all happened so slowly that we were hardly aware of the change ourselves. On my periodic visits to the Royal Ear Hospital and University College, London, the tests of my ability to understand speech when my lipreading is assisted by my implant have shown a continuous improvement over the 5½ years that I have worn the implant.

Although I have benefited enormously from having the implant, there is a loss; the horizon continues to move up and down when I walk and I am more unsteady, especially in the dark. A visit to the REH for some more tests of vestibular function 9 months after the operation confirmed that I had lost the small amount of balance that I had had. Now, 5 years later, things have settled down a bit and I have become more accustomed to the loss of my balance. I certainly do not regret having the operation because of this and even hope that perhaps one day, now there is no balance to damage, I might be able to hear even better with a multichannel implant.

All these gains have also meant that I am able to do more and feel more confident socially. I am no longer a passive member of the congregation of my church; I read the lesson at regular intervals and have joined the fund-raising committee. Our children have grown up in the last 5 years and gone out into the world but I have more than filled the time I used to spend with my family by voluntary work. In particular, I have been very active in founding the National Association of Deafened People of which I was the chairperson for 4 years. But for the implant I am not sure I would have been able to do this. Although I still need the assistance of a lipspeaker or, if I am lucky, palantype if I am to be an effective committee member, it is the implant which tells me when I can make my contribution. I have not been able to change my job or get promotion but I have tried and secured several interviews in pursuit of this. I was in the habit of going to the theatre from time to time with the script of the play, but now my enjoyment of such visits has increased two-fold especially if I can secure a front seat. There have even been visits to the opera of which my husband is very fond.

The real improvements are in being able to hear environmental sounds. When I start the day by going down to feed our horses, I hear the scrunch of my boots on the gravel, the sound of an approaching car and the nicker of welcome from the horses when they see that breakfast is coming – little things that few of us appreciate until we lose them. The joy of being able to converse in one-to-one situations without strain is, perhaps, the biggest gain. There are few people who really defeat me once they have been made aware of my deafness and even then they tend to forget and speak without looking at me. However, now I am able to rectify the situation quickly and ask for a repetition of what was said when I was not looking, that is, if I do not hear and understand and – sometimes I do!

Index